EUROPEAN
SOCIETY OF
CARDIOLOGY®

Cardiovascular imaging

A handbook for clinical practice

THE ESC EDUCATION SERIES

EUROPEAN SOCIETY OF CARDIOLOGY®

Cardiovascular imaging

A handbook for clinical practice

EDITED BY

Jeroen J. Bax
Christopher M. Kramer
Thomas H. Marwick
William Wijns

Blackwell
Publishing

© 2005 European Society of Cardiology
2035 Route des Colles-Les Templiers, 06903 Sophia-Antipolis, France
For further information on the European Society of Cardiology,
Visit our website: www.escardio.org

Published by Blackwell Publishing
Blackwell Publishing, Inc., 350 Main Street, Malden, Massachusetts 02148-5020, USA
Blackwell Publishing Ltd, 9600 Garsington Road, Oxford OX4 2DQ, UK
Blackwell Publishing Asia Pty Ltd, 550 Swanston Street, Carlton, Victoria 3053, Australia

First published 2005

Library of Congress Cataloging-in-Publication Data

Cardiovascular imaging : a handbook for clinical practice / edited by Jeroen J. Bax . . . [et al.].
    p. ; cm. — (ESC educational series)
  Includes index.
  ISBN-13: 978-1-4051-3131-5 (alk. paper)
  ISBN-10: 1-4051-3131-4 (alk. paper)
  1. Heart—Imaging—Handbooks, manuals, etc. 2. Cardiovascular system—Imaging—
Handbooks, manuals, etc.
  [DNLM: 1. Diagnostic Techniques, Cardiovascular. 2. Diagnostic Imaging—methods.
3. Risk Assessment. WG 141 C2688 2005] I. Bax, Jeroen J. II. European Society of
Cardiology. III. Series.

  RC683.5.I42C378 2005
  616.1′20754—dc22

                                                                          2005007226

ISBN-13: 978-1-4051-3131-5
ISBN-10: 1-4051-3131-4

A catalogue record for this title is available from the British Library

Set in 9.5/12pt Meridien by SNP Best-set Typesetter Ltd., Hong Kong
Printed and bound in India by Replika Press Pvt., Ltd

Commissioning Editor: Gina Almond
Development Editor: Helen Harvey
Production Controller: Kate Charman

For further information on Blackwell Publishing, visit our website:
http://www.blackwellpublishing.com

Contents

Section three: Heart failure

Section four: Uncommon entities

Video clips 1–61 can be found on the accompanying CD in the back of this book. They are referred to in the text by 👁.

List of contributors

Editors

Jeroen J. Bax, MD, PhD, Department of Cardiology, University Hospital Leiden, Albinusdreef 2, 2333A Leiden, The Netherlands

Christopher M. Kramer, MD, Departments of Radiology and Medicine, University of Virginia Health System, Box 800170, Charlottesville, VA 22908, USA

Thomas H. Marwick, MD, PhD, Professor of Medicine, University of Queensland, Princess Alexandra Hospital, Brisbane, Q4102, Australia

William Wijns, MD, PhD, Cardiovascular Centre, OLV Hospital, Moorselbaan 164, Aalst, 9300, Belgium

Contributors

Ravi G. Assomull, MRCP, Cardiovascular Magnetic Resonance Unit, Royal Brompton Hospital, Sydney Street, London SW3 6NP, UK

Helmut Baumgartner, MD, Medical University of Vienna, Department of Cardiology, Vienna General Hospital, Währinger Gürtel 18–20, A-1090 Vienna, Austria

George A. Beller, MD, Cardiovascular Division, Department of Internal Medicine, University of Virginia Health System, PO Box 800158, Charlottesville, VA 22908-0158, USA

Frank M. Bengel, MD, Nuklearmedizinische Klinik der TU München, Klinikum rechts der Isar, Ismaninger Str. 22, 81675 München, Germany

Gabe B. Bleeker, MD, Department of Cardiology, Leiden University Medical Centre, Leiden, The Netherlands

Ole-A. Breithardt, MD, I. Medizinische Klinik, Department of Cardiology, Klinikum Mannheim, University of Heidelberg, Theodor-Kutzer-Ufer 1–3, D-68167 Mannheim, Germany

Eric Brochet, MD, Department of Cardiology, Hôpital Bichat, 46 rue Henri Huchard, Paris 75018, France

Darryl J. Burstow, MB, BS, FRACP, The Prince Charles Hospital, Rode Road, Chermside, Brisbane, Queensland, Australia 4032

Agnès Cachier, MD, Department of Cardiology, Hôpital Bichat, 46 rue Henri Huchard, Paris 75018, France

Benedetta De Chiara, MD, CNR Clinical Physiology Institute—Milan, Niguarda Ca' Granda Hospital, Piazza Ospedale Maggiore, 3-20162 Milan, Italy

Pim J. de Feyter, MD, PhD, Erasmus Medical Center, Department of Cardiology (Thorax Center), Room BD 410, PO Box 2040, 3000 CA, Rotterdam, The Netherlands

Albert de Roos, MD, PhD, Department of Radiology, Leiden University Medical Center, C2-S, Albinusdreef 2, 2300 RC Leiden, The Netherlands

Kim A. Eagle, MD, Internal Medicine, North Ingalls Building, 300 North Ingalls, Room NIB 8B02, Ann Arbor, MI 48109-0047, USA

Brett E. Fenster, MD, Department of Medicine, Division of Cardiovascular Medicine, Stanford University Medical Center, Stanford, CA, USA

Frank A. Flachskampf, MD, FESC, FACC, Med. Klinik II, Universitätsklinikum Erlangen Ulmenweg 18, 91054 Erlangen, Germany

Maria Frigerio, MD, Struttura Complessa Cardiologia II, Dipartimento Cardiologico, Ospedale Niguarda Ca' Granda, Piazza Ospedale Maggiore, 3-20162 Milan, Italy

Heynric B. Grotenhuis, MD, Department of Radiology, Leiden University Medical Center, C2-S, Albinusdreef 2, 2300 RC Leiden, The Netherlands

Jong-Won Ha, MD, PhD, Cardiology Division, Yonsei University College of Medicine, Seoul, Korea

Charles B. Higgins, MD, University of California, 505 Parnassus Avenue, Suite L308, Department of Radiology, Box 0628, San Francisco, CA 94143-0628, USA

Eduard R. Holman, MD, PhD, Department of Non-Invasive Cardiology, Leiden University Medical Center, C2-S, Albinusdreef 2, 2300 RC Leiden, The Netherlands

Miklos D. Kertai, MD, PhD, Departments of Cardiothoracic Surgery, Semmelweis University Varosmajor Str 68, H-1122 Budapest, Hungary

Serge Kownator, MD, Cardiology Center, 1 Allee Poincare, 57100 Thionville, France

Lucia J.M. Kroft, MD, PhD, Department of Radiology, Leiden University Medical Center, C2-S, Albinusdreef 2, 2300 RC Leiden, The Netherlands

Joshua Lehrer-Graiwer, MD, University of California, 505 Parnassus Avenue, Suite L308, Department of Radiology, Box 0628, San Francisco, CA 94143-0628

Gerald Maurer, MD, Medical University of Vienna, Department of Cardiology, Vienna General Hospital, Währinger Gürtel 18-20, A-1090 Vienna, Austria

Michael V. McConnell, MD, MSEE, Department of Medicine, Division of Cardiovascular Medicine, Stanford University Medical Center, Stanford, CA, USA

Debabrata Mukherjee, MD, Gill Heart Institute and Division of Cardiovascular Medicine, University of Kentucky, 900 S Limestone, 326 Wethington Building, Lexington, KY 40536-0200, USA

Koen Nieman, MD, PhD, Massachusetts General Hospital, CIMIT, 100 Charles River Plaza, Suite 400, Boston, MA 02114, USA

Petros Nihoyannopoulos, MD, FRCP, FESC, FACC, FAHA, Cardiology Department, Hammersmith Hospital, National Heart and Lung Institute, Imperial College London, London W12 0NN, UK

Jae K. Oh, MD, Division of Cardiovascular Diseases and Internal Medicine, Mayo Clinic College of Medicine, 200 First Street SW, Rochester, MN 55905, USA

Jaap Ottenkamp, MD, PhD, Department of Pediatric Cardiology, Leiden University Medical Center, C2-S, Albinusdreef 2, 2300 RC Leiden, The Netherlands

Catherine M. Otto, MD, Division of Cardiology, Box 356422, University of Washington, Seattle, WA 98195, USA

Oberdan Parodi, MD, CNR Clinical Physiology Institute—Milan, Niguarda Ca' Granda Hospital, Piazza Ospedale Maggiore, 3-20162 Milan, Italy

Dudley J. Pennell, MD, FRCP, FACC, FESC, Cardiovascular Magnetic Resonance Unit, Royal Brompton Hospital, Sydney Street, London SW3 6NP, UK

Fausto J. Pinto, MD, PhD, FESC, FACC, University Hospital Santa Maria, Lisbon University Medical School, Division of Cardiology, Avenida Professor Egas Moniz, 1649-035 Lisbon, Portugal

Don Poldermans, MD, PhD, Department of Vascular Surgery, Room H921, Erasmus Medical Center, Dr. Molewaterplein 40, 3015 GD Rotterdam, The Netherlands

Sanjay K. Prasad, MD, MRCP, Cardiovascular Magnetic Resonance Unit, Royal Brompton Hospital, Sydney Street, London SW3 6NP, UK

Frank E. Rademakers, Department of Cardiology, University Hospitals Leuven, Herestraat 49, B-3000 Leuven, Belgium

Manojkumar Rohit, MD, Department of Cardiology, Postgraduate Institute of Medical Education & Research, Chandigarh, India, 160 012

Benjamin M. Schaefer, MD, Division of Cardiology, Box 356422, University of Washington, Seattle, WA 98195, USA

Kewal Krishnan Talwar, MD, DM, FAMS, Department of Cardiology, Postgraduate Institute of Medical Education & Research, Chandigarh, India, 160 012

Alec Vahanian, MD, Department of Cardiology, Hôpital Bichat, 46 rue Henri Huchard, Paris 75018, France

Ernst E. van der Wall, MD, Department of Cardiology, Leiden University Medical Center, PO Box 9600, 2300 RC Leiden, The Netherlands

Preface

As part of The European Society of Cardiology Education Series, this book is focused on the use of non-invasive imaging in clinical cardiology. Currently, the main non-invasive imaging modalities include echocardiography, nuclear imaging, cardiac magnetic resonance (CMR), and (multi-slice) computed tomography (MSCT). Rather than providing another textbook on imaging techniques, the central theme in this book is how to use these different imaging modalities to solve clinical problems that physicians encounter on a regular basis. A variety of clinical syndromes are discussed, including valvular disease, coronary artery disease, and myocardial and pericardial disease. In these various pathologies, the incremental value of echocardiography, nuclear imaging, CMR and MSCT are highlighted. Timely issues are discussed, for example the use of all imaging modalities in the assessment of myocardial viability in ischemic heart failure, the use of tissue Doppler echocardiography in cardiac resynchronization therapy, non-invasive angiography using MSCT in the evaluation of coronary artery disease, and the use of CMR in the evaluation of adult congenital heart disease.

All the chapters are clinically oriented, illustrating the contribution of different imaging techniques to the management of these clinical issues. The chapters reflect the expertise of the authors in managing the clinical problems, and can serve as a guide to physicians as to how these clinical issues can be addressed. The majority of the chapters are also illustrated with representative case histories and the moving images are available on the accompanying CD-Rom. The cases in particular offer excellent examples of how to use the imaging modalities in clinical cardiology.

The authors were selected based on their knowledge and experience in the field, and represent a broad panel of expertise both from a scientific and clinical point-of-view. Contributors are active members of the various Working Groups and Association of the European Society of Cardiology, including the Working Groups on CMR and Nuclear Cardiology respectively and the Association of Echocardiography. Besides contributors from Europe, additional authors from the United States and Asia have been included to provide a global perspective on the use of non-invasive imaging in clinical cardiology. Not necessarily all imaging modalities are discussed in each chapter, since different imaging modalities are more or less useful in the clinical scenarios discussed. The contributors have provided their own view on how to approach the different clinical problems and which techniques to use. It is possible that other imaging modalities will emerge to be as useful in the future; yet we trust that the current state of the art is adequately described.

The editors (each representing different imaging modalities) are grateful to all the authors for their excellent contributions. With this goal in mind, we sincerely hope that this book will be seen by clinicians as a useful handbook and help them to make the best usage of cardiovascular imaging modalities.

Jeroen J. Bax
Christopher M. Kramer
Thomas Marwick
William Wijns

Foreword

Over the last decade, we have witnessed an exponential development in imaging technology. Today, imaging plays a pivotal role in clinical management and decision making in patients with nearly every disease of the cardiovascular system. Accurate information on anatomy, perfusion, function, tissue viability, and even on molecular mechanisms of the disease process, can be obtained non-invasively through various techniques, all contributing to refined diagnosis and prognosis, and to better understanding of the pathophysiology.

However, the large volume of information can be overwhelming for the clinician who finds it increasingly difficult to select the most appropriate technique to be used in a specific disease. As a result, patients are often submitted to multiple imaging modalities, which may provide redundant information, contributing to the rapidly increasing costs of health care.

This new book in the "The ESC Education Series" intends to provide the reader with the answer to the most critical question that we ask ourselves every day: "Which imaging modality should I use for this particular patient with this specific clinical presentation?". Thus, it is not another technique-driven textbook, but rather a practical guide on optimal use of non-invasive cardiovascular imaging. We trust that this practical, case-based approach, presented by the leading experts in imaging, will make this book an interesting and useful tool to most clinical cardiologists.

Michal Tendera, FESC
President, European Society of Cardiology, 2004–2006

Section one
Valve disease

CHAPTER 1
Mitral stenosis

Kewal Krishan Talwar and Manojkumar Rohit

Introduction

Mitral stenosis (MS) is a progressive disease that can result in serious complications which may be fatal unless an intervention enlarges the mitral valve orifice enough to permit adequate cardiac output. The predominant cause of MS is rheumatic heart disease. Approximately 25% of all patients with rheumatic heart disease have pure MS, and an additional 40% have combined MS and mitral regurgitation.[1]

When MS is symptomatic, the anatomic features consist of thickened mitral cusps, fusion of the valve commissures, shortening and fusion of the chordae tendineae, or a combination of these features. Characteristically, mitral valve cusps fuse at their edge, and fusion of the chordae tendineae results in thickening and shortening of these structures. Although the major obstruction in patients with MS is usually caused by fusion of commissures, it may be below the valve itself, secondary to fusion of the chordae, and this assessment is important because significant subvalvular involvement leads to suboptimal results with mitral commissurotomy or balloon dilatation.

Other rare cause of MS include congenital mitral stenosis (e.g. supramitral ring, cor triatriatum), mitral annular calcification, systemic lupus erythematosus, rheumatoid arthritis, and mucopolysaccharidoses.

Although there are multiple clues to the presence of MS by physical examination, they are often subtle and likely to be overlooked during a routine physical examination of an asymptomatic patient. The diagnosis of MS is often made when the patient presents with a complication (e.g. atrial fibrillation, embolism, acute pulmonary edema, or massive hemoptysis).

The various imaging modalities that are useful in confirming the diagnosis and assessing the severity of MS are discussed in this chapter.

Case Presentation

A 25-year-old woman was referred to our Institute with progressive shortness of breath for 6 months, with chest X-ray as shown in Fig. 1.1. This chest X-ray shows straightening of left heart border with pulmonary venous hypertension. How consistent is this with a diagnosis of MS?

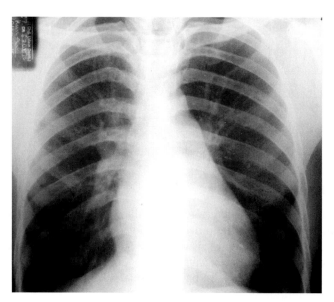

Figure 1.1 Chest X-ray posteroanterior (PA) view showing straightening of left heart border, cephalization of pulmonary veins, and double atrial shadow.

The most frequent roentgenographic findings in MS include left atrial enlargement, redistribution of blood flow to the upper lobes of the lung, Kerley B lines, and enlarged pulmonary artery. Although their cardiac silhouette may be normal in the frontal projection, patients with hemodynamically significant MS almost invariably have evidence of left atrial enlargement.

Left atrial enlargement is one of the earliest signs of mitral stenosis; however, its presentation may be subtle and limited to enlargement of the left atrial appendage, causing a straightening of the left heart border. In more advanced cases, the left atrium is recognized as a double density and elevation of main stem bronchus on the postanterior film. Radiologic changes in the lung fields indirectly reflect the severity of MS. Redistribution of blood flow to the upper lobes correlates best with the degree of mitral valve obstruction. The presence of Kerley B lines is an important finding in patients with MS. These are fine parallel densities in the peripheral lung fields which are perpendicular to a pleural surface and are most frequently seen in the costophrenic sulci. The lines are caused by thickened interlobar septa and signify chronic pulmonary venous hypertension.

This finding is present in 30% of patients with resting pulmonary arterial wedge pressures less than 20 mmHg and in 70% of patients with pressures greater than 20 mmHg.

Case Presentation (Continued)

Although the chest X-ray is strongly suggestive of MS, management decisions need to be informed by details of anatomy and severity, so echocardiography remains the examination of choice for evaluating MS. Indeed, the chest X-ray may be unnecessary, and of course should be avoided in a pregnant woman. The patient's M-mode showed a decreased E-F slope and the posterior mitral leaflet moved anteriorly during diastole, indicative of MS (Fig. 1.2). Is the M-mode still useful?

Although a decreased E-F slope is almost always present in severe MS, it is not diagnostic of MS and it is an unreliable indicator of its severity. The specificity of the diagnosis of MS by M-mode echocardiography is greatly improved by visualizing the initial diastolic movement of the posterior mitral leaflet.[2] In the normal mitral valve, the posterior leaflet moves away from the anterior leaflet during early diastole. In MS, the posterior leaflet moves anteriorly during early diastole.

Case Presentation (Continued)

The patient's two-dimensional (2D) imaging in the short axis view showed a typical "fishmouth" appearance of severely stenotic mitral valve with a mitral valve area of 0.6 cm^2 (Fig. 1.3). Does this confirm the diagnosis of MS on 2D imaging, and how should we evaluate severity of MS and suitability for percutaneous mitral commissurotomy?

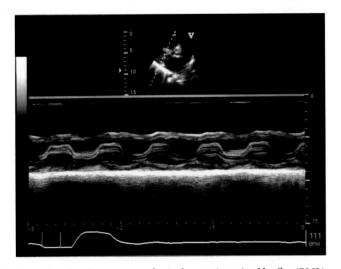

Figure 1.2 M-mode echo showing paradoxical posterior mitral leaflet (PML).

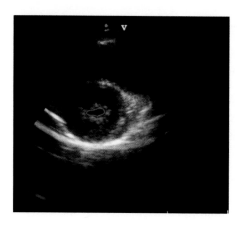

Figure 1.3 Parasternal short axis view showing typical "fishmouth" appearance of severely stenotic mitral valve (mitral valve area [MVA] 0.6 cm^2).

The short axis view allows the mitral valve area (MVA) to be measured by planimetry, although technical factors may compromise the accuracy of this method—not least the difficulty in ensuring that imaging is being performed at the tips of the leaflets. Heavily calcified leaflets may have indistinct borders that are difficult to trace, and there may also be dropout of echoes, leaving gaps in the area to be traced. The hallmark of MS on 2D echocardiography is thickening and restriction of motion of both mitral valve leaflets, with the predominant pathologic process being at the tips of the leaflets and proximal chordae. The abnormal motion of the leaflets is apparent in early diastole. Fusion of the commissures causes restriction in the motion of the tip of the anterior leaflet. The commissural fusion usually causes the posterior leaflet to move anteriorly during diastole with the larger anterior leaflet rather than moving posteriorly.

Doppler echocardiography assesses the severity of the stenotic lesion and color flow imaging is instrumental in determining associated mitral regurgitation. This is important because moderate mitral regurgitation (more than 2+) would be a contraindication to perform a closed procedure. MS produces characteristic changes in the mitral flow velocity pattern, involving an increase in the early diastolic peak velocity of flow and slower than normal rate of fall in velocity. The transvalvular pressure gradient can be measured continuously throughout diastole and correlates well with mean pressure gradient measured by cardiac catheterization. However, the pressure gradient is affected by heart rate, cardiac output, and valvular regurgitation in addition to orifice area, and hence it provides only a rough estimate of severity.

The pressure half-time is the time required for the instantaneous gradient across the valve to fall to half of the peak value (Fig. 1.4). This means of assessing MVA is usually sufficiently accurate for clinical use. The pressure half-time method is not valid for several days after mitral balloon valvuloplasty, probably because of a decrease in left atrial pressure without a commensurate improvement in left atrial compliance.

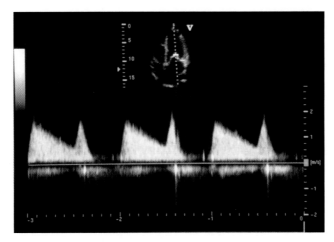

Figure 1.4 Continuous wave Doppler showing gradient across severely stenotic mitral valve.

Case Presentation (Continued)

Pressure half-time measurement in this case showed a mean gradient of 16 mmHg at the heart rate of 66 b/min (Fig. 1.4). Color Doppler performed on our index patient confirmed the stenotic mitral valve and fortunately showed no mitral regurgitation. Is the patient suitable for percutaneous intervention?

An echocardiographic scoring system developed by Wilkins *et al.*[3] has been used widely for assessment of suitability for percutaneous mitral commissurotomy. Leaflet rigidity, thickening, valvular calcification, and subvalvular involvement are each scored from 0 to 4. A score of 8 or less is usually associated with excellent immediate and long-term results, whereas scores exceeding 8 are associated with less impressive results. In our experience, slight commissural calcium is not a contraindication for percutaneous mitral commissurotomy, but when the calcium score is more than 2+, the incidence of restenosis is higher and thus surgical repair of the mitral valve is preferable. Significant subvalvular pathology is a more important determinant of suboptimal results following percutaneous mitral commissurotomy.

In addition to determining the presence and severity of MS, it is important to evaluate the heart for secondary effects of MS. These include left atrial enlargement, stasis, thrombus formation, and secondary pulmonary hypertension. The aortic, tricuspid, and pulmonic valves can likewise be directly evaluated for evidence of rheumatic involvement.

Case Presentation (Continued)

According to the Wilkins scoring system, our patient's mitral valve score was 6. There was no calcium on the mitral valve. This is an ideal candidate for percutaneous transmitral commissurotomy (PTMC) and a good result could be anticipated. What other steps are required before PTMC?

Transesophageal echocardiography

Transesophageal echocardiography (TEE) provides excellent images of the mitral valve leaflets, the left atrium, and the left atrial appendage (Fig. 1.5). Transthoracic imaging is usually diagnostic of MS and can accurately assess the severity of the stenosis. However, in some cases the transthoracic accoustic window may be inadequate. Multiplane TEE visualizes most of this anatomically complex structure and thrombus in the appendage can be accurately diagnosed, although experience is needed to avoid mistaking the pectinate muscle for thrombus.

TEE is well established as the gold standard for detecting thrombi in the left atrium (LA) and LA appendage, with a sensitivity and specificity of 100% and 99%, respectively.[4] The semi-invasive nature and safety of the test make it ideal for serial follow-up of thrombi in the LA body and appendage. TEE is also indicated if there is doubt regarding the presence or severity of mitral regurgitation and assessment of subvalvular pathology, if this is unclear on transthoracic echocardiography (Fig. 1.6). In our practice, all patients undergoing balloon valvuloplasty with atrial fibrillation and suspicion of clot on transthoracic echocardiography undergo TEE before the procedure. Finally, TEE may be used to guide the atrial trans-septal puncture during the balloon valvuloplasty procedure,[5] although we do not use TEE during the procedure at our institution.

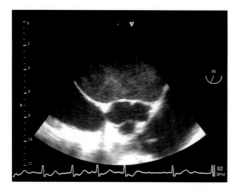

Figure 1.5 Transesophageal echocardiography (TEE) showing large left atrium with dense spontaneous contrast and amputated left atrial appendage.

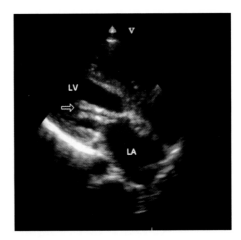

Figure 1.6 Parasternal long axis showing stenotic mitral valve and significant subvalvular thickening.

Case Presentation (Continued)

In this case, TEE was performed before PTMC. TEE showed dense spontaneous contrast but there was no clot in the left atrium (Fig. 1.5).

At cardiac catheterization before PTMC, left heart pressure was measured by retrograde catheterization of the left ventricle. Left atrial pressure was initially measured by pulmonary artery (which is accurate) and later by direct entry into the left atrium through trans-septal puncture. The mean gradient across the mitral valve was 15 mmHg before the PTMC (Fig. 1.7). The mitral valve was successfully dilated with a 26-mm Inoue balloon and the mean gradient across the mitral valve after the procedure was 4 mmHg with mitral valve area of 1.7 cm^2 and trivial mitral regurgitation.

Recently, there has been much interest in cardiac magnetic resonance imaging (MRI) and three-dimensional echocardiography in the assessment of valve lesions. We do not believe that MRI gives any additional information over echocardiography for MS, and MRI is expensive, time-consuming, and may be compromised by atrial fibrillation, which is not uncommon in MS. Three-dimensional echocardiography is a newer imaging modality and, in selected cases, will be useful, especially to assess the subvalvular apparatus.

Three-dimensional echocardiography

Real-time three-dimensional (R3D) echocardiography is a novel technique that permits visualization of mitral valvular anatomy in any desired plane of orientation. The use of R3D echocardiography in evaluation of mitral stenosis has been studied by Zamorano et al.[6] In 76 patients with significant MS, these

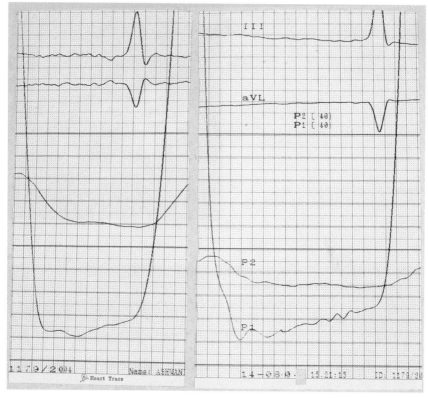

Figure 1.7 Left heart catheterization of left ventricle (LV) and left atrium (LA) tracing showing gradient across mitral valve before and after percutaneous transmitral commissurotomy (PTMC).

authors demonstrated that R3D echocardiography is a feasible, accurate, and highly reproducible technique for assessing MVA. MVA calculation with R3D echocardiography has the best agreement with invasive methods (average difference between both methods: $0.08cm^2$). R3D echocardiography may improve the assessment of MS severity in patients with discordant results between different methods and in clinical scenarios where these methods have limitations, particularly after balloon valvoplasty.[7]

Magnetic resonance imaging

Magnetic resonance imaging can be used to identify the presence of valvular stenosis. The high-velocity flow across the narrow valvular orifice may be recognized as a signal void on cine MRI. Imaging may be performed with steady-state free precession (SSFP) imaging for semi-quantitative assessment of valvular dysfunction or with a standard breath-hold segmented gradient–recalled echoplanar imaging sequence (GE-EPI) (Fig. 1.8). A study by

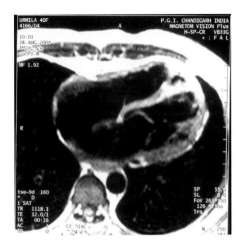

Figure 1.8 Magnetic resonance image (MRI) showing typical thickened doming mitral valve.

Krombach *et al.*[8] demonstrated both SSFP and GE-EPI sequences to share a high sensitivity (100%), although the image quality of SSFP was rated higher than GE-EPI. Peak flow velocity across MS can be quantified using velocity-encoded cine MRI (VE-MRI), analogous to echocardiography.[9] Lin *et al.*[9] reported excellent correlation of MVA by VE-MRI and Doppler echocardiography in 17 patients with MS ($r = 0.86$). An important strength of MRI for evaluation of mitral stenosis is that visualization of the spatial configuration of the mitral valve is excellent and quantification of transvalvular flow jet is unrestricted by echo windows. None the less, the MRI measurement is subject to several potential inaccuracies related to marginal temporal resolution, slice thickness, and signal loss.

Conclusions

In summary, 2D Doppler echocardiography gives sufficient information for imaging of MS. TEE has additional value for the evaluation of LA clot, and in some cases for assessment of mitral regurgitation and subvalvular pathology that is not clear on 2D echo. Of the newer imaging modalities, MRI and 3D echocardiography appear promising, and in selected cases they will avoid invasive (transesophageal or catheterization) studies.

References

1 Braunwald E. Valvular heart disease: mitral stenosis. In: Braunwald E, Zipes DP, Libby P, eds. *Heart Disease: A Textbook of Cardiovascular Medicine*, 6th edn. Philadelphia, PA: WB Saunders, 2001: 1643–53.
2 Dalen JE, Fenster PE. Mitral stenosis. In: Alpert JS, Dalen JE, Rahimtoola SH, eds. *Valvular Heart Disease*, 3rd edn. Philadelphia, PA: Lippincott Williams & Wilkins, 2000: 75–112.

3 Wilkins GT, Weyman AE, Abascal VM. Percutaneous mitral valvotomy: an analysis of echocardiographic variables related to outcome and the mechanism of dilatation. *Br Heart J* 1988;**60**;299–304.

4 Manning WJ, Weintraub RM, Waksmonski CA, *et al.* Accuracy of transesophogeal echocardiography for identifying left atrial thrombi. *Ann Intern Med* 1995;**123**:817–22.

5 Goldstein SA, Campbell AN. Mitral stenosis: evaluation and guidance of valvuloplasty by transesophageal echocardiography. *Cardiol Clin* 1993;**11**:409–25.

6 Zamorano J, Cordeiro P, Sugong L, *et al.* Real-time three-dimensional echocardiography for rheumatic mitral valve stenosis evaluation: an accurate and novel approach. *J Am Coll Cardiol* 2004;**43**:2091–6.

7 Langerveld J, Valocik G, Plokker HW, *et al.* Additional valve of three-dimensional transesophageal echocardiography for patients with mitral valve stenosis undergoing balloon valvoplasty. *J Am Soc Echocardiogr* 2003;**16**:841–9.

8 Krombach GA, Kunl H, Bucker A, Mahnker AH, Spuntrup E, Lipke C, *et al.* Cine MR imaging of heart valve dysfunction with segmented true fast imaging with steady state free precession. *J Magn Reson Imaging* 2004;**19**:59–67.

9 Lin SJ, Brown PA, Watkins MP, *et al.* Quantification of stenotic mitral valve area with magnetic resonance imaging and comparison with Doppler ultrasound. *J Am Coll Cardiol* 2004;**44**:133–7.

CHAPTER 2
Mitral regurgitation

Frank A. Flachskampf and Fausto Pinto

Introduction

Mitral regurgitation (MR) is the most frequent adult valvular lesion and the second most frequent reason for valvular surgery (after aortic stenosis). This chapter illustrates the evaluation of the patient with an asymptomatic pansystolic murmur. However, other typical clinical scenarios in which evaluation of MR is critical are the following:

1 The patient presenting with chronic dyspnea and a murmur suggesting MR.

2 The patient with severe dyspnea of abrupt new onset and a new murmur suggesting MR, with or without fever and signs of infection.

3 The patient with acute or chronic dyspnea, chronic coronary artery disease, an impaired left ventricle, and clinical or invasive evidence of MR.

4 The patient with acute severe dyspnea in the context of an acute coronary syndrome.

As in all forms of valvular regurgitation, assessment of severity is difficult, and no single parameter exists that is both easy to obtain and reliable for grading MR. Clinical assessment of MR therefore relies on gathering information on several characteristics and parameters, including mechanism, severity, duration, impact on the left ventricle, cardiac rhythm, amenability to repair, and other clinical data. These issues can almost always be resolved by careful clinical evaluation and application of modern imaging techniques (Table 2.1). Additionally, clinical and echocardiographic signs of the underlying etiology of MR should be sought systematically (Table 2.2).

Case Presentation

A 55-year-old man presents to his family physician for a routine check-up examination. He is physically active, completely asymptomatic, and in regular heart rhythm. A pansystolic murmur is heard over the apex, radiating to the axillary region. MR is suspected on clinical grounds and he is referred to a cardiologist for further evaluation.

Table 2.1 Imaging goals in mitral regurgitation.

Assessment of severity: mild, moderate, severe, and intermediary degrees, based on qualitative (color jet configuration, Doppler saturation, pulmonary venous flow) or quantitative (effective regurgitant orifice, regurgitant fraction, regurgitant volume) evaluation

Assessment of mechanism: normal/excessive/restricted mobility, degenerative changes (thickening, calcification, shortening), signs of endocarditis (vegetations), dilated annulus, structural damage, hypertrophic obstructive cardiomyopathy with systolic anterior motion, congenital anomaly

Assessment of location of regurgitant lesion (Fig. 2.4): anterior/posterior leaflet, anterolateral, central, posteromedial scallops (Carpentier nomenclature: P1–3, A1–3)

Assessment of left ventricular function: ejection fraction, left ventricular end-diastolic and end-systolic diameter (or volume), contractile reserve during stress

Other echocardiographic signs of underlying etiology: wall motion abnormalities for ischemic MR, leaflet thickening for mitral valve prolapse and systolic displacement, doming and thickening for rheumatic valvular disease

Table 2.2 Etiology of mitral regurgitation.

Degenerative chordal rupture with consecutive flail leaflet, typically in mitral valve prolapse
Degenerative fixation of a leaflet (in particular the posterior leaflet)
Ischemic:
• Impaired left ventricular function with dilatation causing eccentric pull of papillary muscles, restricted leaflet motion, and incomplete closure, together with mitral annular dilatation
• Papillary muscle rupture following myocardial infarction
Dilated cardiomyopathy (similar mechanism as in ischemic impaired left ventricular function)
Infective endocarditis with valvular destruction
Rheumatic valve disease
Hypertrophic obstructive cardiomyopathy
Congenital disease, e.g. mitral valve cleft
Mitral prosthetic dysfunction:
• Postoperative suture dehiscence/paravalvular leak
• Bioprosthetic degeneration
• Bioprosthetic endocarditis with leaflet destruction
• Ring abscess with large paraprosthetic leak or prosthetic dehiscence
• Prosthetic thrombosis with fixed position of occluder
• Fracture of mechanical prosthetic valve with occluder embolization
Rare causes: trauma, postvalvotomy regurgitation, Libman–Sacks endocarditis (systemic lupus erythematosus)

Chest X-ray

In a patient with dyspnea, a chest X-ray usually is performed as part of the basic work-up. Although heart and heart chamber enlargement resulting from MR (e.g. left ventricular and left atrial enlargement) can be diagnosed on chest X-ray, echocardiography is much more specific and accurate for these findings. Thus, nowadays the main information from a chest X-ray in MR is assessment of pulmonary congestion, ranging from mild pulmonary hypervolemia to frank pulmonary edema and pleural effusion. The absence of at least some degree of pulmonary congestion makes severe MR an unlikely cause for symptoms.

Case Presentation (Continued)

A chest X-ray demonstrates cardiac enlargement and mild pulmonary congestion. Kerley lines and pleural effusions are absent.

Which imaging modality for definite diagnosis?

In clinical practice, two imaging modalities are used to evaluate MR: echocardiography and contrast ventriculography by cardiac catheterization. Contrast ventriculography is invasive, costly, carries a small risk, is operator-dependent, and subject to large interobserver variabilities in interpretation.[1] Nevertheless, a well-performed ventriculogram showing no or minimal MR excludes substantial regurgitation. With higher degrees of regurgitation, the influence of injection technique, amount of contrast, catheter position, left ventricular function, and premature ventricular beats become more pronounced. It is particularly difficult to separate moderate from moderate-to-severe or severe degrees of regurgitation. Ventriculography should not be considered a "gold standard," and evaluation of MR per se is only very rarely the indication for cardiac catheterization. Nonetheless, a left ventriculogram is usually part of coronary angiography.

Echocardiography, while operator-dependent and having substantial interobserver variability, is now the dominant imaging technique to evaluate severity of MR, identify its mechanism, and devise therapy. Every patient with substantial MR should have an echocardiogram, and the decision to send a patient to surgery (especially if mitral repair is considered) mandates a thorough echocardiographic work-up, often with transesophageal echocardiography (Figs 2.1 & 2.2). Transesophageal echocardiography also is essential intraoperatively during repair surgery to assess results before the chest is closed.[2]

The use of three-dimensional (3D) echocardiography can improve the anatomic visualization of the different mitral valve scallops. For example, the location of prolapsing or flail leaflet segments is often immediately recognizable on 3D echocardiography, but requires expertise to pinpoint by conventional 2D echocardiography (Fig. 2.3). Communication with the surgeon may be aided by displaying "surgeon's views" from 3D data sets. Other benefits that may prove extremely useful, not only for diagnostic purposes, but also to help the surgeon in defining the feasibility and type of valve repair include a better appreciation

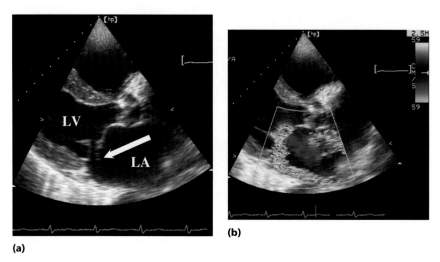

(a)

(b)

Figure 2.1 (a) Severe mitral regurgitation caused by a flail anterior mitral leaflet. Echocardiographic parasternal long axis view. The arrow points at the systolic position of the tip of the anterior mitral leaflet within the left atrium, thus creating a large regurgitant opening between anterior and posterior leaflet. (b) Color Doppler echocardiography, same patient and view as in (a). A large eccentric, posteriorly directed (away from the flail leaflet) turbulent, high-velocity jet is visible in the left atrium. LA, left atrium; LV, left ventricle.

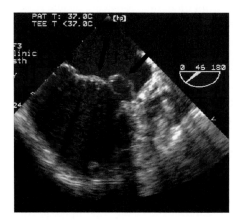

Figure 2.2 Mitral valve prolapse of both leaflets (arrows). Transesophageal view.

of the extension of the prolapse above the mitral annulus plane, the precise location of the diseased portion of the leaflets, its relation to important anatomic landmarks such as the valve commissures, and even the quantification of the volume of prolapsing tissue.[3] Furthermore, 3D echo is superior to 2D echo in calculating left ventricular volumes and ejection fraction.[4]

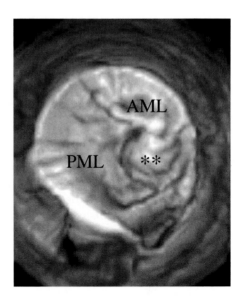

Figure 2.3 Three-dimensional echocardiography of a patient with prolapse (**) of the anterior leaflet of the mitral valve. AML, anterior mitral leaflet; PML, posterior mitral leaflet.

Magnetic resonance imaging (MRI) is the most recent imaging technique in the field. The morphologic and functional information MRI can provide is very similar to echocardiography, with somewhat lesser time and space resolution than transesophageal echocardiography. Atrial fibrillation substantially degrades image quality. Morphologic abnormalities of the leaflets can be detected, as well as high-velocity regurgitant jets. Regurgitant fraction can be calculated as the difference between left ventricular inflow and outflow, or between the difference of end-diastolic and end-systolic left ventricular volume on the one hand and aortic stroke volume on the other hand.[5] Left ventricular volumes and ejection fraction are assessed very accurately by MRI. Moreover, MRI can potentially provide much supplemental information in one examination, such as data on the presence and extent of myocardial scar, regional perfusion, and non-invasive coronary angiography (which, although currently rudimentary, is steadily improving). While these advantages, often summarized in the concept of "one-stop shopping" are impressive, practical reasons, apart from cost, nowadays and most likely in the future too will prevent MRI from superseding echocardiography, which will remain the first, and most often also the only, imaging technique needed. MRI at this time may be seen as an alternative technique if echocardiography cannot provide the necessary data. MRI can be safely performed in the presence of prosthetic valves, but is hazardous in the presence of a pacemaker.

Echocardiography in mitral regurgitation

Mitral valve morphology

Severe MR is always accompanied by morphologic abnormalities of the mitral valve structure or configuration. Specific morphologic assessment of the mitral valve apparatus includes the following:

• *Leaflet morphology:* leaflets are thickened in myxomatous (classic) mitral valve prolapse, degenerative disease, and rheumatic disease. Endocarditic lesions may manifest as vegetations, pseudoaneurysms (a form of abscess), defects, and rupture of subvalvular structures as chordae. Calcification, especially of the posterior annulus and leaflet, occurs in advanced age, hypertension, renal insufficiency, and rheumatic valve disease.

• *Leaflet mobility:* mobility can be conceptually divided into normal, excessive, and restricted.[6,7] Excessive mobility is present in prolapse and flail (Fig. 2.3), while restricted mobility is caused by calcification or rheumatic disease. The most important cause of restricted mobility is eccentric pull (tethering) via the papillary muscles in a dilated ventricle resulting from coronary heart disease with ventricular remodeling (ischemic cardiomyopathy) or dilated cardiomyopathy, leading to incomplete closure of the mitral leaflets. In these circumstances, the mitral annulus is usually also dilated to some degree. Importantly, ischemic MR may be dynamic (i.e. may dramatically increase from minor to severe during acute ischemia).[8,9] This mechanism can be unmasked by exercise stress.

• *Damage to the subvalvular apparatus:* typical examples are (degenerative or endocarditic) chordal or (ischemic) papillary muscle rupture, leading to a flail leaflet or scallop with severe regurgitation. In rheumatic heart disease, the subvalvular apparatus, in particular the chordae, are thickened, calcified, and shortened.

Morphologic assessment should include not only the type of damage, but also the location of the lesion (Fig. 2.4). The posterior leaflet can be subdivided into three scallops, and the anterior leaflet can also be divided in three corresponding segments, although these are anatomically less well-defined than the posterior leaflet scallops. The nomenclature is either anatomic or follows the Carpentier classification (P1–3 and A1–3). The scallops of the posterior leaflet are usually designated anterolateral (P1, adjacent to the A1 region of the anterior leaflet), central (P2, adjacent to A2), and posteromedial (P3, adjacent to A3). The location of mitral valve pathology (e.g. a prolapse) has important implications for repairability.[2] It is also important to correlate morphologic findings with Doppler findings. Restricted leaflet motion leads to regurgitant jets directed towards the side of the affected leaflet, while excessive leaflet motion leads to regurgitant jets directed away from the affected leaflet.

Doppler assessment of hemodynamics

MR should be evaluated by color Doppler using all available windows, especially the apical views. Mitral regurgitant jets are often eccentric (Fig. 2.1b). Visual estimation of the maximal color Doppler jet and relating it to left atrial area yields a rough estimate of severity, but moderate and severe degrees cannot be reliably separated in this way, and eccentric, wall-hugging jets are severely underestimated by the jet area method. While very small and very large jets are

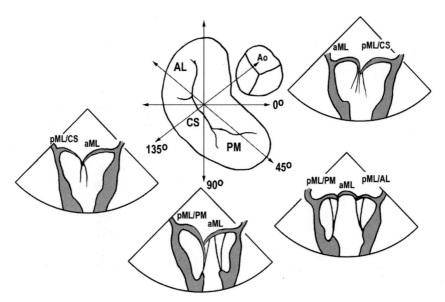

Figure 2.4 Mapping of the mitral valve by multiplane transesophageal echocardiography (schematic drawing). Four cross-sections from a transesophageal transducer position centered on the mitral valve are shown in a "surgeon's view" of the mitral valve, together with the relationship of the mitral leaflets as they are seen in these cross-sections: at 0°, corresponding to a four-chamber view; at 45°, representing an intermediate view; at 90°, corresponding to a two-chamber view; and at 135°, corresponding to a long axis view of the left ventricle. Different scallops of the posterior leaflet (pML) are visualized in the different views: the central scallop (pML/CS, corresponding to P2 in the Carpentier nomenclature) is seen in the four-chamber and the long axis view; the anterolateral scallop (pML/AL, corresponding to P1) in the 45° intermediate view; and the posteromedial (pML/PM, corresponding to P3) in the two-chamber and in the intermediate view. AML, anterior mitral leaflet; AO, aortic valve. (Reproduced with permission from Flachskampf FA, Decoodt P, Fraser AG, Daniel WG, Roelandt JRTC. Recommendations for performing transesophageal echocardiography. *Eur J Echocardiogr* 2001;**2**:8–21.)

usually well identified, the intermediate severities are impossible to grade reliably by color jet area. An important sign of severe MR that should always be evaluated is reduced or reversed systolic pulmonary venous flow (Fig. 2.5). In eccentric jets, it may be useful to sample both upper pulmonary veins to detect flow reversal.

Several quantitative approaches to evaluating MR severity have been validated and are clinically feasible, if image quality is good.[10]

1 Measurement of the proximal jet diameter, which evaluates the regurgitant orifice by measuring the smallest diameter of the regurgitant jet immediately downstream from its passage through the leaflet.

2 The proximal convergence zone method (PISA method). This technique

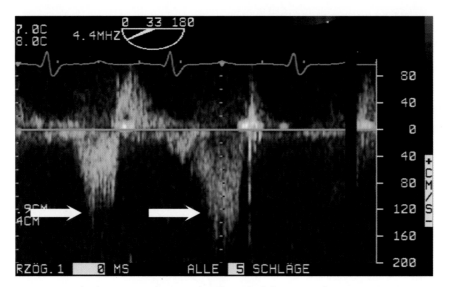

Figure 2.5 Pulsed wave Doppler recording from the left upper pulmonary vein in severe mitral regurgitation (MR) (same patient as Fig. 2.1). Systolic backward flow is present (arrows), indicating severity of regurgitation.

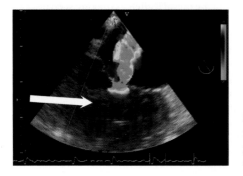

Figure 2.6 Transesophageal view of mitral regurgitation with large central jet and prominent proximal convergence zone (arrow).

analyzes the flow field upstream from the regurgitant orifice (i.e. on the ventricular side of the mitral valve; Fig. 2.6).

3 Calculation of regurgitant fraction based on the difference between transmitral stroke volume, calculated from pulsed-wave Doppler and mitral annular diameter, and transaortic stroke volume or the difference between ventricular stroke volume (end-diastolic minus end-systolic left ventricular volume) and transaortic stroke volume.

Right ventricular systolic pressure as assessed by measuring tricuspid regurgitation velocities is elevated in substantial MR, sometimes to severe pulmonary hypertension levels.

Evaluation of left heart morphology and left ventricular function

Quantitative morphologic parameters of the left ventricle important for the management of severe MR are as follow:

1 *End-systolic and end-diastolic left ventricular diameters (or volumes):* chronic (but not acute!) MR of more than mild severity leads to end-diastolic enlargement (dilatation) of the left ventricle as a consequence of volume overload. Initially, end-systolic diameter remains unaffected, thus leading to an increased shortening fraction, reflecting a hyperkinetic, volume-loaded ventricle. Increase in the end-systolic left ventricular dimension signals contractile impairment. A cutoff of 45 mm has been shown to predict persistent impaired left ventricular function after surgical correction of MR.[11]

2 *Left atrial enlargement:* more than mild chronic regurgitation leads to left atrial enlargement. In chronic severe MR, atrial fibrillation inevitably ensues, further promoting left atrial dilatation. The anteroposterior systolic diameter classically measured by M-mode is a relatively insensitive measure of left atrial enlargement. Left atrial enlargement is best assessed by planimetry of the left atrium in the four-chamber view.

3 *Left ventricular ejection fraction,* similar to fractional shortening, is of paramount importance in assessing MR and identifying candidates for surgical correction, especially in asymptomatic patients. Because MR initially leads to a hyperkinetic ventricle by increasing preload and decreasing afterload, even a low-normal ejection fraction (less than 60%) should be taken as a sign of beginning contractile dysfunction. Exercise ejection fraction may be used to unmask latent contractile dysfunction. Patients with severe MR who are unable to raise their ejection fraction in response to physical exercise (i.e. lacking contractile reserve) are candidates for surgical repair even in the presence of a normal ejection fraction.[12]

With state-of-the-art echocardiographic equipment most if not all these data can be acquired from the transthoracic echo. In patients difficult to image or with questionable results, transesophageal echocardiography is the next diagnostic step. Confirmation of the underlying mitral pathology and its location by transesophageal echocardiography, especially if the patient is a surgical candidate, will usually be sought to give the surgeon as much preoperative information as possible.

Ejection fraction calculation by echocardiography has considerable interobserver, intraobserver, methodologic (e.g. monoplane or biplane disk summation method), and day-to-day variability, the latter mostly resulting from changes in loading conditions such as arterial blood pressure. This variability needs to be kept in mind. Substantially more accurate and reproducible measurements of left ventricular volumes and ejection fraction are possible with 3D echoechocardiography or MRI, although this does not address the problem of load dependency of ejection fraction. Thus, in a few selected patients difficult to image or with inconclusive echocardiographic findings, an MRI may be clinically helpful.

Transthoracic echocardiography reveals a dilated left ventricle (end-diastolic diameter 59 mm; end-systolic diameter 41 mm). The ejection fraction is calculated to be 54%. The mitral valve is mildly and diffusely thickened, with a flail portion of the posterior leaflet well visible in the apical four-chamber view, indicating flail of P2 (central scallop of the posterior leaflet). There is an anteriorly directed, eccentric jet of MR with a proximal diameter of 8 mm, a reproducible proximal convergence zone on the left ventricular side of the mitral valve, and clearly reduced systolic forward pulmonary venous flow in the right upper pulmonary vein. The left atrium is mildly enlarged. There is moderate tricuspid regurgitation, with right ventricular systolic pressure calculated from the peak tricuspid regurgitant velocity to be 38 mmHg plus right atrial pressure.

In summary, this patient has asymptomatic, severe MR with low normal left ventricular function, sinus rhythm, and a presumably repairable lesion. Following the guidelines,[13,14] this constitutes a recommendation for mitral valve repair.

If ejection fraction was clearly in the upper normal range (more than 60%), stress echocardiography might be useful to determine whether ejection fraction increases during exercise. Failure to increase ejection fraction would indicate incipient impairment in myocardial contractility in spite of normal resting function.[12] A transesophageal echocardiogram would be additionally useful to confirm location and repairability of the regurgitant lesion.

Other important clinical situations

Acute severe mitral regurgitation

Acute MR is usually ischemic (e.g. papillary muscle rupture) or endocarditic in origin. Some typical features of severe chronic MR are missing in severe acute regurgitation:

1 Regardless of the severity of regurgitation, neither the left atrium nor the left ventricle are necessarily enlarged. At least initially, sinus rhythm is often preserved. However, the presence of enlargement does not exclude acute regurgitation, because concomitant or previous disease may have led to previous chamber enlargement.

2 Global left ventricular dysfunction is not a typical feature of acute MR, and typically there is left ventricular hyperkinesis as a response to the volume loading of acute regurgitation. However, left ventricular dysfunction does not exclude this condition, because there may be concomitant myocardial disease.

Mitral prosthetic regurgitation

With ever-increasing numbers of patients with mitral valve replacement, this scenario is becoming increasingly important. Importantly, the size of the left atrium and ventricle, as well as the level of pulmonary hypertension are influenced by pre-existing disease and therefore have to be interpreted with caution with respect to the severity of MR. Because of the difficulties inherent in imaging valve prostheses, transesophageal echocardiography is usually necessary for evaluation. Mitral prosthetic regurgitation can have several etiologies:

1 *Bioprosthetic degeneration:* the wear-and-tear lesions of bioprostheses may remain entirely clinically silent before a large tear suddenly manifests as torrential regurgitation.

2 *Infective endocarditis:* endocarditis often leads to ring abscesses which destroy the anchoring of the prosthesis in its bed. Regurgitation may range from paravalvular leakage to dehiscence, defined as abnormal mobility ("rocking") of the whole prosthesis, to embolism of the entire prosthesis. Furthermore, endocarditis can affect bioprosthetic leaflets in a similar manner as native valve leaflets.

3 *Paravalvular leakage or dehiscence* (Fig. 2.7): may occur as the result of suture insufficiency.

4 *Mechanical (and rarely, biological) prosthetic thrombosis or pannus interference:* may fix the occluder or leaflets in a half-open, half-shut position, leading to both severe stenosis and regurgitation.

5 *Prosthetic strut fracture:* this is a very rare cause of acute massive prosthetic regurgitation, leading to embolization of the occluder.

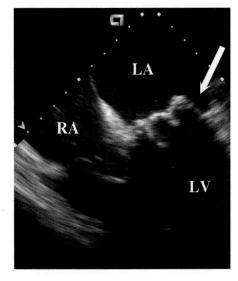

Figure 2.7 Lateral dehiscence (arrow) of a mitral bioprosthesis. Transesophageal four-chamber view in systole, showing displacement and tilting of the prosthesis towards the left atrium. RA, right atrium. (Reproduced with permission from Lambertz H, Lethen H. *Atlas der Transösophagealen Echokardiographie*. Stuttgart: Thieme, 2000.)

Role of imaging in management decisions in mitral regurgitation

The decision to treat MR surgically depends on careful appreciation of the following issues:[13,14]

- Presence of severe MR, at least if MR is the principal reason for surgery.
- Symptom status (dyspnea).
- Left ventricular function. Even mildly impaired or borderline left ventricular function constitutes an indication for valve surgery, even in the absence of symptoms. On the other hand, severely impaired left ventricular function (ejection fraction less than 30%) carries a high surgical risk for valve replacement.
- Amenability of mitral pathology to repair surgery, especially if sinus rhythm can likely be preserved.

These issues can almost always be resolved by careful clinical and echocardiographic evaluation of the patient. In a few cases, contrast ventriculography, together with right heart catheterization, or MRI may be helpful.

References

1 Croft CH, Lipscomb K, Mathis K, *et al.* Limitations of qualitative angiographic grading in aortic or mitral regurgitation. *Am J Cardiol* 1984;**53**:1593–8.

2 Gillinov AM, Cosgrove DM, Blackstone EH, *et al.* Durability of mitral valve repair for degenerative disease. *J Thorac Cardiovasc Surg* 1998;**116**:734–43.

3 Macnab A, Jenkins NP, Bridgewater BJM, *et al.* Three dimensional echocardiography is superior to multiplane transesophageal echo in the assessment of regurgitant mitral valve morphology. *Eur J Echocardiogr* 2004;**5**:212–22.

4 Kuhl HP, Schreckenberg M, Rulands D, *et al.* High-resolution transthoracic real-time three-dimensional echocardiography. *J Am Coll Cardiol* 2004;**43**:2083–90.

5 Hundley WG, Li HF, Willard JE, *et al.* Magnetic resonance imaging assessment of the severity of mitral regurgitation: comparison with invasive techniques. *Circulation* 1995;**92**:1151–8.

6 Carpentier A. Cardiac valve surgery: the "French correction". *J Thorac Cardiovasc Surg* 1983;**86**:323–37.

7 Stewart WJ, Currie PJ, Salcedo EE, *et al.* Evaluation of mitral leaflet motion by echocardiography and jet direction by Doppler color flow mapping to determine the mechanism of mitral regurgitation. *J Am Coll Cardiol* 1992;**20**:1353–61.

8 Lancellotti P, Lebrun F, Pierard LA. Determinants of exercise-induced changes in mitral regurgitation in patients with coronary artery disease and left ventricular dysfunction. *J Am Coll Cardiol* 2003;**42**:1921–8.

9 Pierard LA, Lancellotti P. The role of ischemic mitral regurgitation in the pathogenesis of acute pulmonary edema. *N Engl J Med* 2004;**351**:1627–34.

10 Zoghbi WA, Enriquez-Sarano M, Foster E, *et al.* Recommendations for evaluation of the severity of native valvular regurgitation with two-dimensional and Doppler echocardiography. *J Am Soc Echocardiogr* 2003;**16**:777–802.

11 Enriquez-Sarano M, Tajik AJ, Schaff HV, *et al.* Echocardiographic prediction of left ventricular function after correction of mitral regurgitation: results and clinical implications. *J Am Coll Cardiol* 1994;**24**:1536–43.

12 Leung DY, Griffin BP, Stewart WJ, Cosgrove DM III, Thomas JD, Marwick TH. Left ventricular function after valve repair for chronic mitral regurgitation: predictive value of preoperative assessment of contractile reserve by exercise echocardiography. *J Am Coll Cardiol* 1996;**28**:1198–205.

13 Bonow RO, Carabello B, de Leon AC Jr, *et al.* ACC/AHA guidelines for the management of patients with valvular heart disease: a report of the American College of Cardiology/American Heart Association Task Force on practice guidelines (committee on management of patients with valvular heart disease). *J Am Coll Cardiol* 1998;**32**:1486–588.

14 Iung B, Baron G, Butchart EG, *et al.* A prospective survey of patients with valvular heart disease in Europe: The Euro Heart Survey on Valvular Heart Disease. *Eur Heart J* 2003;**24**:1231–43.

CHAPTER 3
Aortic stenosis

Benjamin M. Schaefer and Catherine M. Otto

Case Presentation

A 79-year-old man was admitted with syncope after walking up an incline. He felt progressively weak, sat down, and subsequently lost consciousness, fully regaining all capacity when the ambulance arrived. On examination there is a 3/6 late-peaking systolic murmur radiating to the carotids, a single second heart sound, and carotid upstrokes are diminished and delayed. The electrocardiogram (ECG) demonstrates left ventricular hypertrophy. He is thought to have severe aortic stenosis and admitted to hospital for further management.

Etiology

Valvular aortic stenosis is caused either by progressive calcification of a trileaflet valve, a process thought to be similar but not identical with atherosclerosis, calcification of a congenitally bicuspid valve, or rheumatic valve disease. Other causes are rare and include a congenitally unicuspid valve, and supravalvular and subvalvular stenosis.[1]

A normal aortic valve has three mobile, thin leaflets designated as the right, left, and non-coronary cusps. A bicuspid valve has two leaflets in either right–left or anterior–posterior configuration. The normal, non-stenotic aortic valve has an opening area of 3–4 cm^2; which is equivalent to the area of the left ventricular outflow tract (LVOT) or aortic annulus. Acquired valvular stenosis is characterized by leaflet thickening and calcification that can be detected using various imaging modalities. As calcification and fibrosis (or commissural fusion with rheumatic disease) progress, leaflet motion becomes restricted, eventually resulting in restriction of valve opening area. This progressive narrowing results in an increasing antegrade velocity of blood flow across the valve, corresponding to a pressure gradient between the left ventricle and aorta during systole. The constrained orifice and the high-velocity jet form the basis for assessment of aortic stenosis severity.

Assessment of aortic stenosis

The evaluation of aortic stenosis can be divided into several components:
1 The anatomy and pathologic features of the valve leaflets
2 The severity of valve obstruction
3 The effect of chronic pressure overload on the left ventricle and pulmonary vasculature
4 Associated dilatation of the ascending aorta
5 In selected cases, the dynamic changes in valve area with exercise or pharmacologic intervention

Imaging of the valve

Direct imaging of the diseased aortic valve allows determination of the number of valve leaflets, the etiology of stenosis, and the severity of leaflet calcification.[2] Imaging also is important to exclude other causes of outflow obstruction, such as a subaortic membrane or obstructive hypertrophic cardiomyopathy. Transthoracic two-dimensional (2D) echocardiography is the standard clinical approach for imaging the aortic valve, although the basic principles apply to any imaging modality including three-dimensional (3D) echocardiography, magnetic resonance imaging (MRI) and computed tomography (CT).

On echocardiography, the transthoracic parasternal long axis view is used to determine the diameter of the LVOT and ascending aorta, and for visualization of valve motion (Fig. 3.1) The right and the non-coronary cusps are usually seen in this view and the degree of valve calcification can be assessed. A bicuspid valve often has an asymmetric closure line, slight doming of the leaflets in systole, and a flat closure line or frank prolapse in diastole (Fig. 3.2). Calcific stenosis shows increased leaflet thickness and echogenicity with reduced systolic motion. In the short axis view, a trileaflet valve can be distinguished from a

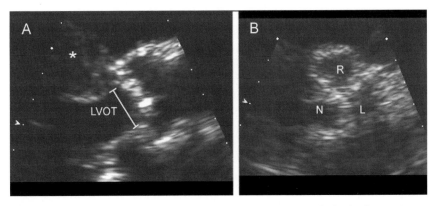

Figure 3.1 Parasternal (A) long and (B) short axis views of a calcified trileaflet aortic valve. The valve is shown closed in diastole. L, left coronary cusp; LVOT, left ventricular outflow tract; N, non-coronary cusp; R, right coronary cusp.

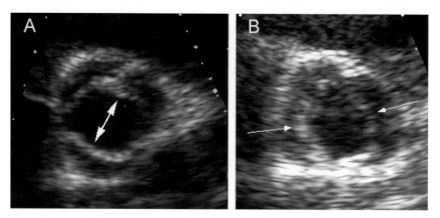

Figure 3.2 Bicuspid aortic valve. Two examples of a bicuspid valve are shown. (A) Leaflet orientation is anterior–posterior with a prominent raphe in the anterior leaflet. (B) Leaflet orientation is left–right.

bicuspid valve by the number of leaflets in systole. Many bicuspid valves have a prominent raphe in one leaflet so that frame-by-frame analysis and identification of the number of commissures is needed for diagnosis of bicuspid valve. In addition, once severe calcification is present it may not be possible to identify the number of leaflets. Rheumatic disease is diagnosed based on commissural fusion and calcification with a central triangular orifice, in contrast to the stellate orifice in calcific disease (Fig. 3.3).

Direct images of the valve are seldom used for planimetry of valve area because of inaccuracy resulting from reverberations from valve calcification and the complex 3D shape of the valve orifice. In some patients, a valve orifice can be visualized with transesophageal echocardiography (TEE), but caution is needed to ensure the image plane is at the smallest valve orifice. Three-dimensional echocardiographic or MRI of the valve may provide better delineation of the stenotic orifice in systole,[3] but these approaches are rarely used because the critical clinical information is obtained from the Doppler data (Fig. 3.4). Multislice CT quantification of aortic valve calcification volume correlates with valve gradients and area,[4] which provides a new parameter for assessment of disease severity, although the clinical utility of valve calcium scores is as yet unknown. Valve calcification can be visualized on fluoroscopy and may initially be noted at the time of coronary angiography.

Severity of valve obstruction
Jet velocity and pressure gradient
Doppler echocardiography is the standard clinical approach for assessing stenosis grade, as maximum aortic jet velocity can be used to calculate mean systolic gradient and also contributes to the calculation of valve area, using the continuity equation. As the valve narrows, the velocity of blood flow increases with jet

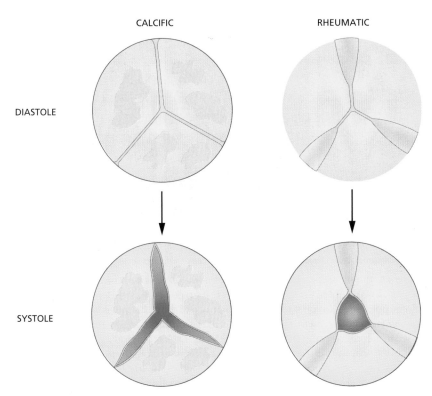

CALCIFIC   RHEUMATIC

DIASTOLE

SYSTOLE

Figure 3.3 Schematic diagrams of valve anatomy is a short axis orientation of calcific aortic stenosis showing the complex stellate orifice in systole (left) and rheumatic stenosis (right) with a central triangular orifice with commissural fusion. Rheumatic disease typically is accompanied by mitral valve involvement.

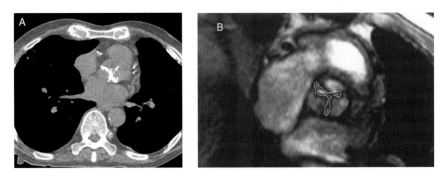

Figure 3.4 Electron beam tomographic and cardiac magnetic resonance images of stenotic aortic valves. (A) Short axis electron beam view at the level of the aortic valve showing severe valve calcification. (E-speed Electron Beam Angiography, General Electric, San Francisco, CA; Image courtesy of Matt Budoff, MD.) (B) Cardiac magnetic resonance imaging showing a cross-sectional view of a moderately stenotic aortic valve; the gray line denotes the aortic valve area (AVA). (With permission from John *et al.* 2003[3].)

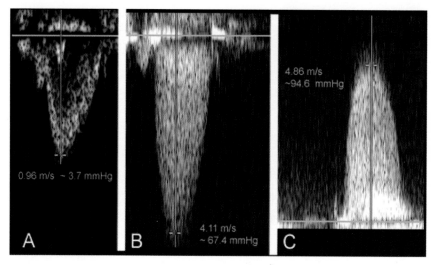

Figure 3.5 Doppler echocardiography of a stenotic aortic valve. The outflow tract velocity (A) is recorded from an apical view using a pulsed wave Doppler sample volume positioned just on the left ventricular side of the aortic valve (at the same site at the diameter measurement as shown in Fig. 3.1). Continuous wave Doppler (B and C) is used to determine the maximum aortic velocity. Lack of alignment between the ultrasound beam and direction of flow can lead to underestimation of the velocity. Note that the maximum velocity from an apical approach (B) is only 4.1 m/s corresponding to a maximum gradient of 67 mmHg, whereas the maximum velocity from a high right parasternal position (C) is 4.9 m/s, corresponding to a maximum pressures gradient of 95 mmHg. The higher velocity represents a more parallel alignment. Also notice that the maximum velocity is measured as the edge of the more intense envelope of flow, avoiding the faint signals resulting from the transit time effect.

velocity being a strong predictor of clinical outcome (Fig. 3.5). Aortic jet velocities (v) are converted to pressure gradients (ΔP), using the simplified Bernoulli equation as:

$$\Delta P = 4v^2$$

using the maximum jet velocity to calculate the maximum gradient and averaging the instantaneous pressures gradients during systole for mean gradient. Note that the maximum Doppler velocity corresponds to maximum instantaneous gradient across the aortic valve, which should not be confused with the peak-to-peak gradient measured by cardiac catheterization, a non-physiologic measure, because these peaks do not occur simultaneously (Fig. 3.6).

Aortic jet velocity is measured with continuous wave Doppler, taking care to use optimal patient positioning, several acoustic windows, and careful transducer angulation to obtain a clear signal with a parallel intercept angle between the ultrasound beam and aortic jet. Because the Doppler equation includes a

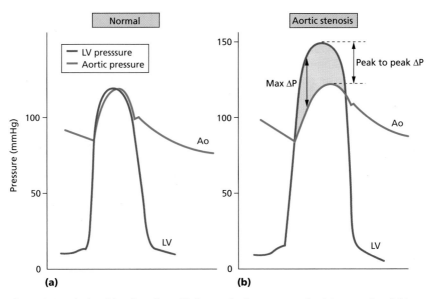

Figure 3.6 Relationship of aortic and left ventricular pressures for (a) normal and (b) stenotic aortic valve. The rate of rise aortic pressure in patients with aortic stenotic is notably decreased, corresponding to a slow carotid upstroke. The maximum instantaneous gradient (*) corresponds to the maximum Doppler gradient and typically is greater that the peak left ventricular to peak aortic ("peak-to-peak") gradient (+) measured with cardiac catheterization.

term for the cosine of the intercept angle, any deviation from a parallel intercept angle results in underestimation of jet velocity (Fig. 3.4). In general, an intercept angle less than 20° is acceptable (error less than 6%). Underestimation of jet velocity because of poor signal strength or a non-parallel intercept angle is the most common pitfall in assessment of stenosis severity; avoidance of this source of error depends on experienced examiners and correct interpretation of the flow signals.

Overestimation of the jet velocity or pressure gradient occurs less often. Causes of an inaccurate velocity signal include measuring the faint signals at the edge of the velocity curve as a result of the transit time effect or misidentification of the mitral regurgitant jet signal. Pressure gradient is overestimated if there is an elevated velocity proximal to the stenosis; in this situation, proximal velocity is included in the Bernoulli equation as:

$$\Delta P = 4 \left(v_{jet}{}^2 - v_{prox}{}^2 \right)$$

The phenomenon of pressure recovery may be an issue in comparing Doppler with invasive pressure gradient data for prosthetic valves (see Chapter 6) but is less of a problem with native valve stenosis; the magnitude of this effect is only a few mmHg and is most pronounced with a large valve area and small ascending aorta.

Aortic valve area

A limitation of velocity and pressure gradient data is that a relatively low velocity, and pressure gradient, may be present if transaortic volume flow rate is decreased, for example with associated left ventricular systolic dysfunction, mitral regurgitation or a small, hypertrophied ventricle. In these situations, aortic valve area (AVA) is calculated from Doppler data using the continuity equation based on the concept that the stroke volume across the narrowed aortic valve orifice is equal to the stroke volume proximal to the valve (Fig. 3.7)

$$SV_{AVA} = SV_{LVOT}$$

because stroke volume is the product of the cross-sectional area (CSA) and velocity time integral (VTI) of flow (e.g. the temporal and spatial mean flow velocity):

$$AVA \times VTI_{AS\text{-}Jet} = CSA_{LVOT} \times VTI_{LVOT}$$

Solving for aortic valve area (Fig. 3.7):

$$AVA = (CSA_{LVOT} \times VTI_{LVOT}) / VTI_{AS\text{-}Jet}$$

In clinical practice, maximum velocities may be substituted for velocity time integrals as the ratio of both are similar, so that the simplified continuity equation is:

$$AVA = (CSA_{LVOT} \times V_{LVOT}) / V_{AS\text{-}Jet}$$

Thus, the measurements needed for calculation of valve area are:

1 LVOT diameter measured from a parasternal long axis view for calculation of a circular cross-sectional area.

2 LVOT velocity measured with pulsed wave Doppler from an apical view (for a parallel intercept angle) with the sample volume positioned immediately adjacent to the aortic valve closure plane (to ensure that diameter and flow are measured at the same place).

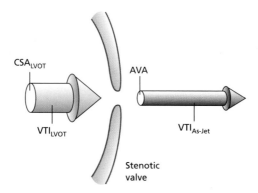

Figure 3.7 Schematic diagram of the continuity equation to calculate the aortic valve area. AVA, aortic valve area; CSA, cross-sectional area; LVOT, left ventricular outflow tract; VTI, velocity time integral.

3 Aortic jet velocity, taking care to obtain the highest velocity signal, indicating a parallel intercept angle.

An accurate valve area calculation depends on attention to technical details for each of these measurements. Slight errors in LVOT diameter measurement translate into larger errors in valve area. However, LVOT diameter does not change with changes in flow rate or over time in adults. In addition, the ratio of LVOT to aortic velocity provides a simple measure of stenosis severity that is independent of body size.

Other approaches

In the past, cardiac catheterization was used to measure the pressure gradient across the stenotic valve and, in conjunction with measurement of transaortic volume flow rate, to calculate valve area using the Gorlin formula. However, catheterization is expensive and entails some risk, because it requires either a transeptal puncture for simultaneous left ventricular and aortic pressure measurements, or retrograde passage of a catheter across the stenotic valve, which is associated with cerebral embolization. Cardiac MRI has the potential to visualize and measure blood flow and allows calculation of valve area, analogous to the Doppler method. However, this approach is not yet established for routine clinical care.

Chronic left heart pressure overload

Pressure overload of the left ventricle leads to concentric left ventricular hypertrophy. Women tend to develop a small, thick-walled chamber with diastolic dysfunction but preserved systolic function. In contrast, men tend to have increased left ventricle (LV) mass resulting from dilatation and are more likely to have a decreased ejection fraction. Most patients with aortic stenosis have a normal ejection fraction until very late in the disease course.

Echocardiography allows measurement of wall thickness and chamber dimensions, and calculation of 2D ejection fraction. LV mass can be determined by echocardiography but is not routinely measured clinically.[5] Both 3D echocardiography and cardiac MRI allow more accurate determination of LV ejection fraction and mass; however, these approaches are largely limited to research applications.

Diastolic function is evaluated with standard Doppler techniques including transmitral flow velocities, pulmonary vein flow patterns, and tissue Doppler velocities to evaluate diastolic relaxation, compliance, and filling pressures.[6]

In patients with long-standing aortic stenosis, pulmonary pressures may become elevated. Pulmonary systolic pressure can be accurately assessed by echocardiography. Measurement of pulmonary vascular resistance requires right heart catheterization.

Associated dilatation of the ascending aorta

In patients with aortic valve disease, it is especially important to image the aorta. Bicuspid aortic valve is associated with aortic dilatation in many patients, probably as the result of a systemic connective tissue disorder.[7] Patients with trileaflet calcified valves also may have aortic involvement resulting from atherosclerosis. The echocardiographic examination should include imaging and measurement of the sinuses of Valsalva, sinotubular junction, and ascending aorta. If an abnormality is present, further evaluation with CT or MRI is warranted. CT imaging is especially helpful as it allows 3D reconstruction of the entire aorta (Fig. 3.8).

Dynamic changes in valve area

In patients with aortic stenosis and severe left ventricular systolic dysfunction, it may be difficult to distinguish whether reduced valve leaflet opening is a result of severe valve stenosis or primary myocardial disease with only mild to moderate stenosis. In these rare patients, evaluation of valve area at different flow rate, with exercise or dobutamine infusion, may be helpful. If AVA increases significantly, the principal problem is myocardial dysfunction, not aortic stenosis. Patients in whom the ventricle fails to demonstrate contractile reserve to stress have a particularly poor prognosis. However, stress evaluation of aortic stenosis is technically difficult and should only be performed in experienced laboratories.

Clinical relevance

Aortic stenosis severity is classified as:
- *Mild:* jet velocity <3 m/s, mean gradient <20 mmHg, valve area >1.5 cm^2
- *Moderate:* jet velocity 3–4 m/s, mean gradient 20–40 mmHg, valve area 1.0–1.5 cm^2
- *Severe:* jet velocity >4 m/s, mean gradient >40 mmHg, valve area <1.0 cm^2

Patients with symptomatic severe aortic stenosis should proceed to aortic valve replacement because the prognosis with medical therapy is very poor.

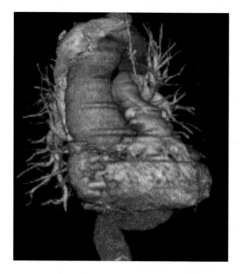

Figure 3.8 Three-dimensional reconstruction of the aorta from computed tomography (CT) imaging in a patient with a bicuspid aortic valve and dilated aorta.

Recently, attention has been focused on the natural history of asymptomatic aortic stenosis using Doppler data to follow disease progression. Predictors of symptom onset in initially asymptomatic patients include age over 50 years, known coronary artery disease, and moderate or severe valve calcification.[8,9] There also is interest in the use of echocardiographic Doppler data and electron beam CT quantitative assessment of valve calcification for assessing potential therapeutic interventions.[10]

Case Presentation (Continued)

The patient was found to have a heavily calcified valve with concentric left ventricular hypertrophy and an ejection fraction of 46%. Aortic jet velocity was 5.3 m/s, mean gradient 65 mmHg, and continuity equation valve area 0.8 cm^2. Because he had severe symptomatic aortic stenosis, valve replacement was recommended. Preoperative coronary angiography was normal and he did well postoperatively.

References

1 Otto CM. Aortic stenosis. In: Otto CM, ed. *Valvular Heart Disease*, 2nd edn. Saunders–Elsevier, Philadelphia, 2004: 197–246.

2 Otto CM. Valvular stenosis. In: Otto CM. *The Textbook of Clinical Echocardiography*, 3rd edn. Elsevier–Saunders, Philadelphia, 2004: 277–314.

3 John AS, Dill T, Brandt RR, *et al*. Magnetic resonance to assess the aortic valve area in aortic stenosis: how does it compare to current diagnostic standards? *J Am Coll Cardiol* 2003;**42**:519–26.

4 Morgan-Hughes GJ, Owens PE, Roobottom CA, Marshall, AJ. Three-dimensional volume quantification of aortic valve calcification using multislice computed tomography. *Heart* 2003;**89**:1191–4.

5 Aurigemma GP, Douglas PS, Gaasch WH. Quantitative evaluation of left ventricular structure, wall stress and systolic function. In: Otto CM, ed. *The Practice of Clinical Echocardiogaphy*, 2nd edn. W.B. Saunders, Philadelphia, 2002: 65–87.

6 Redfield MM, Jacobsen SJ, Burnett JC Jr, Mahoney DW, Bailey KR, Rodeheffer RJ. Burden of systolic and diastolic ventricular dysfunction in the community: appreciating the scope of the heart failure epidemic. *JAMA* 2003;**289**:194–202.

7 Fedak PW, Verma S, David TE, Leask RL, Weisel RD, Butany J. Clinical and pathophysiological implications of a bicuspid aortic valve. *Circulation* 2002;**106**:900–4.

8 Rosenhek R, Klaar U, Schemper M, Scholten C, *et al*. Mild and moderate aortic stenosis: natural history and risk stratification by echocardiography. *Eur Heart J* 2004;**25**:199–205.

9 Rosenhek R, Binder T, Porenta G, *et al*. Predictors of outcome in severe, asymptomatic aortic stenosis. *N Engl J Med* 2000;**343**:611–7.

10 Pohle K, Maffert R, Ropers D, *et al*. Progression of aortic valve calcification: association with coronary atherosclerosis and cardiovascular risk factors. *Circulation* 2001;**104**:1927–32.

CHAPTER 4

Aortic regurgitation

Helmut Baumgartner and Gerald Maurer

Case Presentation

A 33-year-old man had a routine health check-up to get permission for competitive sport. He was completely asymptomatic and had good exercise capacity. On examination, his blood pressure was 160/60 mmHg and ausculation revealed a 3/6 diastolic murmur at the left sternal edge. The electrocardiogram (ECG) showed left ventricular hypertrophy and chest X-ray left ventricular enlargement. The patient was referred to the cardiac outpatient department for further evaluation.

Diagnosis and grading of severity

In general, aortic regurgitation (AR) is detected by physical examination or incidentally by echocardiography. Clinical presentation includes a characteristic decrescendo diastolic murmur and—as soon as moderate to severe—increased systolic pressure, widened pulse pressure, and bounding pulses. Although widened pulse pressure in the absence of other etiologies is a reliable indicator of hemodynamically relevant AR, conversely the lack of this sign does not reliably exclude severe AR, particularly during advanced adult life where other disorders associated with abnormal systemic vascular distensibility may be present. Symptoms usually develop slowly and comprise mostly shortness breath and less commonly angina with exertion.

Diagnostic tools

The results of **ECG** (left ventricular [LV] hypertrophy with or without strain pattern) and **chest X-ray** (LV enlargement, eccentric hypertrophy or dilatation of the ascending aorta) are non-specific.

At present, **echocardiography** is the mainstay for diagnosing AR and grading its severity. The sensitivity and specificity of color Doppler for detection of AR with demonstration of the regurgitant jet (Fig. 4.1) approach 100%. Aortic root angiography or cardiac magnetic resonance imaging (CMRI) may be required in rare instances when echocardiography is technically impossible.

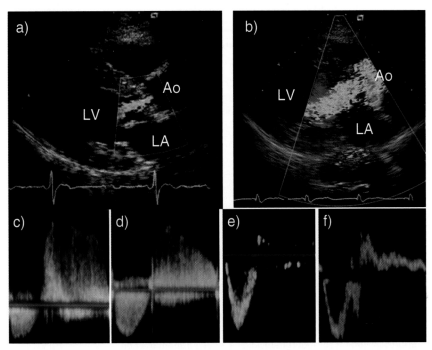

Figure 4.1 Echocardiographic evaluation of aortic regurgitation (AR). (a) Narrow color jet in mild AR (parasternal long axis view); (b) broad color jet and large convergence zone in severe AR (parasternal long axis view); (c) continuous wave (CW) Doppler tracing in mild AR (slow velocity decay); (d) CW Doppler tracing in severe AR (steep velocity decay); (e) pulsed wave (PW) Doppler tracing from the decending aorta (suprasternal approach) in mild AR (minimal diastolic flow reversal); (f) PW Doppler tracing from the decending aorta (suprasternal approach) in severe AR (holodiastolic flow reversal). Ao, aorta; LA, left atrium; LV, left ventricle.

Grading aortic regurgitation severity

While echocardiography has a key role in grading AR severity, the issue of quantification by this technique has not been sufficiently resolved. As there is still no single measurement that can be used for reliable quantitative assessment, an integrative approach incorporating the sum of information obtained from two-dimensional echocardiography (2D echo), color Doppler, and conventional continuous wave (CW) and pulsed wave (PW) Doppler must be recommended.[1] Table 4.1 summarizes the most important parameters to be considered and has been adapted from a consensus paper recently published in the American[1] and European literature. Specific signs having a specificity of more than 90%, supportive signs with more modest predictive accuracy, and quantitative parameters for AR severity are listed. The consensus is that the process of grading AR should be comprehensive, using a combination of these features. When the evidence from the different parameters is congruent, it is

Table 4.1 Grading of aortic regurgitation.

Mild		Moderate	Severe	
Specific signs for AR severity				
			Flail or wide coaptation defect	
Vena contracta < 0.3 cm*		Intermediate values	Vena contracta > 0.6 cm*	
Central jet width < 25% of LVOT*		Intermediate values	Central jet ≥ 65% of LVOT*	
No or brief early diastolic flow reversal in Ao desc.			Holodiastolic flow reversal in Ao desc.	
Supportive signs				
PHT > 500 ms			PHT < 200 ms	
No/minimal flow convergence*			Large flow convergence*	
			Moderate or greater LV enlargement†	
Quantitative parameters‡				
R vol mL/beat	< 30	30–44	45–59	≥ 60
RF %	< 30	30–39	40–49	≥ 50
EROA cm²	< 0.10	0.10–0.19	0.20–0.29	≥ 0.30

AR, aortic regurgitation; Ao desc., aorta descending; EROA, effective regurgitant orifice area; LV, left ventricle; LVF, left ventricular function; LVOT, left ventricular outflow tract; PHT, pressure half-time; R vol, regurgitant volume; RF, regurgitant fraction.
* At a Nyquist limit of 50–60 cm/s.
† In the absence of other etiologies of LV dilatation.
‡ Quantitative parameters can help subclassify the moderate group into mild-to-moderate and moderate-to-severe regurgitation as shown. However, numbers have to be viewed with caution and only in the context of the other signs of severity because of the intrinsic limitations of quantitative measurement techniques.

easy to grade AR severity. However, when different parameters are contradictory, one must look carefully for technical and physiologic explanations for these discrepancies, and rely on the components showing the best quality primary data and that are the most accurate in the context of the underlying clinical condition.

2D echo signs

The clear demonstration of a flail cusp or of a wide coaptation defect is rather rare. However, if present these signs are already highly specific for severe AR. Moderate or greater enlargement of the left ventricle together with well-preserved contractility reflects significant volume overload and is, in the absence of other pathologies that cause LV volume overload (e.g. mitral regurgitation, ventricular septal defect), also a highly specific sign of severe AR. Likewise, moderate or greater enlargement of the LV without clear volume overload in the absence of other etiologies explaining LV dilatation is a supportive sign of severe AR but less specific.

Doppler echocardiographic signs

Measurement of the narrowest width of the proximal jet (**vena contracta**) is a simple valuable measurement for grading AR (Fig. 4.1).[2] Using a Nyquist limit of 50–60 cm/s, a jet width less than 0.3 cm is highly specific for mild AR, whereas a width of more than 0.6 cm is highly specific for severe AR.[1] A cut-off of ≥0.5 cm has high sensitivity but markedly less specificity. In highly eccentric jets this simple measurement becomes unreliable. The ratio of jet width and left ventricular outflow tract width has also been proposed with a cut-off of less than 0.25 for mild and ≥0.65 for severe AR.[1] However, this measurement has no apparent advantage over simple jet width measurement and is therefore less commonly used.

PW Doppler recordings of the flow in the proximal descending aorta have been found to yield additional important information.[1] No or only brief **diastolic flow reversal** indicates mild AR, whereas holodiastolic flow reversal is specific for severe AR (Fig. 4.1). Conversely, severe AR may be present in the absence of holodiastolic flow reversal, particularly when the ascending aorta is dilated.

CW Doppler can be used to record the flow velocity of the regurgitant jet. The **rate of deceleration** and the derived pressure half-time reflect the rate of equalization of aortic and LV diastolic pressure. With increasing severity of AR, aortic diastolic pressure decreases more rapidly. The late diastolic jet velocity is lower and pressure half-time shorter. Although this is rather considered to be a supportive sign and not highly specific, a pressure half-time of more than 500 ms is usually consistent with mild AR, whereas values of less than 200 ms (some would rather use less than 300 ms) is considered compatible with severe AR (Fig. 4.1).[1] In particular, other etiologies of higher end-diastolic LV pressure but also those of low diastolic pressure can cause a steep velocity decay and yield false-positive results of severe AS. Conversely, a pressure half-time of more than 500 ms is much more specific for mild AR.

Considerably less experience exists with the **PISA** (proximal isovelocity surface area) method for the assessment of AR compared with mitral regurgitation. The interposition of valve tissue when using the usual apical approach also limits the application of this technique. Minimal or no flow convergence nevertheless indicates mild AR, whereas a larger flow convergence is consistent with severe AR. Although rarely used, the PISA method has also been applied for AR[3] and has been reported to yield regurgitant volume and when combined with CW Doppler measurements of jet velocity effective regurgitant orifice area (EROA). Thresholds of ≥60 mL and ≥0.30 cm^2 have been reported for severe AR.

Quantitation of flow with PW Doppler for the assessment of AR is based on comparison of measurements of aortic stroke volume at the LVOT with mitral or pulmonic stroke volume.[1] Total stroke volume can also be derived from quantitative 2D measurements of LV end-diastolic and end-systolic volumes. EROA can again be calculated from the regurgitant stroke volume and the regurgitant jet velocity time integral by CW Doppler. As with the PISA method, a regurgitant volume ≥ 60 mL and EROA ≥ 0.30 cm^2 are consistent with severe AR.

These two quantitative methods have also been proposed to subclassify the moderate regurgitation group into mild-to-moderate and moderate-to-severe regurgitation. However, both methods are controversial. There are a considerable number of sources of error resulting from intrinsic limitations. Instead of adhering too much to calculated numbers for the grading of AR, many believe that it is advisable to use the integrative approach with all the signs described above to provide accurate judgment as a basis of clinical decision-making.

Alternative imaging tools

Although grading is possible by Doppler echocardiography in the vast majority of patients, uncertainty may remain in some, particularly when ultrasound imaging quality is poor. In this case, cardiac catheterization is still commonly used. However, invasive evaluation does also not provide true quantitation because it mostly relies on aortic root angiography, which is graded semi-quantitatively, as well as on hemodynamic measurements. In case of uncertainty of echocardiographic grading, CMRI may be a useful next step. Although regurgitant volume and regurgitant fraction can be calculated from stroke volume measurements derived from LV and RV volume estimates, the currently preferred approach involves quantification of forward and backward flow in the ascending aorta (Fig. 4.2).

Additional information needed from imaging procedures

Mechanism of aortic regurgitation

Understanding the etiology and mechanisms leading to regurgitation is essential for proper management. Aortic valve repair, while performed infrequently at this point, may be considered in suitable cases, such as bicuspid aortic valves with leaflet prolapse.

Conversely, there may be severe AR with intact aortic leaflets in some cases of aortic root dilation or of aortic dissection, where prolapse of the dissection membrane prevents valve closure. In such instances, the valve may not require replacement at the time of surgery for dissection. Obtaining information about the mechanism of AR and its etiology is currently the domain of echocardiography, particularly using the transeophageal approach (Table 4.2, Figs 4.3 and 4.4). Newer imaging tools such 3D echo (Fig. 4.4) and MRI may contribute to the assessment of the complex spatial relationships of the aortic valve structures and may ultimately improve the facility of aortic valve repair.

Ascending aorta

In all instances information about morphology and size of the ascending aorta are needed. Aortic root and annular dilatation may cause AR even when leaflets are normal. In presence of a bicuspid aortic valve, the aortic root is frequently dilated, probably because of an abnormality of the wall, which may also explain

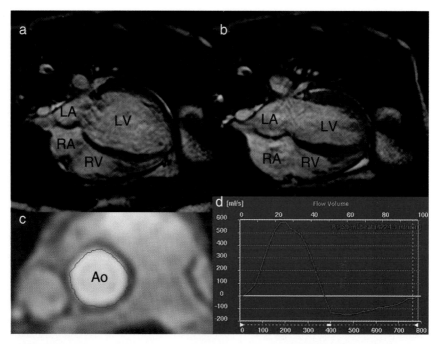

Figure 4.2 Evaluation of AR by magnetic resonance imaging. (a) End-diastolic frame of four-chamber view; (b) end-systolic frame of four-chamber view; (c) velocity image acquired in a plane perpendicular to the proximal ascending aorta; (d) flow volume curve in the ascending aorta indicating a large regurgitant volume and regurgitant fraction. Ao, aorta; LA, left atrium; LV, left ventricle; PA, pulmonary artery; RA, right atrium; RV, right ventricle.

Table 4.2 Etiology of aortic regurgitation (AR).

Primary valve disease
Congenital: Bicuspid aortic valve
Outlet supracristal ventricular septal defect
Discrete subaortic stenosis
Rheumatic
Endocarditis*
Other inflammatory disorders
Degenerative
Traumatic leaflet rupture*
Secondary aortic regurgitation
Aortic root dilatation
Aortic dissection*

* Disorders leading to acute AR.

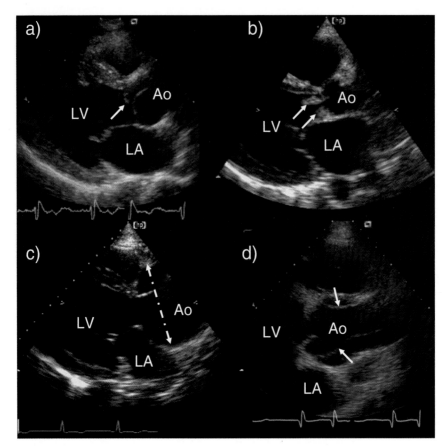

Figure 4.3 Etiology of AR. (a) Bicuspid valve with prolapse of the anterior cusp (arrow); (b) infective endocarditis of the aortic valve with large vegetations (arrows); (c) aortic root aneurysm; (d) dissection of the descending aorta (arrows indicate intimal flap). Ao, aorta; LA, left atrium; LV, left ventricle.

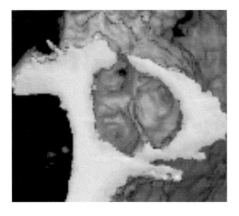

Figure 4.4 Three-dimensional echocardiographic image of a bicuspid aortic valve.

the increased association with aortic dissection. The aortic root dilatation may be independent of hemodynamics and can progress further even after valve surgery. As in other types of aortic dilatation, elective surgical correction is recommended when the diameter exceeds 55 mm.[4]

Additional pathology

Information about additional findings is also needed, including presence of abnormalities of other valves and of endocarditis. Knowledge about possible coexistent congenital abnormalities is also essential, especially in view of the fact that some are associated with AR, such as subaortic stenosis and some forms of ventricular septal defect (VSD).

Left ventricular function

Assessment of LV function is crucial for managing the patient with AR. Knowledge of global LV function is required, as well as of end-diastolic and end-systolic LV size. A diminished LV ejection fraction (below 50–55%) is associated with reduced prognosis even in asymptomatic patients (Fig. 4.5).[5,6] LV dysfunction of short duration is, however, usually reversible; thus serial evaluation LV function is recommended on a routine basis in these patients and surgery should be considered as soon as a drop in ejection fraction occurs. LV enlargement in itself also constitutes an indication for surgery (Fig. 4.5).[7,8] The most commonly used parameters are echocardiographic end-systolic and end-diastolic diameters.[7] At present, ejection fraction is most commonly measured using 2D echo or radionuclide ventriculography. For assessment of LV size, actual volume measurements instead of single-dimensional measurements may gain increasing utility in the future, particularly using accurate and reproducible techniques, such as MRI and 3D echo.

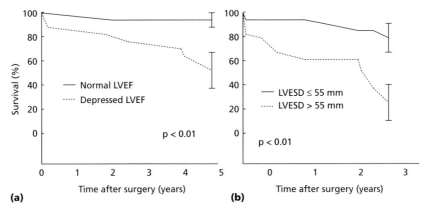

Figure 4.5 Postoperative survival of patients with preoperative normal versus reduced left ventricular function (a) and of patients with preoperative left ventricular end-systolic diameter ≤55 mm versus >55 mm (b). (Redrawn from Dujardin *et al.* 1999[5] and Bonow *et al.* 1985.[6])

Management strategy of aortic regurgitation—a stepwise approach using imaging

Figure 4.6 summarizes a management strategy for AR, which relies heavily on imaging. The ultimate goal of valvular heart disease management is no longer the relief of symptoms caused by these disorders. Optimal management should instead provide optimal long-term outcome with regard to mortality as well as morbidity. This is critically dependent on preservation of LV function. Accomplishment of this goal requires surgical repair in some patients before symptoms even occur. In AR, criteria for early detection of myocardial damage focus on ventricular size and function. Current practice guidelines for the timing of surgery in asymptomatic patients use cut-offs derived from the published literature (Table 4.3).[8,9]

Table 4.3 Indication for surgery in patients with severe aortic regurgitation.

Indication class*	ACC-AHA Guidelines	ESC Guidelines†
I	Any patient in NYHA class III or IV	LVEDD > 70 mm or
I	NYHA class II with normal LVF but progressive	LVESD > 50 mm or
	LV dilatation or declining EF or declining exercise	LVESI > 25 mm/m^2
	tolerance on serial studies	
I	EF 25–49%	Asc. Aorta > 55 mm
I	CCS class II angina	
IIa	NYHA class II with normal LVF and stable LVF	Rapid increase in LV
	LV size and exercise tolerance on serial studies	diameters
IIa	Asymptomatic patient with normal LVF but	Bicuspid aortic
	LVESD > 55 mm	valve or
	or LVEDD > 75 mm (consider body size)	Marfan with aorta
IIb	EF < 25%	> 50 mm
IIb	Asymptomatic patient with normal LVF but LVESD	
	50–55 mm or LVEDD 70–75 mm (consider body size)	
IIb	Asymptomatic patient with decreased EF with	
	exercise	

* Class I indicates that there is evidence or general agreement that the procedure is useful. Class II indicates that there is conflicting evidence or opinion: IIa indicates that the weight of evidence favors surgery, whereas class IIb indicates that the efficacy of surgery is less well established.

† Guidelines are only for asymptomatic patients.

NYHA, New York Heart Association; CCS, Canadian Cardiac Society; EF, ejection fraction; LV, left ventricle; normal LVF, normal left ventricular function defined by EF ≥ 50%; LVEDD, left ventricular end-diastolic diameter; LVESD left ventricular end-systolic diameter; LVESI, left ventricular end-systolic diameter index.

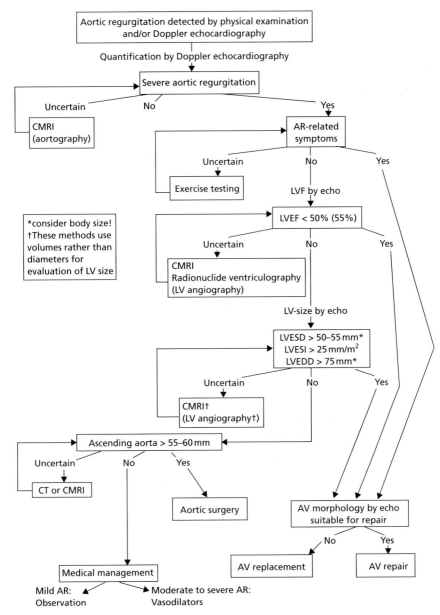

Figure 4.6 Management strategy of aortic regurgitation (AR): a stepwise approach using imaging (see text). AV, aortic valve; CMRI, cardiac magnetic resonance imaging; CT, computed tomography; LV, left ventricle; LVEDD, left ventricular end-diastolic diameter; LVEF, left ventricular ejection fraction; LVESD, left ventricular end-systolic diameter; LVESI, left ventricular end-systolic index; LVF, left ventricular function.

As soon as AR is detected by physical examination and/or Doppler echocardiography the next step is to assess its severity. This is in general provided by echocardiography. In the case of uncertainty, CMRI should preferably be used. Aortography can be an alternative. Even in the absence of severe AR, prophylactic surgery may be needed for aortic root aneurysm, and this requires further evaluation of the ascending aorta. Surgery is recommended when the maximum diameter reaches 55–60 mm. If echo cannot provide reliable measurements, CMRI or computed tomography (CT) should be performed.

In the case of severe AR, the next question concerns symptoms. In their presence, surgery is indicated. Exercise testing may help to assess symptom status. In a definitely asymptomatic patient, the next step is to assess LV function (LVF). In the case of reduced LVF as defined by ejection fraction of less than 50% (some recommend even 55%), surgery should be performed. In the case of

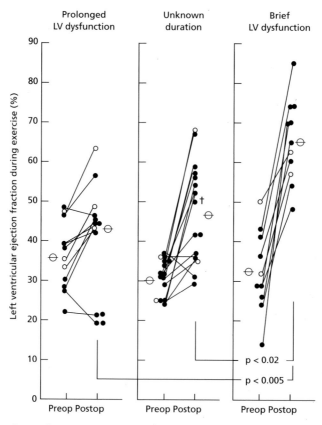

Figure 4.7 Change from preoperative to postoperative left ventricular (LV) ejection fraction at rest in patients with severe aortic regurgitation and prolonged LV dysfunction (more than 14 months), unknown duration, and brief duration of LV dysfunction (≤14 months). (Redrawn from from Bonow *et al.* [1984].[10])

uncertainty by echocardiography, CMRI, radionuclide ventriculography, or LV angiography can be used.

Asymptomatic patients with normal LVF should be considered for valve surgery for preservation of myocardial function when end-systolic diameter exceeds 55 mm[8] (50 mm by European guidelines[9]) or when end-diastolic diameter of the LV exceeds 75 mm. These cut-off values must take body size into account. They are valid for average-sized men but may be too large for women, especially if the patient is small. For this reason, some prefer a cut-off LV end-systolic index of more than 25 mm/m^2. However, indexing has its own limitations and both the absolute value and index must always be viewed on the background of individual patient size. Uncertain echo measurements may again require CMRI or LV angiography.

If surgery is indicated for any of the above-mentioned reasons, echocardiography should evaluate whether a valve repair is feasible or whether valve replacement must be performed. In addition, aortic size and morphology must be assessed in order to evaluate the need for concomitant aortic surgery.

If surgery is not indicated, serial echocardiographic evaluation is required in patients who remain asymptomatic. In stable patients 1-year intervals may be appropriate, as studies have shown that LV dysfunction developing over 12–14 months is usually reversible (Fig. 4.7).[10] Patients with moderate-to-severe AR appear to benefit from vasodilator therapy, particularly when the ventricle is already dilated.

Case Presentation (Continued)

On echocardiographic examination, the patient was found to have a bicuspid aortic valve with severe prolapse of the anterior cusp causing severe AR. There was no calcification of the valve. The left ventricule was enlarged (LV end-systolic diameter 50 mm) and LVF mildly reduced with an ejection fraction of 46%. CMRI confirmed abnormal LVF with an ejection fraction of 44%. Therefore, surgery was thought to be indicated although the patient was asymptomatic. He underwent successful repair of his aortic valve. After the operation he continued to be asymptomatic and LVF normalized (ejection fraction 55%).

References

1 Zoghbi WA, Enriquez-Sarano M, Foster E, *et al*. Recommendations for evaluation of the severity of native valvular regurgitation with two-dimensional and Doppler echocardiography. *J Am Soc Echocardiogr* 2003;**16**:777–802.

2 Tribouilloy CM, Enriquez-Sarano M, Bailey KR, Seward JB, Tajik AJ. Assessment of severity of aortic regurgitation using the width of the vena contracta: a clinical color Doppler imaging study. *Circulation* 2000;**102**:558–64.

3 Tribouilloy CM, Enriquez-Sarano M, Fett SL, Bailey KR, Seward JB, Tajik AJ. Appli-

cation of the proximal flow convergence method to calculate the effective regurgitant orifice area in aortic regurgitation. *J Am Coll Cardiol* 1998;**32**:1032–9.

4 Davies RR, Goldstein LJ, Coady MA, *et al.* Yearly rupture or dissection rates for thoracic aortic aneurysms: simple prediction based on size. *Ann Thorac Surg* 2002; **73**:17–28.

5 Dujardin KS, Enriquez-Sarano M, Schaff HV, Bailey KR, Seward JB, Tajik AJ. Mortality and morbidity of aortic regurgitation in clinical practice: a long-term follow-up study. *Circulation* 1999;**99**:1851–7.

6 Bonow RO, Picone AL, McIntosh CL, *et al.* Survival and functional results after valve replacement for aortic regurgitation from 1976 to 1983: impact of preoperative left ventricular function. *Circulation* 1985;**72**:1244–56.

7 Bonow RO, Rosing DR, Kent KM, Epstein SE. Timing of operation for chronic aortic regurgitation. *Am J Cardiol* 1982;**50**:325–36.

8 Bonow R, Carabello B, DeLeon AC Jr, *et al.* Guidelines for the management of patients with valvular heart disease: executive summary: a report of the American College of Cardiology/American Heart Association Task Force on Practice Guidelines (Committee on Management of Patients with Valvular Heart Disease). *Circulation* 1998;**98**: 1949–84.

9 Iung B, Gohlke-Barwolf C, Tornos P, *et al.* Recommendations on the management of the asymptomatic patient with valvular heart disease. *Eur Heart J* 2002;**23**:1253–66.

10 Bonow RO, Rosing DR, Maron BJ, *et al.* Reversal of left ventricular dysfunction after aortic valve replacement for chronic aortic regurgitation: influence of duration of preoperative left ventricular dysfunction. *Circulation* 1984;**70**:570–9.

CHAPTER 5

Aortic dissection

Debabrata Mukherjee and Kim A. Eagle

Introduction

Swift diagnosis of aortic dissection is imperative because of the potentially catastrophic nature of the illness and the exceedingly high mortality if not diagnosed early in the course. Aortic dissection should be considered in the differential diagnosis of patients presenting with myocardial ischemia, syncope, chest pain, back pain, abdominal pain, stroke, and acute heart failure. Ideally, rapid and non-invasive diagnostic imaging is preferred to assess the need for immediate intervention, particularly in patients with involvement of ascending aorta. Currently, various imaging modalities are available for the diagnosis of aortic dissection including transthoracic echocardiography (TTE), transesophageal echocardiography (TEE), computed tomography (CT), magnetic resonance imaging (MRI), and contrast aortography. Visualization of an intimal flap separating two lumina is considered diagnostic of aortic dissection. If the false lumen is completely thrombosed, central displacement of the intimal flap, calcification, or separation of intimal layers signals chronic dissection rather than mural thrombosis.

Classification of aortic dissection is based upon the site of the intimal tear and the extent of the dissecting hematoma. In DeBakey type I and type II dissection, the intimal tear is located in the ascending aorta, usually just a few centimeters above the aortic valve. In type I dissection, the hematoma extends for a variable distance beyond the ascending aorta, while in type II the dissecting hematoma is confined to the ascending aorta. In type III, the dissection originates in the descending aorta, typically just beyond the origin of the left subclavian artery, and propagates antegrade into the descending aorta or, rarely, retrogradely into the aortic arch and ascending aorta. In the Stanford classification, type A refers to all dissections that involve the ascending aorta and the entry site may be located anywhere along the course of the aorta. All other dissections are classified as type B. In type B, the dissection is confined to the aorta distal to the left subclavian artery.

In the past, diagnosis of aortic dissection was typically made by contrast angiography. However, technological developments in TTE, TEE, CT, and MRI have changed the approach to diagnosis of aortic dissection. The preferred imaging modality depends on availability in emergency situations as well as the experience of the particular hospital with a particular modality. Sarasin *et al.*[1]

compared diagnostic strategies for the emergency assessment of patients with suspected acute aortic dissection and measured the effect of delays related to the availability of these tests on the selection of the most appropriate one. The investigators performed a decision analysis representing the risks of performing one or two sequential tests, the tests' accuracy, the risks and benefits of treatment, and the time-dependent mortality rate in untreated patients with dissection, which is typically 1% per hour in the first 24–36 h. They determined that the "threshold" clinical probability of aortic dissection above which the benefits of testing outweigh its risks is quite low. It ranges from 2% with the most reliable procedure (MRI) to 9% with the least (TTE). At low probability of dissection (less than 15%), the accuracy of all tests except TTE is sufficient to rule out dissection. Delays have negligible effect on these results. When the pretest likelihood of dissection is higher, the preferred option is to order a second diagnostic test if the results of the first are negative. Excessive delays may affect the selection of tests when the likelihood of dissection is high (e.g. 50%). Thus, although it is less accurate, a CT scan obtained within 2 h or a TEE obtained within 6 h of presentation yields a higher survival rate than an MRI obtained within 9 h.[1] Similarly, the benefits of ordering a second test, if the result of the first is negative or equivocal, outweigh the risks only if the delay in obtaining the test does not exceed 10 h. It appears that all patients for whom aortic dissection is suspected, even if the index of suspicion is very low, should undergo one of the available diagnostic procedures (except TTE). A patient with a moderate to high probability of disease should undergo a second investigation if the findings of the first are negative. When the probability of dissection is high, the physician must consider delays in obtaining specific diagnostic tests and order those that will be the most quickly available. In this chapter, we review the currently available imaging modalities for the diagnosis of aortic dissection including chest X-ray.

Chest X-ray

A chest X-ray is a simple and inexpensive test which may be performed initially and may suggest dissection but lacks specificity for diagnosis of aortic dissection. A chest X-ray will be abnormal in 60–90% of cases of aortic dissection, but a normal chest X-ray is not sufficient to rule out aortic dissection.[2] The classic radiologic sign characteristic of aortic dissection is widening of the mediastinum. Other radiographic signs include a double shadow of the aortic wall or a disparity in the size of the ascending and descending aorta. The International Registry of Acute Aortic Dissection (IRAD) reported that mediastinal widening was present in approximately 63% of patients with type A dissection and 56% with type B dissection. Approximately 11% of patients with type A dissection had no abnormality on chest radiography compared with 16% of patients with type B.[2] Von Kodolitsch et al.[3] recently assessed the diagnostic accuracy of routine chest radiography for the acute aortic syndrome (dissection, intramural hematoma, penetrating ulcer, or non-dissecting aneurysm). During a 6-year period, 216 patients underwent chest X-ray for suspected acute aortic syndrome. Chest films were re-evaluated blindly for aortic disease, based on an overall impression using standard criteria such as widening of the aortic contour and mediastinal shadow. Findings were matched to tomographic images, anatomic inspection, or both, Chest radiography had a sensitivity of 64% and a specificity of 86% for aortic disease. Sensitivity was 67% for overt aortic dissection, 61% for non-dissecting aneurysm, and 63% for intramural hemorrhage or penetrating ulcer. However, sensitivity was lower for involvement of the proximal aorta (47%) compared with disease involving the distal aortic segments (77%). Based on this and other reports, chest radiography is of limited value for diagnosing acute aortic syndromes, particularly for conditions confined to the ascending aorta.

Echocardiography

Echocardiography (TTE and TEE) is a non-invasive and readily available modality for evaluation of aortic dissection. TTE can evaluate the aortic root and arch, but the distal ascending aorta and descending aorta are not well visualized. TTE has low sensitivity for diagnosis of aortic dissection and so TEE is the preferred ultrasound modality. TEE provides significantly enhanced evaluation of the thoracic aorta compared with TTE. TEE does have a blind spot in the ascending aorta because of the presence of the right mainstem bronchus. However, the addition of multiplaner TEE has allowed better assessment of the aortic arch as well as a reduction in blind spots, limited to a small part of the ascending aorta and the proximal aortic arch.[4] The presence of a mobile intimal flap within the aortic lumen that separates the true and false lumen is considered diagnostic for aortic dissection. Other indicative findings include complete obstruction of false lumen, separation of the intimal layers from the thrombus, central displacement of intimal calcification, and shearing of different wall layers during aortic pulsation. Specific criteria for identifying the true lumen include systolic expansion and diastolic collapse of the lumen, the absence or low-intensity of spontaneous echocardiography contrast, systolic jets directed away from the lumen, and systolic forward flow. The false lumen can be identified by diastolic diameter expansion, spontaneous echocardiographic contrast, reversed, delayed, or absent flow, and thrombus formation. Sensitivity and specificity for TTE is in the ranges 77–80% and 93–96%, respectively, for the involvement of the ascending aorta. TEE has sensitivity as high as 100% and specificity as high as 95%.[5] A major advantage of TEE compared with CT and MRI is that it can be rapidly performed in unstable patients who are too ill to be transferred to an imaging center or may have contraindications to CT or MRI. A disadvantage of TEE is limited ability to visualize the distal thoracic and the abdominal aorta. The procedure is also operator dependent, requires sedation, and may be contraindicated in patients with esophageal diseases such as varices, strictures, or tumors. Representative TEE images are shown in Figs 5.1 and 5.2.

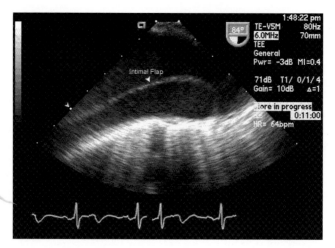

Figure 5.1 A 69-year-old man presented with acute back pain and diaphoresis. Transesophageal echocardiography (TEE) showed acute type A aortic dissection with dissection flap and large false lumen. The patient underwent emergent surgical repair and was discharged home with appropriate follow-up. (Image courtesy of Peter Hagan MD, Department of Cardiology, University of Michigan.)

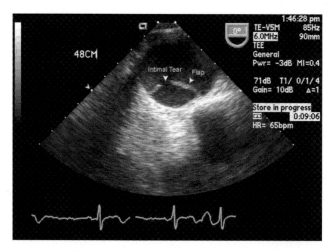

Figure 5.2 A 74-year-old hypertensive woman presented with abdominal pain, nausea, and emesis. TEE showed acute aortic dissection with an intimal tear and dissection flap in the descending thoracic aorta. The patient was treated medically with intravenous beta-blockers and nitroprusside and was discharged home on beta-blockers and appropriate follow-up. (Image courtesy of Peter Hagan MD, Department of Cardiology, University of Michigan.)

Computed tomography

Computed tomography is a fast, accurate, non-invasive method which continues to undergo technical improvements. CT was the most common initial diagnostic test in the IRAD study.[2] Previous studies have demonstrated that the sensitivity of CT ranges from 83% to 100% and the specificity from 87% to 100%.[6,7] Fast CT scanning (CT angiography) represents a significant advance in CT imaging. It permits breath-hold volumetric acquisitions eliminating ventilatory misregistration artifacts. Narrower collimation results in improved through-plane resolution with improved visualization of vascular structures compared with conventional CT. With shorter imaging times, better bolus tracking is accomplished and more images are obtained during peak contrast enhancement, resulting in improved visualization of vascular structures compared with conventional CT. The development of multislice CT has been another major advancement. Multislice CT results in more rapid scanning times with improved spatial resolution and reduced helical artifacts.[8] Multislice CT is useful in identifying the intimal flap, branch vessel involvement, extent of dissection, patency of false lumen, size of aorta, presence of pericardial fluid, evidence of end-organ ischemia, and can visualize the proximal third of the coronary arteries.[7] Intramural hematoma appears as a crescent-shaped, high-attenuation signal within the wall of the aorta on non-contrast CT. It may also present as localized thickening of the aortic wall with internal displacement of intimal calcifications.[6,7] Diagnosis of aortic dissection is made by the identification of the intimal flap separating the true and false lumens. Indirect signs of aortic dissection that may be visualized include compression of the true lumen by the false lumen, displaced intimal calcifications, and aortic lumen widening. Despite rapid recent advances, CT imaging still has several limitations. For example, it cannot detect aortic regurgitation and carries the risk of intravenous contrast administration. Representative CT images are shown in Figs 5.3–5.5.

Magnetic resonance imaging

Magnetic resonance imaging is a dynamic, non-invasive imaging modality which provides high-resolution structural and functional information. It allows visualization of the vascular compartment, the vessel wall, and its surrounding tissue, and provides functional information of the depicted vasculature. Several varieties of pulse sequences are now available. MRI displays vessel lumen as black blood on ECG gated spin-echo and as bright blood with contrast-enhanced techniques. ECG triggered spin echo images provide excellent anatomic detail of the heart and aorta. Cine MRI, using either steady-state free precession or gradient echo techniques, allows visualization of flowing blood, facilitating the differentiation of slow flowing blood and clot, and determination of the presence of aortic insufficiency. The double lumen and intimal flap are readily identified. The sensitivity and specificity of MRI for the diagnosis of aortic dissection has been reported to be between 95 and 100%. For identifying

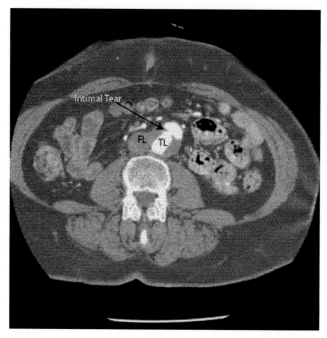

Figure 5.3 A 59-year-old man presented with acute abdominal pain and diaphoresis. CT scan showed acute aortic dissection with intimal tear and large false lumen. The patient was treated medically and discharged home on beta-blockers and appropriate follow-up. FL, false lumen; TL, true lumen. (Image courtesy of Leslie E. Quint, MD, Department of Radiology, University of Michigan.)

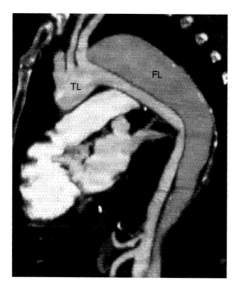

Figure 5.4 An 80-year-old woman presented with severe back pain and diaphoresis. CT scan with 3D reconstruction showed type B aortic dissection with aneurysmal dilatation of the descending thoracic and proximal abdominal aorta, and a large false lumen. The patient underwent surgical repair because of rapid expansion of the false lumen. The postoperative course was complicated by retrograde extension of the dissection after repair, leading to cardiac arrest and death. FL, false lumen; TL, true lumen. (Image courtesy of Leslie E. Quint, MD, Department of Radiology, University of Michigan.)

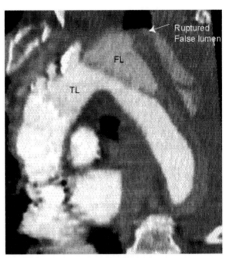

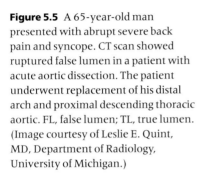

Figure 5.5 A 65-year-old man presented with abrupt severe back pain and syncope. CT scan showed ruptured false lumen in a patient with acute aortic dissection. The patient underwent replacement of his distal arch and proximal descending thoracic aortic. FL, false lumen; TL, true lumen. (Image courtesy of Leslie E. Quint, MD, Department of Radiology, University of Michigan.)

the site of entry, sensitivity was 85% and specificity 100%, and for identifying thrombus and the presence of a pericardial effusion, sensitivity and specificity were both 100%. Newer, gadolinium-enhanced, three-dimensional magnetic resonance angiography (3D MRA) techniques allow rapid acquisition of angiograms of the thoracic and abdominal aorta and their branch vessels. The technique allows coverage of large volumes with and without breath-holding. The 3D data sets may be reconstructed. 3D MRA permits easy identification of both the true and false lumen, enables identification of the type of dissection, and assessment of patency of the false lumen. Contrast-enhanced MRA is superior to black blood MRI in detecting the presence or absence of intimal flaps and is particularly useful in assessing supra-aortic branch vessel involvement.

MRI allows for evaluation of the entire aorta, branch vessel involvement, and associated complications of aortic dissection. Newer technologies in MRI have also increased its speed. Non-enhanced true fast imaging with steady-state precession may allow patients to be evaluated for acute aortic dissection in as little as 4 min.[9] Visualization of a double lumen with intimal flap is required for diagnosis with MRI. Velocity encoded cine MRI may be able to help differentiate the true and false lumen by measuring the velocity of blood flow, assuming flow is slower in the false channel. This is an important feature as it can determine whether the aortic side branches are perfused by the true or false lumen. MRI has the highest sensitivity and specificity for detecting all classes of aortic dissection with the exception of class III lesions.[10] Moreover, MRI takes advantage of the inherent properties of unsaturated protons in the blood, thus obviating the need for contrast dye administration, although currently 3D gadolinium-enhanced MRA is more commonly used. The use of MRI is limited by its contraindication in patients with metallic hardware and may be further restricted by its lack of availability in emergent situations. In addition, unstable patients who are intubated or require other hemodynamic monitoring devices may not be ideal candidates for MRI. Another factor is patient discomfort and dissatisfaction with prolonged imaging sequences within the MRI cocoon. Representative MR images are shown in Figs 5.6 and 5.7.

Aortography

Contrast aortography was the first method of evaluating aortic dissection and has traditionally been considered the gold standard for its diagnosis. Diagnosis requires the identification of two lumina or the presence of an intimal flap. Aortography has high specificity, approximately 94%, but its sensitivity may be lower than that of other techniques, being described as low as 88%.[11] Aortography may be helpful in identifying the site of origin of original dissection, branch artery involvement, aortic regurgitation, and coronary involvement.[11] Currently, arterial digital subtraction angiography (IA-DSA) with a large field of view image intensifier and rapid filming is used most frequently. The high frame rates of arterial DSA facilitate identification of the intimal tear and the degree of aortic insufficiency. If large field of view DSA is unavailable, standard cut film radiography, which has higher resolution than intra-arterial DSA may be used. Cine angiography has been used, but the field of view is usually limited. Intravenous DSA, because of artifacts that obscure the aortic root and ascending

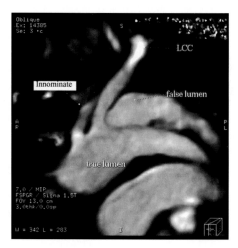

Figure 5.6 A 74-year-old woman presented with severe back and chest pain and syncope. MRI/MRA showed a type A dissection which extended distally into the infrarenal abdominal aorta beginning just superior to the prior ascending aortic graft. The patient underwent distal aortic arch and entire descending thoracic aortic replacement with a Hemashield graft. She had an uneventful recovery and was discharged home on beta-blockers and appropriate follow-up. FL, false lumen; TL, true lumen. (Image courtesy of G. Michael Deeb, MD, Department of Cardiothoracic Surgery, University of Michigan.)

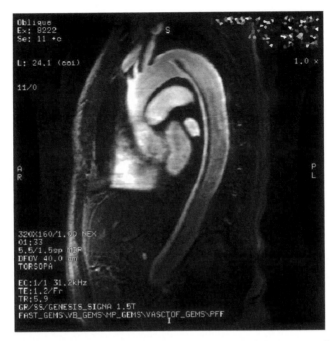

Figure 5.7 A 54-year-old man presented with severe back and chest pain and syncope. MRI/MRA showed acute type B aortic dissection beginning just distal to the left subclavian artery and extending to left renal artery origin. The patient was treated medically and discharged home on beta-blockers and appropriate follow-up. (Image courtesy of G. Michael Deeb, MD, Department of Cardiothoracic Surgery, University of Michigan.)

aorta, is not indicated. False-negative arteriograms may occur when the false lumen is not opacified, when there is simultaneous opacification of the true and false lumen, and when the intimal flap is not seen. Other disadvantages include the length of time to complete the study, the risks of contrast dye, relative expense, and the complications of an invasive procedure. In addition, aortography may also fail to detect intramural hematoma. Advances in imaging modalities have led to the increasing use of non-invasive imaging studies such as CT, MRI, and echocardiography, and contrast aortography is rarely used today for the initial diagnosis of aortic dissection.

Choice of imaging modality

Barbant *et al.*[12] used Bayes theorem to calculate predictive values and accuracies for angiography, CT, MRI, and TEE for the diagnosis of aortic dissection. In high-risk populations (disease prevalence ≥50%), positive predictive values were all greater than 85% for all four diagnostic modalities. In intermediate-risk populations (disease prevalence 10%), positive predictive values were ≥90% for CT,

MRI, and TEE, but were 65% for contrast aortography. In low-risk populations (disease prevalence 1%), positive predictive values were 100% for MRI and ≤50% for contrast aortography, CT, and TEE. In all three populations, negative predictive values and accuracies were ≥85%. Thus, as with other tests in other conditions, diagnostic imaging techniques for aortic dissection do not perform as well in low-risk populations as they do in high-risk populations.[12] Table 5.1 summarizes the overall sensitivity of the four imaging modalities in the IRAD study.[13]

American College of Radiology appropriateness criteria

Imaging studies in the evaluation of suspected aortic dissection should be directed toward confirmation of the presence of dissection, determination of whether the dissection is type A or B, assessment of entry and re-entry sites, identification of thrombus in the false lumen, assessment of aortic valve competency, detection of the presence or absence of aortic branch involvement, and determination of the presence of pericardial and pleural effusions. The American College of Radiology reviewed available data on the sensitivity, specificity, and accuracy of the available imaging modalities and developed appropriateness criteria for the diagnosis of aortic dissection (Table 5.2). Available evidence suggests that in skilled hands the accuracy of TEE, fast CT, and MRI/MRA will be nearly identical. Because patients with aortic dissection are usually critically ill and potentially in need of emergency intervention, the selection of a given modality will depend on clinical circumstances and availability. In centers where experienced cardiologists are available to perform state-of-the-art TEE in the emergency room, TEE may be the preferred first-line imaging modality because it can provide sufficient information to determine whether emergency surgery is needed. However, fast CT is likely to be more readily available on a 24-h basis and can also provide information on branch vessel involvement. Although it does not provide information regarding aortic insufficiency, this can be obtained with TTE or TEE while the operating room is being prepared. When information about branch vessel involvement is required by the surgeon

Table 5.1 Sensitivity of the four imaging modalities for aortic dissection in the IRAD study. Adapted from Moore *et al.*[13]

Imaging study	Overall sensitivity (%)	Stanford classification	
		Type A (%)	Type B (%)
TEE	88	90	80
CT	93	93	93
MRI	100	100	100
Aortography	87	87	89

CT, computed tomography; MRI, magnetic resonance imaging; TEE, transesophageal echocardiography.

Table 5.2 American College of Radiology appropriateness criteria for suspected aortic dissection. (Adapted from Gomes *et al.*[14])

Imaging modality	Appropriateness rating
Chest X-ray	9
CT with contrast including spiral CT and ultrafast electron beam CT	9
MRI/MRA	8
Angiography	8
TEE*	8
TTE	4
Intravascular ultrasound	3

Appropriateness criteria scale
Least appropriate ←1 2 3 4 5 6 7 8 9→Most appropriate

* If skilled operator is available.
CT, computed tomography; MRA, magnetic resonance angiography; MRI, magnetic resonance imaging; TEE, transesophageal echocardiography; TTE, transthoracic echocardiography.

but not provided by fast CT, aortography will be the definitive modality. MRI may be sufficient to replace angiography in stable patients, and those with chronic dissection or uncertain diagnoses. Faster imaging sequences may extend its use to unstable patients. Use of 3D reconstruction algorithms with fast CT and MRI/MRA may provide additional useful information in treatment planning.

Conclusions

In the IRAD study, the first diagnostic test used was TTE and TEE in 33%, CT in 61%, MRI in 2%, and angiography in 4%, reflecting the current use of diagnostic resources around the world. As a secondary technique, TTE/TEE was used in 56%, CT in 18%, MRI in 9%, and angiography in 17%. On average, approximately 1.8 methods were used to diagnose aortic dissection. Of the cases in which three methods were used, CT was used in 40%, MRI in 30%, and angiography in 21%. Hospital and operator preference, availability, and access in the emergency setting may impact the choice of imaging method because overall accuracy for the parameters are similar. Moreover, a high index of suspicion for the problem is more important than the type of test used. If aortic dissection is suspected, patients should be considered for transfer to a center with interventional and surgical back-up. Each institution should ideally establish pathways for diagnosis and early treatment to optimize outcomes in patients with aortic dissection.

References

1 Sarasin FP, Louis-Simonet M, Gaspoz JM, Junod AF. Detecting acute thoracic aortic

dissection in the emergency department: time constraints and choice of the optimal diagnostic test. *Ann Emerg Med* 1996;**28**:278–88.

2 Hagan PG, Nienaber CA, Isselbacher EM, *et al.* The International Registry of Acute Aortic Dissection (IRAD): new insights into an old disease. *JAMA* 2000;**283**:897–903.

3 von Kodolitsch Y, Nienaber CA, Dieckmann C, *et al.* Chest radiography for the diagnosis of acute aortic syndrome. *Am J Med* 2004;**116**:73–7.

4 Sommer T, Fehske W, Holzknecht N, *et al.* Aortic dissection: a comparative study of diagnosis with spiral CT, multiplanar transesophageal echocardiography, and MR imaging. *Radiology* 1996;**199**:347–52.

5 Nienaber CA, Spielmann RP, von Kodolitsch Y, *et al.* Diagnosis of thoracic aortic dissection: magnetic resonance imaging versus transesophageal echocardiography. *Circulation* 1992;**85**:434–47.

6 Ledbetter S, Stuk JL, Kaufman JA. Helical (spiral) CT in the evaluation of emergent thoracic aortic syndromes: traumatic aortic rupture, aortic aneurysm, aortic dissection, intramural hematoma, and penetrating atherosclerotic ulcer. *Radiol Clin North Am* 1999;**37**:575–89.

7 Gotway MB, Dawn SK. Thoracic aorta imaging with multislice CT. *Radiol Clin North Am* 2003;**41**:521–43.

8 Rubin GD. MDCT imaging of the aorta and peripheral vessels. *Eur J Radiol* 2003;**45**(Suppl 1):S42–9.

9 Pereles FS, McCarthy RM, Baskaran V, *et al.* Thoracic aortic dissection and aneurysm: evaluation with non-enhanced true FISP MR angiography in less than 4 minutes. *Radiology* 2002;**223**:270–4.

10 Erbel R, Alfonso F, Boileau C, *et al.* Diagnosis and management of aortic dissection. *Eur Heart J* 2001;**22**:1642–81.

11 Cigarroa JE, Isselbacher EM, DeSanctis RW, Eagle KA. Diagnostic imaging in the evaluation of suspected aortic dissection: old standards and new directions. *N Engl J Med* 1993;**328**:35–43.

12 Barbant SD, Eisenberg MJ, Schiller NB. The diagnostic value of imaging techniques for aortic dissection. *Am Heart J* 1992;**124**:541–3.

13 Moore AG, Eagle KA, Bruckman D, *et al.* Choice of computed tomography, transesophageal echocardiography, magnetic resonance imaging, and aortography in acute aortic dissection: International Registry of Acute Aortic Dissection (IRAD). *Am J Cardiol* 2002;**89**:1235–8.

14 Gomes AS, Bettmann MA, Boxt LM, *et al.* Acute chest pain: suspected aortic dissection. American College of Radiology (ACR) Appropriateness Criteria. *Radiology* 2000;**215**(Suppl):1–5.

CHAPTER 6

Evaluation of prosthetic heart valves

Darryl J. Burstow

Introduction

Transthoracic echocardiography (TTE) is well established as the imaging modality of first choice for the evaluation of prosthetic valve function because of the comprehensive anatomic, functional, and hemodynamic data obtained combined with its excellent safety profile. However, the acoustic properties of prosthetic valves impair the echocardiographic examination and can result in reduced diagnostic accuracy. To reduce errors in interpretation, a meticulous approach is required with integration of all data obtained from two-dimensional, spectral Doppler, and color flow imaging examinations. In addition, knowledge of the limitations of TTE in the assessment of prosthetic valves will enable the appropriate selection of cases where additional imaging procedures, such as transesophageal echocardiography (TEE) and cine fluoroscopy (CF) may be required.

Types of prosthetic valves and their distinctive features

To interpret accurately the appearance of a prosthetic valve with any imaging modality, an understanding of its basic structure and normal hemodynamic performance is required. In addition, knowledge of the complications that can result in prosthetic valve dysfunction is essential for their reliable detection. Prosthetic valves are of two major types:

1 *Mechanical valves:* composed of metal or pyrolytic carbon

2 *Bioprosthetic valves:* composed of porcine or bovine tissue (heterografts), or preserved human cadaveric aortic valves (homografts or allografts)

A selection of commonly used prosthetic valve subtypes is illustrated in Fig. 6.1.

Valve design and normal hemodynamic features
Mechanical
Mechanical valves are further classified according to their occluder structure as ball-cage, single tilting disk, and bileaflet. The ball-cage valves contain a ball oc-

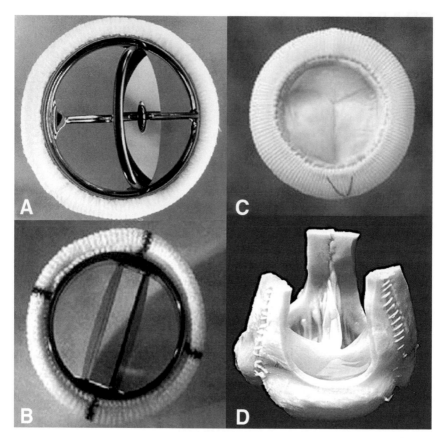

Figure 6.1 Four commonly used subtypes of prosthetic valves. (A) Medtronic–Hall tilting disk mechanical prosthesis. (B) Medtronic Advantage Bileaflet mechanical prosthesis. (C) Hancock porcine heterograft stented bioprosthesis. (D) Cryolife O'Brien porcine heterograft stentless bioprosthesis.

cluder within a wire cage and were the first successful valve replacements. One ball-cage valve, the Starr–Edwards valve, is still in use. The single tilting disk design (e.g. Bjork–Shiley, Lillehei–Kaster, Medtronic–Hall, Omniscience) has a single hinged disk forming major and minor orifices when in the open position. The disk has a defined normal opening angle of 60–80°, varying with the specific valve model. The bileaflet design (e.g. St Jude, ATS, Carbo-Medics, Medtronic Advantage) is now the most common type of prosthetic valve inserted worldwide. Two equal-sized semi-circular disks are attached to central pivot hinges, resulting in the formation of two large lateral orifices and one smaller central orifice when the leaflets are open. The leaflets open to an angle of 80–85° and close to an angle of 30–35° forming a shallow 'V'. All prosthetic valve designs cause obstruction to flow resulting in measurable pressure gradients. The bileaflet design has the best hemodynamic profile followed by the tilting disk and the ball-cage designs.[1] In addition, trivial to mild regurgitation is a characteristic feature of normally functioning mechanical valves with two types being described:

1 *'Closing volume'*: where the regurgitant volume is displaced as the occluder shuts

2 *'Leakage volume'*: where transvalvular regurgitation arises from around the closed occluder with the aim of preventing blood stasis and secondary thrombus formation

Bioprosthetic valves

Heterografts have traditionally been manufactured with the leaflets mounted on a metal support (stented bioprosthesis), but in recent years a number of companies have released designs without metal support (stentless bioprosthesis).

Stented valves (e.g. Hancock, Mosaic, Intact, Perimount) consist of glutaraldehyde-treated (non-viable) leaflets fixed to a molded polypropylene or metal alloy mount consisting of three struts. Stentless valves (e.g. Cryolife–O'Brien, Edwards Prima, Ross Stentless, Medtronic Freestyle, Toronto stentless) are exclusively used in the aortic position and have superior hemodynamics with lower gradients and larger valve areas in comparison to similar sized stented valves.[1] Homograft (allograft) valves are inserted into the aortic or pulmonary position utilizing the valve only or as a valved conduit. As expected, they have an excellent hemodynamic profile.[2] Trivial central regurgitation is common.

Complications

Structural valve degeneration

Excellent durability is a feature of mechanical prosthetic valves, with follow-up studies reporting extremely low rates of structural valve degeneration (SVD). By comparison, bioprosthetic valves develop progressive leaflet calcification with the incidence of significant valvular dysfunction accelerating 10–15 years after implantation. The incidence varies with the age of the patient (SVD following aortic valve replacement [AVR] is 60% at 10 years in patients aged 16–39 years compared with ≤15% in patients aged ≥70 years at 15 years) and is higher in mitral bioprosthetic valves.[3] Allograft aortic valves inserted using the root replacement technique and stentless heterografts may have improved durability, but longer follow-up studies past 15 years are required for confirmation. Regurgitation is the dominant form of dysfunction, with stenosis being quite rare.[3,4]

Valve thrombosis

Mechanical valves are more thrombogenic than bioprostheses, resulting in an increased risk of thromboembolism and thrombotic valve obstruction. The reported incidence of prosthetic valve thrombosis varies widely from 0.1 to 0.6% per patient year for left-sided valves, with major contributing factors being inadequate anticoagulation, a mitral location of the prosthetic valve, and likely other patient-related factors.[3] Much higher rates of thrombosis have been reported in mechanical tricuspid valves. The clinical presentation is dependent on the severity of valve obstruction and may vary from systemic embolism without hemodynamic abnormality to heart failure or even cardiogenic shock.

Infective endocarditis

Although prosthetic valve endocarditis is a fairly rare complication, occurring in approximately 4% of patients during their postoperative life, it is a serious condition with high mortality. It can be further complicated by the development of annular abscess and perivalvular regurgitation with a worsening of prognosis. The incidence of endocarditis is similar for all prosthetic valve subtypes.[3] A summary of prosthetic valve features is provided in Table 6.1.

Table 6.1 Summary of comparative design and clinical features of the major prosthetic valve subtypes. (From Rosenhek *et al.*[1] and Burstow *et al.*[2])

Model	Valve subtype		Hemodynamics		Complications			
			MG (mmHg)	EOA (cm^2)	TE	VT	IE	SVD
S-E	Mech.	A	14–26	NA	+++	++	++	−
	BC	M	4–10	1.3–2.1				
B-S	Mech.	A	7–17	1.5–2.1	++	++	++	+
	TD	M	1–4	1.9–2.5				
St Jude	Mech.	A	8–18	1.4–2.4	++	++	++	−
	BL	M	2–7	1.7–2.3				
Han	Stented	A	8–14	1.3–1.7	+ to ++	+	++	+++
	HET	M	3–8	1.4–1.8				
Med Free	Stentless	A	4–7	1.6–2.4	+ to ++	+	++	++
	HET							
Allo	–	A	4–6	2.9–3.5	+	−	+	++

+ Lower incidence to +++ higher incidence. Allo, allograft; A, aortic; BC, ball-cage; BL, bileaflet; B-S, Bjork–Shiley; EOA, effective orifice area; Han, Hancock; HET, heterograft; IE, infective endocarditis; M, mitral; Mech, mechanical; Med Free, Medtronic Freestyle; MG, mean gradient; NA, data not available; S-E, Starr–Edwards; SVD, structural valve degeneration; TD, tilting disk; TE, thromboembolism; VT, valve thrombosis. Hemodynamic data is for 25 mm aortic prostheses except Starr–Edwards (26 mm) and 31 mm mitral prostheses except Starr–Edwards (30 mm).

Case Presentation

A 73-year-old woman presented with a 2-year history of progressive dyspnea. A 23-mm St Jude aortic prosthesis had been implanted in 1987 for rheumatic valvular disease and the patient had undergone periodic clinical assessments since that time with careful supervision of anticoagulation. How should she be evaluated?

Assessment of prosthetic valve function

Baseline assessment with transthoracic echocardiography

The utility of TTE in the assessment of prosthetic valves has been extensively studied over the last 20 years. TTE provides a comprehensive description of prosthetic valve function and should be considered an integral part of the routine assessment of patients with prosthetic valves.

Two-dimensional imaging

The two-dimensional (2D) imaging component of TTE provides information on prosthetic valve structure. Prior to imaging, the type and size of the prosthetic valve should be established. The characteristic structural features of that device, as outlined earlier in this review, should be prerequisite knowledge. The appearance and motion of the leaflets and/or occluder can then be assessed. Careful attention to imaging planes will help to reduce the problems caused by acoustic shadowing and improve diagnostic yield. If the ultrasound beam can be orientated parallel to the direction of occluder opening, acoustic shadowing across the plane of the valve is reduced with resultant improvement in visualization of occluder motion. This is particularly relevant in the assessment of aortic prostheses where the apical five-chamber view can provide an improved view of the leaflets and/or occluder. In addition to assessing prosthetic valve structure, TTE also provides a complete assessment of native valvular and ventricular function.

Doppler examination (spectral Doppler, color flow imaging)

The Doppler examination adds an accurate hemodynamic assessment of prosthetic valve function to the anatomic assessment provided by 2D imaging. Doppler assessment allows the non-invasive measurement of flow velocities across prosthetic valves from which valve gradients can be calculated using the Bernoulli equation, $\varnothing P = 4 \ (V_2{}^2 - V_1{}^2)$, where V_2 is the peak velocity across the prosthetic valve and V_1 is the peak velocity immediately proximal to the valve. However, as with all stenotic lesions, valve gradients are determined by both volumetric flow and the stenotic valve area. Thus, in addition to valve gradients, the derivation of flow-independent parameters of prosthetic valve function such as effective orifice area (EOA) and dimensionless performance index (DPI) is essential. The Doppler parameters used to assess prosthetic valve function are listed in Table 6.2.

Table 6.2 The measured and derived echocardiographic parameters used for the routine evaluation of prosthetic valve function. The derived parameters, effective orifice area (EOA) and dimensionless performance index (DPI) are flow-independent and thus provide the most accurate assessment of valve hemodynamics.

Aortic prosthetic valves	Mitral prosthetic valves
Aortic flow velocity	*Mitral flow velocity*

Measured parameters

1. Peak velocity across prosthesis (V_2), m/s
2. Peak velocity in LVOT (V_1), m/s
3. Maximum gradient (mmHg) = $4(V_2^2 - V_1^2)$
4. Mean gradient = $\dfrac{4\,[\bullet\,(V_a)^2 + (V_b)^2 + \ldots (V_n)^2]}{n}$ (mmHg)
5. Aortic valve velocity time integral (VTI), cm
6. LVOT VTI, cm., LVOT diameter, cm

Measured parameters

1. Peak velocity across prosthesis(E), m/s
2. Mean gradient = $\dfrac{4\,[\bullet\,(V_a)^2 + (V_b)^2 + \ldots (V_n)^2]}{n}$ (mmHg)
3. Pressure half-time (PHT), ms
4. LVOT VTI, cm; LVOT diameter, cm

Derived parameters

EOA, cm^2

$= \dfrac{\text{LVOT VTI} \times \text{LVOT area}}{\text{AV VTI}}$

DPI = V_1/V_2

Derived parameters

EOA, cm^2

$= \dfrac{\text{LVOT VTI} \times \text{LVOT area}}{\text{MV VTI}}$

Dimensionless performance index

This is a useful flow-independent parameter of aortic prosthetic valve function which is easily derived (V_1/V_2) and does not require the measurement of a dimension such as the left ventricular outflow tract (LVOT) diameter which can be technically difficult. Higher DPI values indicate superior hemodynamic performance. In an individual patient, a baseline DPI value obtained in the early postoperative period can serve as the control value or "valve fingerprint" for future examinations. Providing prosthetic valve function remains normal, the DPI will remain constant even with changes in stroke volume.

Normal Doppler values

A large amount of data now exists documenting the normal values for Doppler parameters of prosthetic valve function.[1] Following completion of the Doppler examination, reference should be made to the normal Doppler data available for that particular prosthetic valve subtype and size.

Diagnosis of specific abnormalities
Obstruction

In mechanical valves, the usual causes of valve obstruction are thrombosis or ingrowth of fibrous tissue called pannus below the inflow orifice of the valve restricting occluder motion. In bioprosthetic valves, SVD is the usual cause. Patient–valve mismatch, a form of non-structural dysfunction, can cause clinically significant obstruction to flow in the presence of a structurally normal prosthetic valve. This usually results from implantation of an inappropriately small prosthesis for the size of the patient.

Role of transthoracic echocardiography

TTE provides an accurate hemodynamic assessment of prosthetic valve function, and the Doppler examination should provide the hemodynamic diagnosis on most occasions. The diagnosis of aortic valve obstruction is suggested by the following:

1 Increased gradients for valve subtype and size
2 Decreased EOA and DPI below the normal reference range
3 Significant deviation of EOA or DPI from the baseline study

Although individual EOA and DPI values should always be referenced against normal values for the valve subtype and size, an EOA less than $0.9 \, cm^2$ and a DPI less than 0.2 will almost always be abnormal and are useful figures to memorize. For the mitral prosthesis, increased gradients (for valve subtype and size), increased PHT over 150 ms and decreased EOA of less than $1.5 \, cm^2$ are indicative of obstruction. Patient–valve mismatch should be suspected if abnormally elevated Doppler gradients are obtained despite the following:

1 No obvious structural abnormality of the prosthesis
2 Normal values for EOA and DPI for valve subtype and size
3 Indexed EOA ″ $0.85 \, cm^2/m^2$.[5]

Typically, the prosthesis is of small size and the patients are of older age and larger body surface area.

High Doppler gradients in normal small bileaflet prostheses

The unique geometry of the bileaflet design is characterized by a larger pressure drop across the divergent central orifice compared with the two larger side orifices. In addition, there is rapid recovery of pressure within the aorta immediately distal to the prosthetic valve orifice and this phenomenon may be especially pronounced if the aorta is of small diameter. Thus, these features can result in high recorded Doppler gradients (typically in 19 and 21mm sizes) which are substantially higher than the equivalent gradients obtained using standard cardiac catheterization techniques and may be an overestimate of LV pressure work. If a high gradient is identified, it is worthwhile scanning the continuous wave Doppler signal across the central and side orifices — a more reliable lower velocity signal may be detected from the side orifice (although this selective sampling can be technically difficult in small aortic prostheses). If a small aortic root is present, equations have been developed to facilitate compensation for this.[6]

If, after comparison with normal reference values, the 2D and Doppler findings remain inconclusive, an additional imaging assessment of occluder motion will be required as discussed below.

Case Presentation (Continued)

Figure 6.2 shows the serial Doppler assessment of the aortic prosthesis from 2002 to 2004 which demonstrated a marked rise in mean gradient and fall in DPI over the last two examinations, confirming significant obstruction. TTE failed to clearly display occluder motion or any associated soft tissue abnormality. What should be done next?

The major limitation of TTE is its inability to reliably detect the etiology of obstruction, particularly in mechanical aortic valves. Delineation of associated soft tissue abnormalities such as thrombus is poor, and in one study was as low as one in eight cases.[7] However, TTE is more accurate in detecting SVD in bioprostheses, presumably because of the lesser amount of reflective material used in their construction.

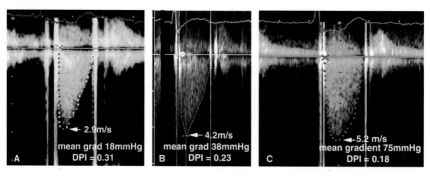

Figure 6.2 The continuous wave (CW) Doppler examination of a 23-mm St Jude aortic prosthesis on three separate occasions: (A) in 2002; (B) in 2003; and (C) in 2004. The values recorded in 2002 are within the normal range for this type and size of prosthesis. Note the subsequent rise in peak velocity and mean gradient while the dimensionless performance index (DPI) progressively falls. The Doppler hemodynamics are consistent with the relatively gradual development of severe prosthetic valve obstruction.

Role of transesophageal echocardiography

TEE has been advocated to clarify the mechanism of prosthetic valve obstruction and also to identify suitable candidates for thrombolysis.[8] First, thrombus needs to be distinguished from pannus and features favoring thrombus include "soft" echogenicity and large size, together with clinical factors such as short duration of symptoms and inadequate anticoagulation.[9] Second, identification of a large thrombus reflects a greater risk of systemic embolism with lytic therapy. TEE provides excellent imaging and a high diagnostic yield for mitral prostheses but the data are less convincing for mechanical valves in the aortic position. In one study,[10] the etiology of mechanical AVR obstruction by TTE was correct in only 10% and increased to just 49% with TEE. Obstructing pannus in the presence of a coexistent mitral prosthesis was especially difficult to identify.

Role of cine fluoroscopy

CF is a safe and relatively rapid method of demonstrating occluder motion in mechanical prosthetic valves.[11] As in the case described above, its main use is in the assessment of aortic prosthetic valves where obstruction is suspected on hemodynamic criteria but echocardiographic visualization of occluder motion has been suboptimal.

Case Presentation (Continued)

TEE also failed to identify the cause of the increasing gradients (Fig. 6.3a). Cine fluoroscopy was then performed which clearly demonstrated reduced leaflet excursion (Fig. 6.3b). Surgery was considered the most appropriate option in view of the likely diagnosis of pannus ingrowth.

Infective endocarditis

Transthoracic versus transesophageal echocardiography

In a large study by Daniel *et al.*,[12] the sensitivity of TEE in detecting vegetations in prosthetic valve endocarditis verified at surgery or autopsy was 82%, compared with 36% for TTE. It was again noted that abnormalities were more easily identified in the mitral than in the aortic position (97% versus 77%). An illustrative case is shown in Fig. 6.4. The superiority of TEE in detecting associated complications such as root abscess is also well documented. Thus, in patients with suspected prosthetic valve endocarditis, TEE should be performed in all cases where there is no contraindication to esophageal intubation.

Role of magnetic resonance imaging

The utility of MRI in assessing prosthetic valves has not been extensively studied. Except for one early Starr–Edwards model, MRI is not considered hazardous for patients with prosthetic valves. At this stage in the evolution of this technology, MRI is unlikely to challenge echocardiography for hemody-

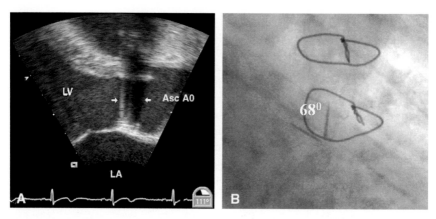

Figure 6.3 (A) The acoustic shadowing (between arrows) generated by the St Jude aortic prosthesis resulting in poor definition of the prosthetic valve leaflets and the anterior margin of the aortic annulus. (B) Cine fluoroscopy, which demonstrated abnormal leaflet motion with an opening angle of 68° compared with a normal opening angle between the leaflets of 10–11°. Asc Ao, ascending aorta; LA, left atrium; LV, left ventricle.

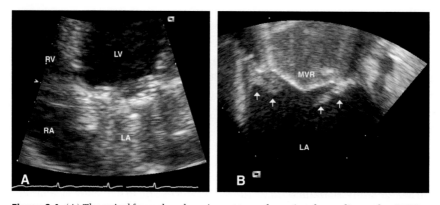

Figure 6.4 (A) The apical four-chamber view at transthoracic echocardiography (TTE) in a patient with an ATS bileaflet mitral prosthesis and suspected infective endocarditis. Acoustic shadowing of the left atrium (LA) prevents adequate anatomic definition. (B) The corresponding view at TEE demonstrating vegetations (arrows) on LA surface of the valve sewing ring. LV, left ventricle; MVR, mitral valve replacement; RA, right atrium; RV, right ventricle.

namic assessment or in its ability to detect small mobile anatomic abnormalities such as vegetations. However, in a recent case at our institution, a patient with a periaortic abscess postaortic root replacement with an ATS valved conduit was successfully imaged by MRI (Fig. 6.5). The extent of the infection was particularly well seen including the anterior margin of the aortic root which is often poorly visualized by TEE. This case suggests that MRI may have a role

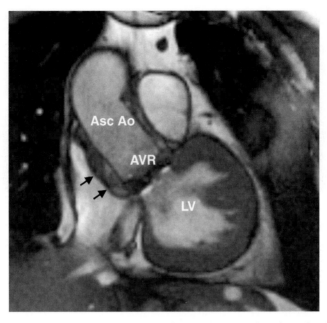

Figure 6.5 Magnetic resonance image (MRI) from a patient with endocarditis following an aortic valve and root replacement. There is a soft tissue collection surrounding the aortic graft consistent with abscess formation (black arrows). The extent of the abscess collection is well seen. Asc Ao, ascending aorta; AVR, aortic valve replacement; LV, left ventricle.

in assessing major anatomic abnormalities of soft tissue that can complicate endocarditis.

Prosthetic valve regurgitation

Regurgitation of prosthetic valves may arise from valvular and/or perivalvular sites. Most mechanical prostheses have mild closing and leakage volume regurgitation which must be recognized and differentiated from pathologic leaks (Fig. 6.6a).

Transthoracic versus transoesophageal echocardiography
Aortic regurgitation TTE usually provides adequate assessment of the severity of aortic prosthetic valve regurgitation utilizing the standard parameters applied to native valve regurgitation. The origin of regurgitation (valvular versus perivalvular) is best assessed in the parasternal short axis view where the full circumference of the annulus can be visualized. 2D imaging may demonstrate the etiology of regurgitation by showing evidence of leaflet degeneration in bioprostheses, abnormal occluder motion in mechanical protheses, or associated abnormalities of the valve bed and vegetations. TEE further improves the detection of these 2D abnormalities[7] but

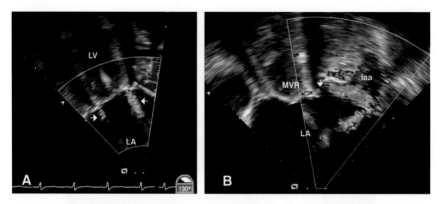

Figure 6.6 (A) Two typical jets of normal leakage volume regurgitation (arrows) from a bileaflet mitral prosthesis at transesophageal echocardiography (TEE). The jets are multiple, narrow, of low turbulence, and transvalvular. By comparison, (B) shows moderately severe (Grade 3–4) perivalvular regurgitation arising from outside the lateral margin of the sewing ring (arrow). LA, left atrium; laa, left atrial appendage; LV, left ventricle; MVR, mitral valve replacement.

may still miss abnormalities of occluder motion as well as pathology of the anterior annular region.

Mitral regurgitation Evaluation of mitral prosthetic valve regurgitation is a major limitation of TTE. The acoustic shadowing of the left atrium by the mitral prosthesis results in a low sensitivity for the detection of mitral regurgitation by color flow imaging. In view of this, studies have focused on a number of spectral Doppler parameters to determine their ability to predict the presence of significant regurgitation. The most useful parameters, all of which indicate high forward flow across the prosthesis, are as follows:

1 Increased early mitral flow velocity, E > 1.9 m/s; sensitivity 90%, specificity 89%

2 Mean gradient >5 mmHg; sensitivity 90%, specificity 70%

3 Mitral inflow VTI ÷ LVOT VTI > 2.5; sensitivity 89%, specificity 91%[13]

When combined with a normal pressure half-time excluding significant stenosis as a cause of the increased flow velocities, these parameters help to identify patients who need to go on to further imaging with TEE. The detection and semi-quantitation of mitral prosthetic regurgitation by TEE was one of the earliest applications of this technology and the increased diagnostic yield compared with TTE was soon apparent. More recently, "quantitative" parameters of mitral regurgitation severity obtained at TEE have been studied and the best parameters at identifying angiographically severe mitral regurgitation are as follows:

1 Regurgitant orifice area by PISA method >0.45 cm²; sensitivity 96%, specificity 90%

2 Proximal jet diameter > 0.6 cm; sensitivity 96%, specificity 95%[14]

Both methods are technically simple requiring relatively few measurements. TEE also provides additional data on site of regurgitation and allows accurate identification of perivalvular regurgitation as shown in the case in Fig. 6.6(b).

Role of cardiac catheterization

Cardiac catheterization is rarely required to obtain a hemodynamic diagnosis. Mechanical prostheses are hazardous to cross and thus accurate assessment will require chamber puncture which further increases the risk of the procedure. This approach is sometimes justified in difficult cases of aortic mechanical valve obstruction or regurgitation where the hemodynamic diagnosis remains in doubt after echocardiographic assessment.

Conclusions

The above review has emphasized the central role of TTE in the evaluation of prosthetic valves, its strengths and weaknesses in assessing complications, and the complementary role played by other imaging modalities in specific patholo- gies. With this information, a logical imaging pathway can be developed for each clinical problem as summarized in Table 6.3. This type of approach should enable the selection of the most appropriate imaging modality to aid in the clin- ical assessment and diagnosis of patients with prosthetic valve dysfunction.

Table 6.3 Summary of the utility of various investigations in evaluating prosthetic valve function and a suggested investigation pathway for various pathologies.

Clinical indication	TTE		TEE		CF	CC	MRI	Investigation pathway
	Hem	Anat	Hem	Anat				
Routine assessment	•••	••	—	—	—	—	—	TTE
Bioprosthetic AVR obstruction	•••	••	••	•••	—	—	?	TTE ± TEE
Mechanical AVR obstruction	•••	•	••	••	•••	••	?	TTE + CF ± TEE ± CC
Bioprosthetic MVR obstruction	•••	••	•••	•••	—	—	?	TTE ± TEE
Mechanical MVR obstruction	•••	••	•••	•••	••	•	?	TTE + TEE
Infective endocarditis	•••	••	••	•••	—	—	••	TTE + TEE ± MRI
MVR regurgitation	•	••	•••	•••	—	•	—	TTE + TEE
AVR regurgitation	••	•	••	••	—	••	?	TTE + TEE ± CC

• Low clinical utility to ••• excellent clinical utility. Anat., anatomy; AVR, aortic valve replacement; CC, cardiac catheterization; CF, cine fluoroscopy; Hem, hemodynamics; MRI, magnetic resonance imaging; MVR, mitral valve replacement; TEE, transesophageal echocardiography; TTE, transthoracic echocardiography.

References

1 Rosenhek R, Binder T, Maurer G, *et al.* Normal values for Doppler echocardiographic assessment of heart valve prostheses. *J Am Soc Echocardiogr* 2003;**16**:1116–27.

2 Burstow DJ, Shameem R, Smith I, *et al.* Echo/Doppler evaluation of 137 normal aortic allografts: comparison with new generation bileaflet mechanical and stentless xenograft prostheses. *J Am Coll Cardiol* 2002;**39**(Suppl):427A.

3 Rahimtoola SH. Choice of prosthetic heart valve for adult patients. *J Am Coll Cardiol* 2003;**41**:893–904.

4 Palka P, Harrocks S, Lange A, *et al.* Primary aortic valve replacement with cryopreserved aortic allograft: an echocardiographic follow-up study of 570 patients. *Circulation* 2002;**105**:61–6.

5 Pibarot P, Dumesnil JG. Hemodynamic and clinical impact of prosthesis–patient mismatch in the aortic valve position and its prevention. *J Am Coll Cardiol* 2000;**36**: 1131–41.

6 Baumgartner H, Stefenelli T, Niederberger J, *et al.* "Overestimation" of catheter gradients by Doppler ultrasound with aortic stenosis: a predictable manifestation of pressure recovery. *J Am Coll Cardiol* 1999;**33**:1655–61.

7 Daniel WG, Mugge A, Grote J, *et al.* Comparison of transthoracic and transesophageal echocardiography for detection of abnormalities of prosthetic and bioprosthetic valves in the mitral and aortic positions. *Am J Cardiol* 1993;**71**:210–5.

8 Tong AT, Roudaut R, Ozkan M, *et al.* Transesophageal echocardiography improves risk assessment of thrombolysis of prosthetic valve thrombosis: results of the international PRO-TEE registry. *J Am Coll Cardiol* 2004;**43**:77–84.

9 Barbetseas J, Nagueh S, Pitsavos C, *et al.* Differentiating thrombus from pannus formation in obstructed mechanical prosthetic valves: an evaluation of clinical, transthoracic and transesophageal echocardiographic parameters. *J Am Coll Cardiol* 1998;**32**:1410–7.

10 Girad SE, Miller FA Jr, Orszulak TA, *et al.* Reoperation for prosthetic aortic valve obstruction in the era of echocardiography: trends in diagnostic testing and comparison with surgical findings. *J Am Coll Cardiol* 2001;**37**:579–84.

11 Vogel W, Stoll HP, Bay W, *et al.* Cineradiography for determination of normal and abnormal function in mechanical heart valves. *Am J Cardiol* 1993;**71**:225–32.

12 Daniel WG, Mugge A, Martin RP, *et al.* Improvement in the diagnosis of abscesses associated with endocarditis by transesophageal echocardiography. *N Engl J Med* 1991;**324**:795–800.

13 Olmos L, Salazar G, Barbetseas J, *et al.* Usefulness of transthoracic echocardiography in detecting significant prosthetic mitral valve regurgitation. *Am J Cardiol* 1999; **83**:199–205.

14 Vitarelli A, Conde Y, Cimino E, *et al.* Assessment of severity of mechanical prosthetic mitral regurgitation by transesophageal echocardiography. *Heart* 2004;**90**:539–44.

CHAPTER 7

Echocardiography in infective endocarditis

Eric Brochet, Agnès Cachier, and Alec Vahanian

Case Presentation

A 61-year-old man was admitted because of acute pulmonary edema and aortic regurgitation. He had no history of valvular or cardiac disease but he did have a history of débridement of an infected total knee arthroplasty 2 years previously, with recurrent drainage. Fifteen days before admission, he reported fever and local pain and swelling of the knee and was referred to another institution. Blood cultures were positive for coagulase-negative *Staphylococcus*. Intravenous antibiotics were begun and initial progress was favorable, with regression of fever and normalization of biologic markers of inflammation. However, in the course of this recovery, the patient complained of acute onset dyspnea. On physical examination, his temperature was 39°C, blood pressure was 140/50 mmHg, and a diastolic murmur of aortic regurgitation was heard for the first time. Inspiratory crackles were audible half way up both lung fields. There were peripheral signs of aortic regurgitation. No jugular distension or peripheral edema was seen. There were no peripheral stigmata of endocarditis. Electrocardiography showed sinus tachycardia, without arrhythmia or conduction disturbances. Chest X-ray showed diffuse alveolar and interstitial infiltrates consistent with congestive heart failure and a cardiac silhouette at the upper limits of normal. Laboratory data revealed 18,000 leukocytes, with 15,000 neutrophils, no anemia; elevated C-reactive protein (297 mL/L), and normal renal function. He was referred to our institution and an echocardiogram was requested.

In this situation of likely endocarditis, what is the value of echocardiography?

Introduction

In patients with infective endocarditis (IE), echocardiography provides important information for diagnosis, detection of complications, and identification of valvular dysfunction, all of which may guide the management of these patients.[1]

Diagnosis of infective endocarditis

The now well-accepted Duke criteria incorporate echocardiographic findings as major criteria for the definite diagnosis of IE in combination with clinical and bacteriologic parameters. The three following echocardiographic findings are considered as major criteria in the diagnostic strategy:

1 Characteristic vegetations, defined as mobile echo-dense masses attached to the valvular or mural endocardium, or to the implanted prosthetic material

2 Periannular abscess

3 New dehiscence of a valvular prosthesis[2]

Detection of vegetations

Echocardiographically defined vegetations are classically described as shaggy, irregular masses of echoes attached to the leaflet tips or non-valvular endocardium, with varying degrees of independent motion. Pedunculated or fixed, they may vary in size from less than 1 mm to several centimeters. Characteristics of vegetations may vary according to the underlying valvular abnormalities. Multiple vegetations, involving different valves, are not uncommon.

Transthoracic echocardiography (TTE) is generally the first non-invasive technique performed in patients suspected of having IE. Although highly specific, especially in native valve IE (98%), the sensitivity of TTE to detect vegetations is only moderate, at 40–80%,[3] despite improvement in the quality of TTE images during recent years, especially with the introduction of harmonic imaging. TTE sensitivity may vary according to the quality of images, size of vegetations, presence of valve prostheses or pre-existing valvular abnormalities. TTE can easily detect vegetations larger than 2 mm in native valve IE, or vegetations on right-sided valves in echogenic patients. However, in other situations, performance of TTE may be limited because of a poor acoustic window (e.g. obesity, underlying lung disease, chest deformation), vegetation size beyond the resolution capability, or, with prosthetic valves, the presence of artifacts. In these situations, a negative TTE may not be sufficient to rule out IE.

Case Presentation (Continued)

TTE showed a pedunculated vegetation of the posterior aortic cusp, measuring 7 mm (Fig. 7.1). Vegetation was highly mobile, prolapsing into the left ventricular outflow tract (LVOT). Marked thickening of the subaortic region suggested the presence of an abscess of the mitral–aortic intervalvular fibrosa (Fig. 7.2). Color and spectral Doppler identified severe aortic regurgitation, with a large jet width in the LVOT, and steep deceleration rate of aortic velocity (Fig. 7.3a). Premature closure of the mitral valve was also present (Fig. 7.3b). Left ventricular ejection was normal. Estimated systolic pulmonary pressure was 45 mmHg. Other valves were structurally normal, without vegetations.

Is a transesophageal echocardiogram of value?

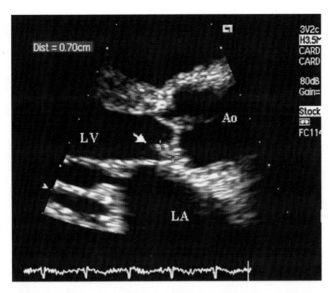

Figure 7.1 Transthoracic echocardiogram (long axis parasternal image) showing a pedunculated vegetation on the posterior aortic cusp.

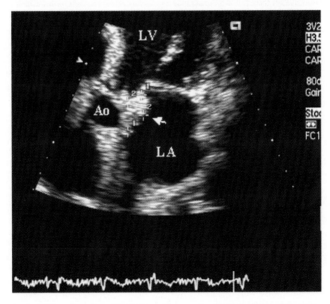

Figure 7.2 Apical five-chamber view showing marked thickening of the subaortic region suggesting the presence of an abscess of the mitral–aortic intervalvular fibrosa.

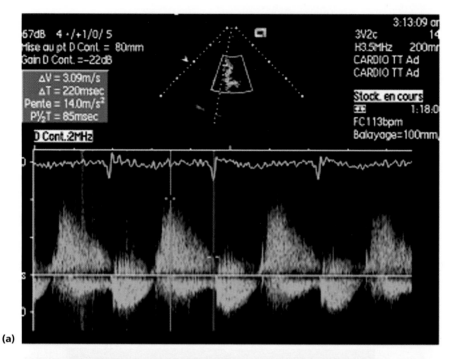

(a)

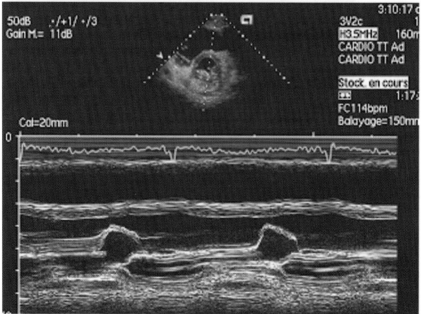

(b)

Figure 7.3 Evidence of severe aortic regurgitation — continuous wave Doppler showing: (a) steep deceleration rate of aortic velocity; and (b) premature closure of the mitral valve.

Table 7.1 Comparative value of transthoracic echocardiography (TTE) and transesophageal echocardiography (TEE) in the diagnosis of valvular vegetations.

Reference	n	Prostheses (%)	Transthoracic echo		Transesophageal echo	
			Sensitivity (%)	Specificity (%)	Sensitivity (%)	Specificity (%)
Mügge et al. (1989)[4]	91	24	58	–	90	
Shively et al. (1991)[5]	66	18	44	94	98	100
Daniel et al. (1993)[6]	33	100	36	–	82	
Shapiro et al. (1994)[7]	68	–	68	91	87	91

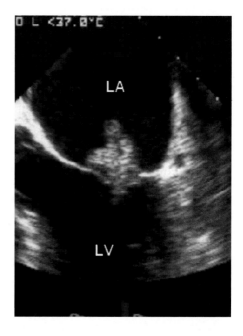

Figure 7.4 Transesophageal echocardiography demonstrating large mitral vegetation. LA, left atrium; LV, left ventricle.

Transesophageal echocardiography (TEE) overcomes many of these limitations and has been shown in many studies to be far superior to TTE for the identification of vegetations (Table 7.1). The higher resolution of TEE, multiplane capabilities, and proximity to the valves explain the better sensitivity of TEE in detecting vegetations compared with TTE in both native valve IE (90–100%) and prosthetic valve IE (86–94%).[1,3,8] TEE allows a complete assessment of vegetation characteristics, such as location, size, and number of vegetations (Fig. 7.4). TEE is also superior to TTE in the detection of pacemaker lead vegetations.[1]

A negative TEE examination has a very high negative predictive value for IE in patients with native heart valve (over 90%).[3] The rare false-negative results may be related to an incomplete TEE examination, TEE performed very early in the infectious process before the development of vegetations, or vegetations that are too small to be detected or have already embolized. Careful multiplane TEE examination might reduce the likelihood of false-negative results.

In patients with prosthetic valves, false-negative results are more prone to occur, possibly because of incomplete visualization, presence of artifacts, and interference. In these patients, a negative TEE does not completely exclude the diagnosis of IE.

Although TEE specificity for IE vegetations is high (88–100%), possible false-positive findings may occur in certain situations. Underlying native valvular abnormalities such as myxomatous mitral valve disease, non-specific valvular thickening, Lambl's excrescences, or fibroelastomas may mimic vegetations. Echocardiography does not permit differentiation between active versus healed vegetations or between bacterial versus non-bacterial thrombotic vegetations, such as those observed in systemic lupus erythematosus, antiphospholipid syndrome, or marantic endocarditis. In patients with prosthetic valve, common findings such as sutures or prosthetic strands should not be confused with vegetations. Distinction between vegetations and prosthetic thrombus is often impossible, and other prosthetic abnormalities such as bioprosthetic leaflet degeneration can be also difficult to differentiate from vegetations.

Detection of abscesses and perivalvular complications

Aortic location, prosthetic valve IE, and staphylococcal infection are the best predictive factors for IE associated perivalvular complications. TEE is strongly indicated in these high-risk patients to identify perivalvular complications. The presence and size of vegetations do not seem helpful in predicting perivalvular extension of the infection.[9] Abscesses may extend into contiguous tissue, especially the mitral–aortic intervalvular fibrosa, resulting in the formation of cavities, pseudoaneurysms, and fistulas. Mitral annular abscesses are less frequent, and almost always in patients with mitral prostheses.

Echocardiographically, these abscesses appear as a perivalvular region of increased thickness (greater than 10 mm) and reduced echo-density, without evidence of flow with color Doppler (Fig. 7.5). A pseudoaneurysm is defined as a pulsatile, echo-free, perivalvular cavity with flow communicating with the cardiovascular lumen. A fistula is defined as a color Doppler tract communicating two adjacent cardiac chambers (Fig. 7.6).[9]

The superiority of TEE over TTE in the diagnostic of periannular complications is well established.[9,10] Only approximately 25% of paravalvular abscesses are detected by TTE, whereas sensitivity and specificity are very high with TEE (87% and 95%, respectively, in the Daniel series[10]). Combined with spectral and color Doppler techniques, TEE can also identify the abnormal communicating flow in pseudoaneurysms and fistulae. TEE also provides information about the localization and extension of paravalvular abscesses. Intervalvular fibrosa abscesses and pseudoaneurysms are more frequently detected by TEE than by TTE.

False-positive and false-negative TEE results may occur in some cases.

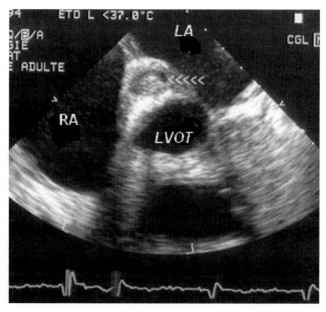

Figure 7.5 Transesophageal echocardiography demonstrating a region of reduced echo density with no flow in the periannular aortic ring (arrows). Abscess was confirmed on surgery. LA, left atrium; LV, left ventricle; LVOT, left ventricular outflow tract.

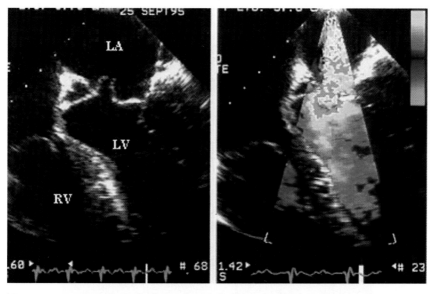

Figure 7.6 Transesophageal echocardiography demonstrating perforation of an aneurysm of the anterior mitral leaflet (left) secondary to infection of the mitral–aortic intervalvular fibrosa in an aortic endocarditis. Color flow Doppler shows the large eccentric jet of mitral regurgitation through the perforation (right). LA, left atrium; LV, left ventricle; RV, right ventricle.

Abscesses may be missed when they are too small. Diagnostic accuracy of TEE is better for pseudoaneurysms than for abscesses.[9] Although periannular complications are frequent in patients with prosthetic valve IE, their identification — even with TEE — may be challenging. Prostheses, especially mechanical valves, may create confusing images because of artifacts and shadows of the prosthetic material and eccentric color Doppler jets. Anterior aortic abscesses may be missed with TEE in patients with prosthetic valves.

Case Presentation (Continued)

TEE showed a large vegetation attached to the tip of the non-coronary aortic valve with complete prolapse of the cusp (Fig. 7.7). Severe aortic regurgitation was confirmed with color flow Doppler (Fig. 7.8). A large abscess was observed at the level of the posterior aortic root, with no flow (Fig. 7.9a). This abscess extended to the subaortic region of mitral–aortic intervalvular fibrosa (Fig. 7.9b). The patient underwent cardiac surgery the same day. At the time of surgery, there was complete destruction of the non-coronary aortic valve, with multiple vegetations. The periannular abscess, extending to the intervalvular fibrosa, was confirmed. The patient underwent aortic valve replacement with a homograft and exclusion of the abscess.

Cultures of the aortic valves grew coagulase-negative *Staphylococcus* which responded to 6 weeks of rifampicin and oxacillin therapy. The patient did well after 6 weeks of treatment.

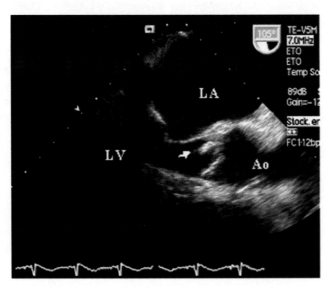

Figure 7.7 Transesophageal echocardiography (TEE) showing a large vegetation attached to the tip of non-coronary aortic valve with complete prolapse of the cusp.

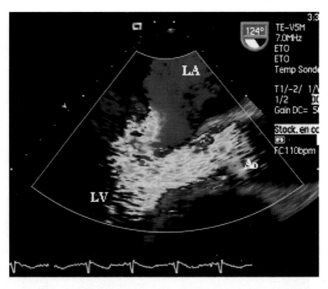

Figure 7.8 Confirmation of severe aortic regurgitation with color flow Doppler.

New valvular dysfunction

The assessment of valvular regurgitation is based on a comprehensive utilization of both TTE and TEE, coupled with pulsed, color flow, and continuous wave Doppler. This allows a complete evaluation of underlying valve disease, mechanism, and severity of valvular regurgitation.

In typical situations, diagnosis of acute, severe, valvular regurgitation is strongly suggested by the mechanisms of valve dysfunction, destruction, or perforation, with flail leaflet, associated with typical Doppler findings of severe regurgitation. Valvular perforation, especially in the aortic position is associated with an adverse outcome. TTE can detect or suggest valvular perforation in IE, but TEE better defines this complication.

Identification of new paraprosthetic regurgitation is a major echocardiographic finding in patients suspected of having IE. Because of its superiority in determining the spatial location of regurgitant jets, TEE is the modality of choice for the diagnosis of paravalvular regurgitation. However, small intraprosthetic regurgitant jets, present in the majority of normal prostheses, should not be confused with paraprosthetic leakage.

Prognosis of infective endocarditis

Echocardiography provides important prognostic information in patients with IE that can help medical or surgical decisions.

Prognosis related to the presence and size of the vegetations

The presence and morphology of echocardiographically documented vegetations are associated with a higher rate of complications in IE. Several studies

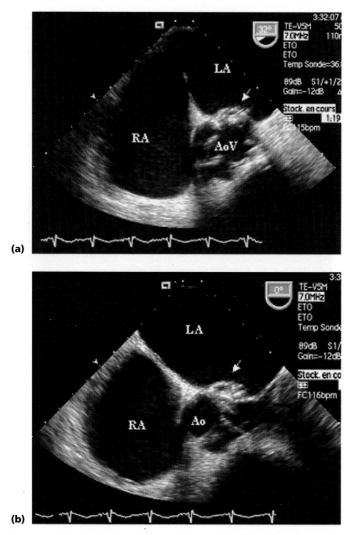

Figure 7.9 Transesophageal echocardiogram (TEE) showing a large abscess at the level of the posterior aortic root: (a) with no flow; (b) with extension to the subaortic region of mitral–aortic intervalvular fibrosa.

have shown a significant association between morphologic characteristics of the vegetations and the incidence of embolic events. Both vegetation size and mobility are predictive of embolic events. The risk of embolization is particularly high in large and highly mobile mitral valve IE and in staphylococcal infection. In a recent study of 178 consecutive patients with definite IE as established by the Duke criteria, patients with vegetations larger than 10 mm had a 60% incidence of emboli, while severely mobile vegetations larger than 15 mm had an

83% incidence of emboli.[11] Embolism before initiation of antimicrobial treatment, or increase in vegetation size during treatment, may also predict later embolism.[12] A high incidence of embolic events is also observed in patients with right heart IE.[11] The indication for early surgery in patients with large vegetations should be discussed individually for each patient. Although large and highly mobile vegetations, especially on the mitral valve, are more prone to embolize, indications for surgery should not be purely based on echocardiographic parameters,[1,13] but should also take into account the causative agent, the presence of complications such as heart failure, the feasibility of valve repair, and the extracardiac condition of the patient.

Early detection of complications

Periannular extension of the infection is associated with more complications, poor clinical outcome, and frequent need for surgery.[9]

Early and accurate identification of periannular extension or prosthetic dehiscence in patients suspected of having IE are critical for appropriate patient management and surgical decisions. Surgical repair is more difficult when these complications are diagnosed at too late a stage.

Evaluation of hemodynamic consequences of valvular regurgitation

Besides the identification and quantification of valvular regurgitation, echocardiography allows evaluation of their hemodynamic consequences. Acute, severe aortic or mitral regurgitation with signs of ventricular failure is associated with an adverse outcome and requires early surgical management.

When acute regurgitation is superimposed on chronic regurgitation, interpretation of echocardiographic data may be more difficult.

A major role of echocardiography in prognostic evaluation is the identification of the causes and severity of congestive heart failure. Chamber size, segmental and global wall motion, ejection fraction, and left ventricular and pulmonary artery pressures should be defined and monitored during follow-up. Although no or moderate left ventricular dilatation favors acute regurgitation, left ventricular enlargement and left ventricular dysfunction may be present in both acute and chronic situations. Assessment of the progression of the impact of regurgitation on left ventricular volumes and function, along with clinical evaluation, is needed for adequate timing of intervention.

Guidelines for the use of echocardiography in suspected or definite infective endocarditis

The diagnostic value of echocardiography in suspected IE differs according to the pretest probability of the disease.[14] Although TTE is often performed to exclude IE in patients with low probability of IE, it has been shown that echocardiography has a low diagnostic yield and low impact on clinical management in these patients.[14] In addition, false-positive results are more likely to occur in these situations. Thus, it could be recommended to perform echocardiography (especially TEE) only in patients with a reasonable probability of the disease. Indeed, recent ACC/AHA and ESC recommendations have emphasized the need for a selective approach to TEE in suspected IE (Fig. 7.10):[1,13]

• When TTE images are of good quality and prove to be negative and there is only a low clinical suspicion of IE, endocarditis is unlikely, TEE is not necessary, and other diagnoses should be considered.[13] In patients with a high or intermediate probability of IE, TEE should be performed if TTE is negative or inconclusive, or in patients with prosthetic valves. Negative predictive value is very high (95%) when both TTE and TEE are negative.[1]

• When TTE is positive, use of TEE is recommended if complications are suspected, or in high-risk patients (prosthetic valve, previous endocarditis, congenital heart disease, staphylococcal IE), or before surgery.[1,13]

• If TTE and TEE results remain negative, but clinical condition still leads to suspicion of IE, in the absence of an alternative source of infection, TEE should be repeated within 1 week.[13]

More generally, skilled operators and good-quality images are required to avoid imaging pitfalls. As often as possible, abnormal findings should be compared with previous examinations, especially in the postoperative period, to avoid false-positive results. Repeated examinations should be performed in difficult cases to follow the progression of images. The time interval between TEE studies should be individualized according to clinical, bacteriologic, and echocardiographic findings.

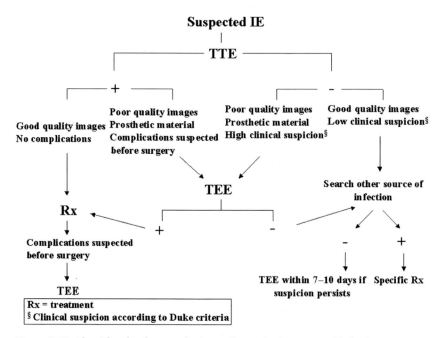

Figure 7.10 Algorithm for the use of echocardiography in suspected infective endocarditis. (Modified from Bayer *et al.* [1998][1] and Graupner *et al.* [2002].[9])

Conclusions

Echocardiography has a major role in the diagnosis, risk stratification, and management of patients with IE. Identification of vegetations, early detection of complications, identification of valvular dysfunction and their hemodynamic consequences are important information provided by echocardiography that can help in risk stratification and clinical decision-making.

References

1 Bayer AS, Bolger AF, Taubert KA, *et al.* Diagnosis and management of infective endocarditis and its complications. *Circulation* 1998;**98**:2936–48.

2 Durack DT, Lukes AS, Bright DK. New criteria for diagnosis of infective endocarditis: utilization of specific echocardiographic findings. Duke Endocarditis Service. *Am J Med* 1994;**96**:200–9.

3 Shively BK, Gurule FT, Roldan CA, Leggett JH, Schiller NB. Diagnostic value of transesophageal compared with transthoracic echocardiography in infective endocarditis. *J Am Coll Cardiol* 1991;**18**:391–7.

4 Mugge A, Daniel WG, Frank G, Lichtlen PR. Echocardiography in infective endocarditis: reassessment of prognostic implications of vegetation size determined by the transthoracic and the transesophageal approach. *J Am Coll Cardiol* 1989;**14**:631–8.

5 Shively BK, Gurule FT, Roldan CA, Leggett JH, Schiller NB. Diagnostic value of transesophageal compared with transthoracic echocardiography in infective endocarditis. *J Am Coll Cardiol* 1991;**18**:391–7.

6 Daniel WG, Mugge A, Grote J, *et al.* Comparison of transthoracic and transesophageal echocardiography for detection of abnormalities of prosthetic and bioprosthetic valves in the mitral and aortic positions. *Am J Cardiol* 1993;**71**:210–5.

7 Shapiro SM, Young E, De Guzman S, *et al.* Transesophageal echocardiography in diagnosis of infective endocarditis. *Chest* 1994;**105**:377–82.

8 Daniel WG, Mugge A, Grote J, *et al.* Comparison of transthoracic and transesophageal echocardiography for detection of abnormalities of prosthetic and bioprosthetic valves in the mitral and aortic positions. *Am J Cardiol* 1993;**71**:210–5.

9 Graupner C, Vilacosta I, SanRoman J, *et al.* Periannular extension of infective endocarditis. *J Am Coll Cardiol* 2002;**39**:1204–11.

10 Daniel WG, Mugge A, Martin RP, *et al.* Improvement in the diagnosis of abscesses associated with endocarditis by transesophageal echocardiography. *N Engl J Med* 1991;**324**:795–800.

11 Di Salvo G, Thuny F, Rosenberg V, *et al.* Endocarditis in the elderly: clinical, echocardiographic, and prognostic features. *Eur Heart J* 2003;**24**:1576–83.

12 Vilacosta I, Graupner C, San Roman JA, *et al.* Risk of embolization after institution of antibiotic therapy for infective endocarditis. *J Am Coll Cardiol* 2002;**39**:1489–95.

13 Horstkotte D, Follath F, Gutschik E, *et al.* Guidelines on prevention, diagnosis and treatment of infective endocarditis executive summary: the task force on infective endocarditis of the European Society of Cardiology. *Eur Heart J* 2004;**25**:267–76.

14 Lindner JR, Case RA, Dent JM, Abbott RD, Scheld WM, Kaul S. Diagnostic value of echocardiography in suspected endocarditis: an evaluation based on the pretest probability of disease. *Circulation* 1996;**93**:730–6.

Section two
Coronary artery disease

CHAPTER 8

Coronary imaging and screening

Koen Nieman and Pim J. de Feyter

Introduction

Non-invasive imaging of the coronary arteries was first demonstrated by magnetic resonance imaging (MRI) in the early 1990s. Since these first images, the capabilities of cardiac MRI have rapidly developed, even though cardiac MRI has proven most useful for functional assessments and infarct imaging. Parallel to these developments, computed tomography (CT) has evolved into a reliable cardiac imaging modality. Electron beam CT, followed by multislice spiral CT have proven able to provide high-resolution imaging of the coronary lumen as well as the diseased coronary artery wall. The time has come to determine the role of non-invasive coronary imaging, merely as an alternative to conventional angiography, or a complementary addition to non-invasive functional imaging.

Magnetic resonance imaging

Of the currently applied non-invasive coronary imaging techniques, MRI is the most attractive in terms of patient safety, because it does not require potentially nephrotoxic contrast media or radiation. High-resolution images of the heart can be obtained in any orientation, and with excellent tissue differentiation.

MRI is a tomographic imaging technique based on the behavior of protons (hydrogen nuclei) in a magnetic field. After excitation by a radiofrequency (RF) pulse, protons will emit an RF signal over a short period of time while they return to their aligned position. The time required for complete relaxation depends on the physical and biochemical environment of the proton, which is exploited by MRI to create images using various pulsing sequence designs. MRI is recognized as an important tool in cardiovascular medicine for imaging of cardiovascular morphology, myocardial perfusion, and myocardial viability. It is considered the gold standard for ventricular function assessment.[1]

Magnetic resonance coronary angiography

Coronary imaging by MRI was first demonstrated in the early 1990s. Using var-

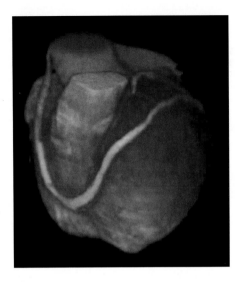

Figure 8.1 Cardiac magnetic resonance imaging (MRI). Volume-rendered MR angiogram showing a venous bypass graft arising from the aortic root along the anterior surface of the heart, with anastomoses to branches of the left coronary artery, which are not well seen.

ious 2D and 3D, breath-hold and free-breathing acquisition protocols, obstructive disease in the coronary arteries and bypass grafts can be visualized (Fig. 8.1). Although initial reports were very promising, comparative studies with numerous MRI techniques against conventional coronary angiography have shown that lesions can be detected in the proximal coronary artery segments with a reasonable sensitivity and specificity, which remained at 38–93% and 42–97%, respectively.[2] Despite steady technologic advancement, MRI has not yet reached a level of robustness that allows high-quality imaging of the entire coronary artery tree with sufficient spatial resolution, temporal resolution, and contrast-to-noise. Additional limitations include the long examination times, inability to scan and/or evaluate patients with implanted metal objects, ECG–signal distortion during scanning, suppression of signal from fat tissue, and motion artifacts resulting from averaging of data that was acquired over several heart cycles.[1]

Magnetic resonance plaque imaging

MRI can express numerous biochemical properties of the tissue being investigated, which make this modality ideal for tissue differentiation. By exposing atherosclerotic tissue to different pulse sequences that focus on different biochemical parameters, various plaque components can be identified, including fibrous or lipid tissue, calcium, and thrombus. Most of these experiences have been acquired in larger vessels, namely the carotid arteries and the aorta. In these vessels accurate measurements of the plaque size can be performed, which allows monitoring of plaque progression or regression.[3] High-resolution coronary plaque imaging is a challenging and time-consuming procedure and only limited coronary sections can be imaged within a reasonable examination time.

Electron-beam computed tomography

Electron-beam computed tomography (EBCT) is a fast CT technology, specifically designed for imaging of the heart. Because of the lack of mechanically moving parts, the time to acquire one image can be as short as 50 ms. The acquisition of images is prospectively triggered by the ECG. Based on the interpretation of the recorded ECG trace, the scan is initiated during the predicted diastolic phase of the next heart cycle.

Non-enhanced imaging of coronary calcium

The presence of calcium in the cardiovascular system is possible with any X-ray modality, as well as ultrasound and MRI. Without the use of contrast media, CT is able to detect small atherosclerotic calcifications in the coronary arteries. Since the early 1990s, EBCT has been used for the detection and quantification of coronary calcium.

By detecting calcium in the coronary arteries, the evidence for atherosclerosis is compelling. An exceptional cause for vessel wall calcification is Mönckeberg media sclerosis. However, the inability to detect calcium does not exclude the possibility of non-calcified atherosclerotic plaque being present. It has been shown extensively that the calcium score is not useful as an reliable indicator of obstructive coronary artery disease.[4] While calcification of the individual lesion may indicate plaque stability, it has been proven that the age-adjusted amount of coronary calcium is correlated to the occurrence of coronary events. It holds additional predictive value over the traditional risk factors for the long-term risk of developing symptomatic coronary artery disease. Whether widespread screening of asymptomatic individuals for coronary calcium is desirable remains a matter of debate. Selective use in those with an intermediate coronary risk, to determine whether intensive risk factor modification and medical intervention is warranted, has been suggested.[5] The use of non-enhanced EBCT as a triage tool has been explored, to exclude coronary involvement in patients with acute chest pain at the emergency department. In a relatively small study no coronary events occurred in those without coronary calcium in the period after they visited the hospital.[6] However, because the absence of coronary calcium does not exclude coronary plaque (rupture), particularly in young patients, these studies had little influence on clinical practice.

EBCT coronary angiography

Minimally invasive imaging of the coronary lumen by EBCT is possible by injecting iodinated contrast medium into a peripheral vein. A number of comparative studies with conventional angiography have been performed since 1997. In most studies, assessment was limited to the proximal and middle coronary segments. After exclusion of segments or vessels with non-diagnostic image quality (10–28%), the sensitivity and specificity to detect significant coronary artery disease was in the range 74–92% and 63–94%, respectively (Fig. 8.2).[4] Contrast-enhanced EBCT has also been used to detect bypass graft

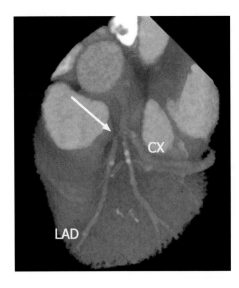

Figure 8.2 Coronary electron beam computed tomography (EBCT). Volume-rendered reconstruction of an EBCT coronary angiogram. The proximal left anterior descending coronary artery is severely stenosed (arrow). CX, left circumflex branch.

occlusion as well as non-complete graft obstruction with a good sensitivity and specificity.

The advantage of EBCT is the high temporal resolution and the relatively low radiation exposure, compared with multislice spiral CT (MSCT). Disadvantages include the lower spatial resolution in the longitudinal axis (3.0 mm detector width), the limited longitudinal coverage or long breath-hold period, and the lower signal-to-noise ratio. Widespread clinical use has further been limited by the intensive maintenance of the system and inferior suitability for non-cardiac examinations. Studies with recently innovated EBCT technology, which includes double 1.5 mm-detector row, multiphasic acquisition protocols, and 50 ms acquisition time, are awaited.

Multislice spiral computed tomography

The most recent non-invasive coronary imaging modality is multislice spiral computed tomography (MSCT), or multidetector-row helical computed tomography (MDCT). Rather than the step-and-shoot approach of sequential scanners, MSCT requires continuous patient propagation while data are acquired by up to 64 detector rows, allowing fast imaging of large body sections. By using an overlapping scan protocol each (longitudinal) position is sampled (by different detectors) during at least one entire heart cycle, and ECG-synchronized images of the entire heart can be created at any temporal position within the heart cycle (Fig. 8.3). Current scanners have a rotation time as short as 330 ms, resulting in a temporal resolution of 165 ms or less. Although this may be sufficient to avoid severe motion artifacts in the majority of patients, use of beta-blocking medication is recommended in those with a heart rate over 65–70 min^{-1}, to optimize image quality. To handle the enormous amount of

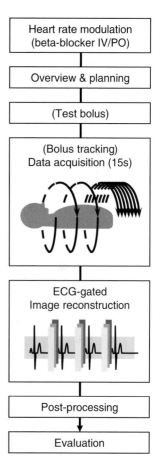

Figure 8.3 Multislice spiral computed tomography (MSCT) data acquisition. Schematic overview of the data acquisition with MSCT. Either a test bolus prior to the acquisition, or tracking the arrival of the bolus followed by the data acquisition can be used to synchronize data acquisition with contrast enhancement. Images are reconstructed from the spiral data (at any time-point within the cardiac cycle), gated to the recorded ECG.

image data (up to 300 axial slices per reconstructed cardiac phase), and present findings to referring physicians, advanced image processing tools have been developed (Figs 8.4–8.7; Video clips 1–7 ⟨👁⟩).

MSCT coronary angiography

Detection of coronary stenoses with four-slice MSCT could be demonstrated with a reasonable diagnostic accuracy compared with conventional angiography.[7] These studies also exposed the limitations of this technique, in terms of motion artifacts, long acquisition times, and the complicated evaluation of calcified coronary arteries. The relatively slow rotation of four-slice scanners, and the inherent poor results in patients with high heart rates, promoted the use of beta-blockers.[8] Comparative studies using 16-slice MSCT incorporated heart rate modulation in their protocol. In combination with the improved scanner performance (i.e. 420 ms rotation time), more and thinner detector rows, general image quality, as well as diagnostic accuracy could be improved (Figs

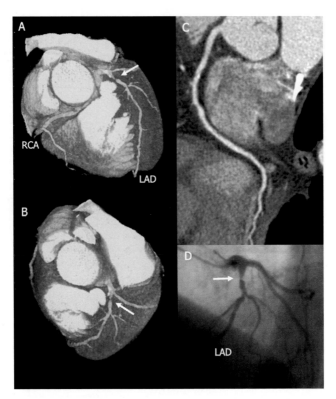

Figure 8.4 MSCT coronary angiography. A severely stenosed, partially calcified lesion can be identified in the left anterior descending coronary artery (LAD) on volume-rendered CT angiography images (A,B) and by conventional coronary angiography (D). The right coronary artery (RCA) shows no significant stenotic disease, on the curved multiplanar reformatted CT angiogram (C). See also Video clips 1–7 👁.

8.4–8.6). By reducing the average heart rate to less than 60 min^{-1}, and limiting the evaluation to larger coronary vessels (≥2.0 mm diameter), a high sensitivity and specificity could be achieved without exclusion of less-interpretable scans (Table 8.1).[9,10] Overestimation of stenosis severity, particularly in calcified vessels, resulted in a substantial number of false-positive diagnoses and a modest positive predictive value. Investigators who extended the evaluation to smaller coronary segments, and included all ≥1.5-mm vessels, found a lower diagnostic accuracy, particularly in these smaller segments.[11,12]

Graft imaging

Imaging of (venous) bypass grafts is gratifying because of their large size and relative immobility. Graft occlusion can be detected with high accuracy, but also stenosis and obstructive disease in specific sequential graft segments can be visualized (Fig. 8.7). Assessment of the native coronary artery system is more

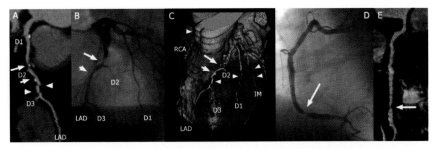

Figure 8.5 MSCT coronary angiography. A CT coronary angiogram in a patient with two-vessel disease. A partially calcified, stenotic lesion (long arrow) can be observed in the left anterior descending coronary artery (LAD), between a small septal and the second diagonal branch (D2) (A,B,C). A large, mostly non-calcified plaque (short arrow) can be identified on CT just distal to the stenotic lesion (A,C). This lesion is poorly visualized on conventional angiography (B). Because of vessel remodeling, the lesion does not cause narrowing of the vessel lumen (A). A significantly stenosed, non-calcified lesion (arrow) was found in the distal right coronary artery (RCA) (D,E). There is discontinuity between the several sets of slices (each set acquired during one heart cycles), causing interruption of the coronary arteries on CT (arrow heads). In this case it is most likely caused by inconsistent breath-holding or other non-cardiac movement. IM, intermediate branch. See also Video clips 1–7.

Table 8.1 Diagnostic performance of 16-slice MSCT to detect coronary stenosis, with conventional coronary angiography as the reference standard. Collimation as the number times the width of the individual detector rows (Coll), study population size (*n*), vessels/segments included in the analysis (Incl), sensitivity (Sens), specificity (Spec), positive (PPV) and negative predictive value (NPV), all with respect to the assessable segments/branches, sensitivity including missed lesions in non-assessable segments/branches (Sens*).

Reference	Coll (mm)	*n*	Incl (%)	Sens (%)	Spec (%)	PPV (%)	NPV (%)	Sens* (%)
Nieman *et al.* (2002)[9]	12×0.75	58	All	95	86	80	97	95
Ropers *et al.* (2003)[10]	12×0.75	77	88	92	93	79	97	85
Mollet *et al.* (2004)[11]	16×0.75	128	All	92	95	79	98	92
Martuscelli *et al.* (2004)[12]	16×0.63	64	84	89	98	90	98	78

complicated because of the often diffuse coronary artery disease and extensive calcification.[13] In the presence of chronic total occlusions, collateral vascularization, and diffuse microvascular disease, CT angiography cannot be well interpreted without functional imaging data.

Limitations and future developments

One of the important technical limitations of MSCT coronary angiography is the

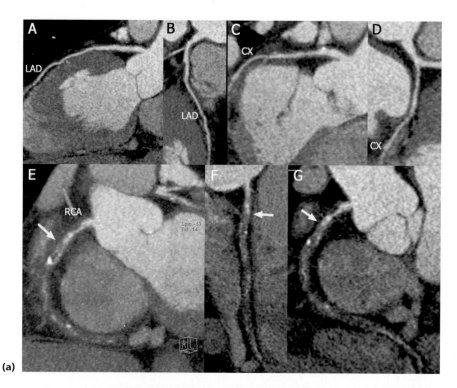

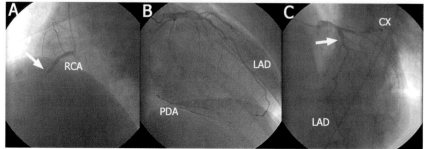

Figure 8.6 (a) MSCT cardiac imaging. A 75-year-old man with multiple risk factors recently suffered an inferior myocardial infarction and was treated with fibrinolysis. After a nuclear scan showed ischemia the patient underwent MSCT coronary angiography. Percutaneous recanalization of the occluded vessel was unfortunately not successful. Curved multiplanar reconstructions of the left main and left anterior descending (LAD) and left circumflex coronary artery (CX) in two orthogonal directions (A,B,C,D). Calcified and non-calcified plaque material and mild luminal obstruction is discernable along the vessel wall, although no high-grade lesions were detected in either branch. The right coronary artery, imaged using maximum-intensity projection (E) and two orthogonal curved multiplanar reconstructions (F,G), shows a complete obstruction at the level of the proximal–middle level with calcified and non-calcified material. (b) Conventional angiography. Conventional coronary angiography showing occlusion of the right coronary artery (RCA) (A), and collateral filling of the distal branches (B). The mid-LAD is mildly stenosed, no lesions were detected in the CX. See also Video clips 1–3 \ominus. *Continued on facing page.*

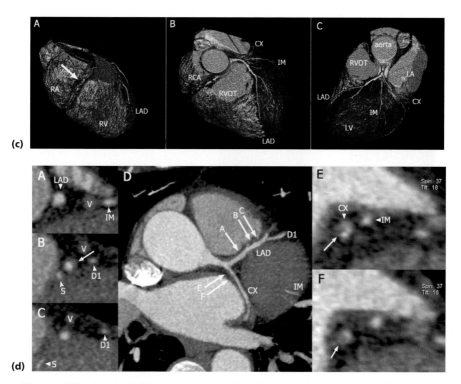

Figure 8.6 *Continued.* (c) 3D reconstruction. 3D volume-rendered reconstructions form a right-oblique (A), anterocranial (B), and latero-cranial perspective (C) of the heart and coronary arteries. The obstructed RCA runs within the right atrioventricular groove (A). The LAD and diagonal and intermediate (IM) branches can be followed along the epicardial surface of the left ventricle (B,C). The small circumflex branch is partially hidden behind the great cardiac vein (C). LA, left atrium; LV, left ventricle; RA, right atrium; RV, right ventricle; RVOT, right ventricular outflow tract. See also Video clips 4–6 👁. (d) Plaque imaging. 2D image of the left coronary artery (D) with arrows corresponding to the locations of cross-sections through the left anterior descending coronary artery (LAD) and left circumflex coronary artery (CX). A non-calcified lesion (arrow) is visible in the LAD, without significant encroachment of the vessel lumen (B), in comparison to the proximal (A) and distal reference image (C). A short, partially calcified lesion (arrows) with intermediate narrowing was found in the proximal CX (E,F). Great cardiac vein (V), intermediate branch (IM), diagonal branch (D1), septal branch (S).

relatively low temporal resolution, which causes motion artifacts in patients with a higher heart rate, and necessitates the use of beta-blockers. Given the spatial resolution of current scanners, the proximal segments can be evaluated but assessment of smaller vessels and calcified lesion is less reliable. Despite the

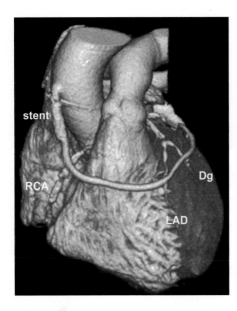

Figure 8.7 Graft imaging. A venous bypass graft arises from the aortic root, runs along the anterior surface of the heart, with anastomoses to the left anterior descending coronary artery (LAD) and a diagonal branch (Dg). A stent has been placed in the proximal graft. RCA, right coronary artery. See also Video clips 1–7 .

implementation of dose modulation protocols, the radiation exposure is still considerable, which prevents unrestricted use of this technology. While it is feasible to further improve the image quality, in terms of signal-to-noise, temporal, and spatial resolution, the true innovative challenge is to achieve this without further increase of the radiation dose.

Patients with arrhythmia are mostly excluded from MSCT coronary angiography. Patients with impaired renal function have a relative contraindication to contrast-enhanced CT.

Interpretation of the hemodynamic significance of particularly intermediate obstructions or total occlusions can be difficult without functional information. One can either gather this information separately, or physically fuse the functional and angiographic data acquisition, for example in CT positron emission tomography (CT-PET).

MSCT plaque imaging

Non-enhanced MSCT can be used for coronary calcium scoring in spiral mode, or in sequential mode to minimize the radiation dose. On contrast-enhanced MSCT coronary angiograms, both calcified and non-calcified tissue can be visualized (Fig. 8.6). No other imaging modality provides more information concerning the coronary plaque distribution, including conventional angiography.[14] In comparative studies with intracoronary ultrasound and histology, lipid, fibrotic, and calcified plaque components have different but overlapping CT attenuation characteristics.[15] Based on current knowledge, it is yet impossible to determine the likelihood of plaque rupture based on the CT appearance of a certain plaque. Considering the use of radiation and contrast medium, our current lack of understanding towards the meaning or therapeutic consequences of findings, unselective screening in asymptomatic individuals seems unjustified. To which extent CT plaque characterization can be used for risk stratification, monitoring of plaque progression and effect of medical intervention, is currently a topic of intensive research.

Clinical role of non-invasive coronary angiography

MRI, MSCT, and EBCT are effective modalities to image coronary anomalies. MRI may be preferred in younger patients because of the lack of radiation. For imaging of the coronary arteries and the non-invasive detection of stenotic disease, MSCT currently seems the most reliable modality. The diagnostic accuracy is best in patients with a low regular heart rate, a modest body size, and minimal coronary calcification. Larger branches are more reliably imaged than smaller (side) branches. The available data have so far come from single-center trials in high-risk populations with a disease prevalence of more than 50%. Given the high negative predictive value, it makes sense to use this technique in patients with a relative low disease likelihood, for instance women and patients with atypical symptoms. CT may also be an option in those who are unsuitable for certain functional tests, or have inconclusive results, before submitting these patients to catheter angiography. Compared with the populations in the literature, these patients have a lower pretest likelihood for coronary artery disease and the diagnostic accuracy may not be the same. While it makes sense to refer patients with a high pretest likelihood straight to the intervention laboratory, MSCT may offer an alternative in centers without interventional facilities to avoid diagnostic angiography in patients with favorable CT characteristics. Alternatively, CT angiography (CTA) could be the initial test in patients with medically treated (mild) stable angina to exclude significant disease in the proximal left anterior descending coronary artery (LAD) or all coronary branches, in which case there would be prognostic benefit from an intervention. Until the specific benefits of CT in specific situations has been validated, the application of CT as a substitute or addition to existing diagnostic modalities is currently decided on a case-by-case basis, depending on the local traditions and logistics.

Conclusions

The achievements in the field of non-invasive coronary imaging are considerable. The diagnostic accuracy of MSCT for the detection of coronary artery stenosis is good, and technical developments are still ongoing. The time has come to define clear indications for CT and determine which role non-invasive coronary angiography will have in clinical cardiovascular medicine.

References

1 Constantine G, Shan K, Flamm SD, *et al*. Role of MRI in clinical cardiology. *Lancet* 2004;**363**:2162–71.

2 Wielopolski PA, van Geuns RJ, de Feyter PJ, *et al*. Coronary arteries. *Eur Radiol* 2000;**10**:12–35.

3 Corti R, Fuster V, Fayad ZA, *et al*. Lipid lowering by simvastatin induces regression of human atherosclerotic lesions: two years' follow-up by high-resolution non-invasive magnetic resonance imaging. *Circulation* 2002;**106**:2884–7.

4 O'Rourke RA, Brundage BH, Froelicher VF, *et al*. American College of Cardiology/American Heart Association expert consensus document on electron-beam computed tomography for the diagnosis and prognosis of coronary artery disease: committee members. *Circulation* 2001;**102**:126–40.

5 Greenland P, LaBree L, Azen SP, *et al*. Coronary artery calcium score combined with Framingham score for risk prediction in asymptomatic individuals. *JAMA* 2004; **291**:210–5.

6 Georgiou D, Budoff MJ, Kaufer E, *et al*. Screening patients with chest pain in the emergency department using electron beam tomography: a follow-up study. *J Am Coll Cardiol* 2001;**38**:105–10.

7 Achenbach S, Hoffmann U, Ferencik M, *et al*. Tomographic coronary angiography by EBCT and MDCT. *Prog Cardiovasc Dis* 2003;**46**:185–95.

8 Giesler T, Baum U, Ropers D, *et al*. Non-invasive visualization of coronary arteries using contrast-enhanced multidetector CT: influence of heart rate on image quality and stenosis detection. *Am J Roentgenol* 2002;**179**:911–6.

9 Nieman K, Cademartiri F, Lemos PA, *et al*. Reliable non-invasive coronary angiography with fast submillimeter multislice spiral computed tomography. *Circulation* 2002; **106**:2051–4.

10 Ropers D, Baum U, Pohle K, *et al*. Detection of coronary artery stenoses with thin-slice multi-detector row spiral computed tomography and multiplanar reconstruction. *Circulation* 2003;**107**:664–6.

11 Mollet NR, Cademartiri F, Nieman K, *et al*. Multislice spiral computed tomography coronary angiography in patients with stable angina pectoris. *J Am Coll Cardiol* 2004;**43**:2265–70.

12 Martuscelli E, Romagnoli A, D'Eliseo A, *et al*. Accuracy of thin-slice computed tomography in the detection of coronary stenoses. *Eur Heart J* 2004;**25**:1043–8.

13 Nieman K, Pattynama PMT, Rensing BJ, *et al*. CT angiographic evaluation of post-CABG patients: assessment of grafts and coronary arteries. *Radiology* 2003;**229**: 749–6.

14 Achenbach S, Moselewski F, Ropers D, *et al*. Detection of calcified and non-calcified coronary atherosclerotic plaque by contrast-enhanced, submillimeter multidetector spiral computed tomography: a segment-based comparison with intravascular ultrasound. *Circulation* 2004;**109**:14–7.

15 Leber AW, Knez A, Becker A, *et al*. Accuracy of multidetector spiral computed tomography in identifying and differentiating the composition of coronary atherosclerotic plaques: a comparative study with intracoronary ultrasound. *J Am Coll Cardiol* 2004;**43**:1241–7.

CHAPTER 9

Diagnosis and prognosis in patients with chest pain

George A. Beller

Case Presentation

A 54-year-old man developed new onset, exertional, left precordial chest pain which was aching in nature and non-radiating. He had a family history of coronary artery disease (CAD) and was on an angiotensin-converting enzyme (ACE) inhibitor for mild hypertension. The previous week he had been physically active in making repairs to his house. On physical examination, his blood pressure was 140/80 mmHg, and his heart rate was 65 b min^{-1} and regular. The cardiovascular examination was entirely normal. A resting electrocardiogram (ECG) was within normal limits (Fig. 9.1a). He was referred for a treadmill exercise test to be performed in conjunction with a technetium-99m (^{99m}Tc)-sestamibi myocardial perfusion scan. At peak exercise, he demonstrated 1.0–1.5 mm horizontal ST-segment depression in the inferolateral leads (Fig. 9.1b). The stress and rest short axis tomograms from the myocardial perfusion scan are shown in Fig. 9.1(c).

Introduction

A host of non-invasive cardiovascular imaging techniques can be employed for the diagnostic and prognostic evaluation of patients with chest pain. Most of the non-invasive diagnostic imaging tests that are available to clinicians are based on the assessment of regional and global function, regional myocardial perfusion, myocardial metabolism, or coronary anatomy. The cardiovascular system can be stressed either by exercise or by administration of pharmacologic agents (e.g. dipyridamole, adenosine, or dobutamine). Vasodilator stress can be combined with low-level exercise to enhance the quality of single-photon emission computed tomography (SPECT) images and reduce side-effects.

The rationale underlying radionuclide, echocardiographic, or cardiac magnetic resonance (CMR) stress tests is the detection of either abnormal flow reserve or ischemia-induced regional systolic function abnormalities in patients who have coronary artery narrowings that are physiologically relevant.

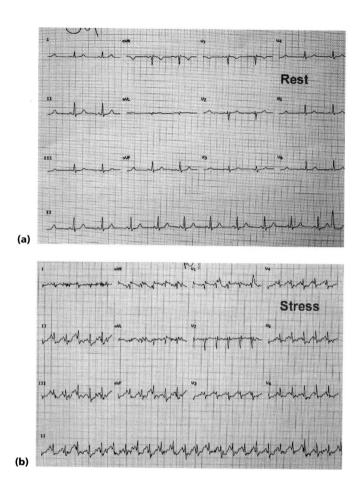

Figure 9.1 (a) Resting electrocardiogram (ECG) showing no abnormalities. (b) ECG at peak stress showing ST-segment changes as described in the text. *Continued on facing page.*

Ischemia can be identified as a defect on a myocardial perfusion scan indicative of flow heterogeneity, whereas regional abnormal systolic thickening or abnormal wall motion represents a mismatch between perfusion and metabolism in a local myocardial region. With respect to contrast echocardiography, the integrity of the microvasculature is simultaneously evaluated with regional function at rest and stress.

Recently, multidetector computed tomography (CT) employing 16, 32 or 64 slices per second has permitted the evaluation of coronary anatomy after intravenous contrast injection. Drawbacks of this approach are the high radiation exposure and the necessity to administer intravenous beta-blockers in order to reduce the resting heart rate prior to imaging.

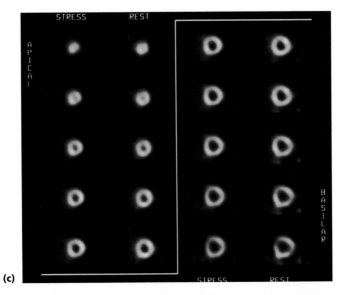

(c)

Figure 9.1 *Continued.* (c) Stress and rest short-axis ^{99m}Tc-sestamibi tomograms with apical slices shown in the upper left corner and basilar slices in the lower right corner. The first column of each pair represents the stress images, and the second column represents rest images. The perfusion pattern in this study is entirely normal.

Exercise electrocardiography

A meta-analysis of all studies in the literature revealed that the sensitivity and specificity of the exercise ECG stress tests for CAD detection were 68% and 77%, respectively.[1] The sensitivity of the exercise ECG is highly dependent on the level of exercise achieved. Patients who fail to achieve at least 85% of age-adjusted maximum predicted heart rate and have a negative exercise ECG response may still have a significant coronary artery stenosis. Specificity of the ST-segment depression response is affected by states that alter the resting ECG including left ventricular (LV) hypertrophy with strain, hyperventilation, digoxin therapy, intraventricular conduction disturbances (e.g. left bundle branch block, Wolff–Parkinson–White syndrome, and electrolyte abnormalities), and a resting ST depression that can occur from a variety of other causes. The specificity of the exercise ECG response has been reported to be suboptimal in women, particularly those who are in the premenopausal age group with a low-to-intermediate pretest likelihood of CAD.

The extent of CAD tremendously influences the sensitivity of the exercise ECG. Its sensitivity is below 50% in patients with single-vessel disease but is higher than 85% for patients with three-vessel or left main CAD. Horizontal or down-sloping ST-segment depression of ≥1.0mm for 80ms at low exercise heart rates has a higher positive predictive value for myocardial ischemia than does ST-segment depression at high heart rates or workloads. Beta-blocking drugs and rate-lowering calcium-blockers should be held in order for an adequate heart rate response to be attained during increasing workloads during testing. Using slow up-sloping ST-segment depression as a criterion for ischemia will enhance the sensitivity of the exercise ECG but at the cost of lower specificity.

Perhaps one of the most powerful predictive variables on exercise ECG testing for identifying high-risk patients is functional capacity reflected by workload achieved. Similarly, absolute peak exercise capacity is perhaps a stronger predictor of subsequent mortality than the percentage of age-predicted maximum heart rate achieved. Frequent ventricular ectopy in the immediate post-exercise period, abnormal post-exercise heart rate recovery, and chronotropic incompetence are other high-risk ECG stress test variables. The Duke Treadmill Score, which incorporates the duration of exercise, maximal ST-segment deviation, and an angina index, can be employed for risk stratification.[2]

Diagnostic and prognostic value of stress radionuclide myocardial perfusion imaging

In the past 15 years, significant advances have been made in the ability to assess myocardial perfusion with radionuclide tracers under stress and rest conditions in patients with chest pain for identifying those with CAD who will manifest inducible myocardial ischemia.[3] For many years, planar imaging and then SPECT with thallium-201 (^{201}Tl) constituted the only scintigraphic techniques available for detecting CAD and assessing prognosis in patients undergoing stress perfusion imaging. The major limitation of ^{201}Tl scintigraphy is the high false-positive rate in many laboratories, which is attributed predominantly to image attenuation artifacts and variance of normal that are interpreted as defects attributed to significant CAD.[3] Breast attenuation artifacts in women are sometimes difficult to distinguish from perfusion abnormalities secondary to ischemia or scar.

In recent years, new ^{99m}Tc-labeled perfusion agents have been introduced into clinical practice to enhance the specificity of SPECT and to provide additional information regarding regional and global LV systolic function accomplished by ECG gating of images. Quality of images obtained with these new ^{99m}Tc-labeled radionuclides was shown to be superior to that of images obtained with ^{201}Tl because of the more favorable physical characteristics of ^{99m}Tc imaging with a gamma camera. With ^{99m}Tc, doses 10–20 times higher than those that are feasible with ^{201}Tl can be administered, yielding images with higher count density. ^{99m}Tc demonstrates less scatter and attenuation than ^{201}Tl and, thus, is associated with fewer image artifacts. Use of ^{99m}Tc-labeled imaging agents permits easy gated acquisition, permitting the simultaneous evaluation of regional systolic thickening or wall motion, global LV function, LV volumes, and myocardial perfusion.

Sensitivity and specificity of stress myocardial perfusion

The sensitivity for detecting CAD (≥50% stenosis) averaged 87% in 33 studies pooled from the literature.[3] Specificity, derived from patients referred for cardiac catheterization who had normal angiograms, averaged 73%. There was a normalcy rate of 91% in this pooled analysis. The normalcy rate, defined as the percentage of patients with less than 5% pretest likelihood of CAD who have normal myocardial perfusion imaging studies, is a variable that reduces the referral bias inherent in specificity determinations that employ patients who are referred for cardiac catheterization and have normal coronary angiograms. This is because the majority of patients referred for angiography have abnormal scans, yielding an exaggerated referral of patients with false-positive nuclear studies. The sensitivity and specificity of pharmacologic vasodilator stress imaging are comparable to those of exercise stress imaging.[3] The sensitivity of vasodilator SPECT is 89%, with a specificity of 75%. The sensitivity, specificity, and accuracy of dobutamine stress myocardial perfusion imaging for diagnosis of CAD is comparable to that observed with vasodilator stress imaging.

One of the challenges of myocardial perfusion imaging is the confounding influence of soft-tissue attenuation of the tracers utilized, leading to diminished diagnostic accuracy. Attenuation artifacts produced by the breasts, lateral chest wall, abdomen, and left hemidiaphragm can cause artifacts that mimic perfusion defects comparable to that seen in patients with CAD, thus decreasing test specificity. Attenuation-corrected, stress-only myocardial perfusion imaging enhances the ability to interpret SPECT studies as definitely normal or abnormal, reducing the need for rest imaging.[4] In this study, attenuation-corrected myocardial perfusion imaging coupled with ECG gated data were compared with perfusion imaging gated data alone and myocardial perfusion imaging without gating or attenuation correction. With stress myocardial perfusion imaging alone, only 37% of studies were interpreted as definitely normal or abnormal, with a perception that rest imaging would be required in 77% of the studies. Attenuation-corrected data increased the number of studies characterized as definitely normal or abnormal to 84%, reducing the perceived need for rest imaging to 43%.

Prognostic value of myocardial perfusion imaging

The major goal of non-invasive risk stratification in patients presenting with chest pain or an angina equivalent is the identification of those at high risk for subsequent cardiac death or non-fatal myocardial infarction who may benefit from prompt referral for invasive strategies. Conversely, patients judged to be at low or low-to-intermediate risk for subsequent hard events based on non-invasive scan findings can be spared unnecessary premature referral for invasive evaluation and, thus, treated medically.

Table 9.1 lists the SPECT imaging variables on exercise or pharmacologic myocardial perfusion imaging that are associated with high-risk CAD and an increased probability of future cardiac events.

A large amount of data published in the literature has accumulated during

Table 9.1 High-risk single-photon emission computed tomography (SPECT) imaging variables.

- Multiple reversible or persistent defects in more than one coronary supply region (multivessel coronary artery disease scan pattern)
- An extensive area of stress-induced hypoperfusion in a single or multivessel disease scan distribution (e.g. proximal left anterior descending coronary artery scan pattern)
- A large ischemic burden reflected by multiple reversible defects or a high summed difference score
- Transient ischemic left ventricular cavity dilatation
- Multiple abnormal regional wall motion or thickening abnormalities
- A gated SPECT ejection fraction of less than 40%
- Increased diastolic and end-systolic volumes on quantitative SPECT
- Increased lung : heart ratio of thallium uptake when ^{201}Tl is employed for exercise imaging

the past 20 years that demonstrate the incremental value of stress myocardial perfusion imaging variables for separating high- and low-risk patient subgroups in determining prognosis.[3,5,6]

The annualized cardiac death or myocardial infarction rate in 39,173 patients from 19 series in the literature who were followed for an average 2.3 years after a normal scan was 0.6% per year.[6] Conversely, the cardiac death and/or non-fatal myocardial infarction rate was 5.9% per annum in patients with high-risk scan variables as derived from 39 published series in the literature comprising 69,655 patients who were followed for an average of 2.3 years.[6] In this latter pooled analysis, low-risk patients had a 0.8% annual hard event rate per year.

Perhaps one of the most powerful predictors of high-risk CAD on stress SPECT imaging is transient ischemic dilatation of the LV cavity.[5] Reversible LV cavity dilatation is thought to be secondary to ischemia-induced subendocardial hypoperfusion, yielding an apparent increase in the LV cavity size on stress scintigrams compared with the rest scintigrams in which resolution of the subendocardial ischemia has occurred. This finding is associated with a higher incidence of multivessel CAD and a worse outcome than in patients not demonstrating this variable.

Gating of SPECT images adds significant prognostic value to the sole evaluation of myocardial perfusion patterns on post-stress and rest SPECT studies. The detection of post-stress wall motion abnormalities increases the sensitivity of detecting high-risk CAD. In addition, measurement of the LV ejection fraction (LVEF) and ventricular volumes by SPECT provides additional prognostic information in the risk stratification process.[3,5,6]

Functional assessment by quantitated gated SPECT with measurement of regional systolic thickening fractions was shown to enhance the identification of three-vessel CAD compared with the evaluation of the extent of myocardial perfusion defects alone.[7] In that study, 25% of patients with angiographic three-vessel disease had either abnormal perfusion or abnormal systolic thickening, or both, in three coronary vascular supply regions on post-stress images, compared with 9.8% who had such abnormalities on perfusion images alone. Some patients may exhibit normal or near-normal scans on post-stress images and still have underlying three-vessel disease, which has been referred to as "balanced ischemia" but more likely is caused by diffusely abnormal flow reserve. Such patients often demonstrate poor exercise tolerance and may exhibit abnormal regional dysfunction despite absence of inducible, localized perfusion defects.

The more extensive and severe the stress perfusion abnormalities are, the worse is the subsequent outcome. For example, in one study from the Cedars-Sinai group,[8] patients with a normal SPECT study had annual mortality and non-fatal infarction rates of 0.3% and 0.5%, respectively (Fig. 9.2). Patients with mildly abnormal post-stress scans had annual death and non-fatal infarction rates of 0.8% and 2.7%, respectively. The patients with the most severely abnormal scans had annual death and infarction rates of 2.9% and 4.2%, respectively. The same group showed substantial incremental value of exercise SPECT perfusion variables over the Duke Treadmill Score.[9] Figure 9.3 depicts the relationship between the percent stress defect and the adjusted risk of subsequent cardiac death in 16,020 consecutive patients who underwent exercise or vasodilator stress ^{99m}Tc-sestamibi SPECT and were followed for 2.1 ± 0.8 years.[10]

A certain subset of patients judged to be at low risk after exercise ECG testing reflected by a low Duke Treadmill Score may still benefit from the addition of myocardial perfusion imaging for risk stratification.[11] In this study, a clinical

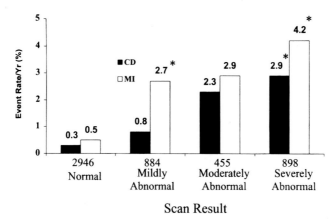

Figure 9.2 Cardiac death (CD) rate and non-fatal myocardial infarction (MI) rate per year in patients with various abnormalities on exercise ^{99m}Tc-sestamibi SPECT myocardial perfusion imaging. Note that patients with a normal scan had a very low hard event rate per year. The cardiac death rate significantly increases with more severe post-stress perfusion defects. (Reproduced with permission from Hachamovitch *et al.* [1998].[8])

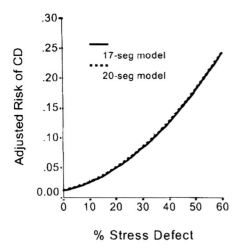

Figure 9.3 Adjusted risk of cardiac death (CD) per year relative to the percent stress defect on stress ^{99m}Tc-sestamibi SPECT myocardial perfusion imaging. Note that for either the 17-segment (seg) model or the two-segment model, the relationship between perfusion defect size and subsequent cardiac death is similar. (Reproduced with permission from Berman *et al.* [2004].[10])

score was useful in deciding which patients at low risk after conventional ECG treadmill testing would benefit from further risk stratification with myocardial stress perfusion imaging. Variables incorporated in the clinical score were male gender, history of prior myocardial infarction, diabetes, typical angina, and advanced age. Patients with a high clinical score and a low Duke Treadmill Score were further successfully risk stratified by myocardial perfusion imaging variables.

Diabetics are a subgroup of patients who may benefit significantly from risk stratification by stress myocardial perfusion imaging.[12] In this multicenter study, diabetic women with ischemia on stress SPECT imaging in two or more coronary vascular regions had only a 60% event-free survival rate over the subsequent 3 years compared with 79% for diabetic men with multivessel ischemia. The higher cardiac event rate in diabetics with either a low-risk or a high-risk scan is depicted in Fig. 9.4.[6] Note that in this pooled analysis, diabetic women had a greater than 10% hard event rate per year with a high-risk scan.

Pharmacologic stress imaging provides comparable prognostic information at exercise stress imaging, although the cardiac event rate in patients with normal pharmacologic stress scans is higher than the event rate seen in patients' normal exercise perfusion studies.[3,5,6] This is because the patient population is a clinically higher risk one, given that referral for pharmacologic stress implies either inability to exercise adequately (e.g. from peripheral vascular disease) or concomitant pulmonary disease with bronchospasm (e.g. requiring dobutamine stress). Adenosine stress SPECT imaging yielded a combined cardiac death or myocardial infarction rate for patients with a normal scan of 1.6% per annum compared with 10.6% per annum in those with a severely abnormal scan.[13]

Myocardial stress SPECT imaging is as useful at assigning risks for future cardiac events in the community outpatient setting as it is in an academic setting environment.[14] In 1612 patients, dual-isotope ^{201}Tl/^{99m}Tc reliably identified

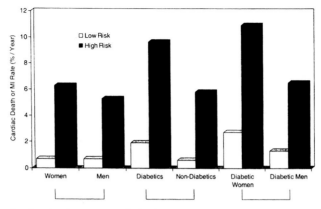

Figure 9.4 Cardiac death or myocardial infarction (MI) rate per year for various groupings of patients as derived from pooled analyses of the literature. Note that patients with high-risk scans (solid bars) had a substantially higher hard event rate per year than patients who were judged to have low-risk scans. Diabetics have a significantly higher event rate with either normal or abnormal scans than non-diabetics, and diabetic women with abnormal scans have the highest annual event rate. (Reproduced with permission from Shaw and Iskandrian [2004].[6])

high-risk patients. The hard event rate was 0.4% per annum for patients with a normal scan versus 2.3% per annum in those with an abnormal scan. Figure 9.5 shows the cumulative 2-year event-free survival stratified by defect extent score (panel A) and reversibility score (panel B). Patients with the highest score (4) had large defects with a moderate-to-severe change in intensity from stress to rest. This subgroup has the worst event-free survival.

Stress SPECT imaging may be useful in determining which CAD patients benefit most from revascularization versus medical therapy, although no randomized studies have been performed regarding this issue. In an analysis of the Cedars-Sinai database,[15] patients with more than 11% of the left ventricle rendered ischemic as assessed on post-stress ^{99m}Tc-sestamibi SPECT, had a more favorable outcome with revascularization versus medical therapy. Patients with lesser degrees of inducible ischemia had no advantage with revascularization compared with medical therapy. It should be pointed out that this study was observational in nature, and patients were not randomized to medical therapy versus revascularization.

Stress perfusion imaging appears to be cost-effective, compared with direct referral to coronary angiography, for patients presenting with stable chest pain. When stress perfusion imaging was used as the initial testing strategy for patients with a stable chest pain syndrome, the cardiac death and non-fatal infarction rates were comparable to patients referred directly for cardiac catheterization for such chest pain evaluation.[16] The cost of care for the direct catheterization strategy compared with stress myocardial perfusion imaging and selective catheterization was substantially higher (Fig. 9.6).

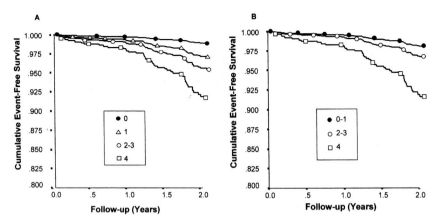

Figure 9.5 Cumulative 2-year event-free survival stratified by the defect extent and severity score (A) and the reversibility score (B). Defect extent and severity ranged from a score of 1 (small, mild-to-moderate intensity defect) to a score of 4 (large, severe intensity defect). The reversibility score comprised elements of defect size with absolute change in tracer activity from stress to rest. (Reproduced with permission from Thomas *et al.* [1998].[14])

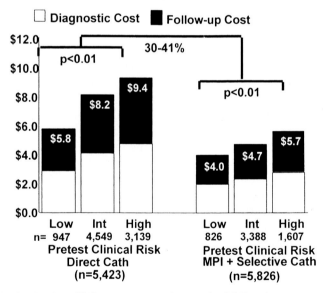

Figure 9.6 Diagnostic and follow-up costs in thousands of dollars for patients referred directly to catheterization for stable chest pain or compared with patients who had myocardial perfusion imaging (MPI) first, followed by selective catheterization (Cath). Note that the total costs are significantly higher for the direct catheterization group for subsets with either low, intermediate (Int), or high pretest clinical risk. The cardiac death and non-fatal myocardial infarction rates were similar for both groups. (Reproduced with permission from Hachamovitch *et al.* [1999].[16])

Diagnostic and prognostic applications of stress echocardiography

Stress echocardiography can be performed with treadmill, upright bicycle or supine bicycle exercise, or by using pharmacologic stressors such as dobutamine or dipyridamole. The weighted mean sensitivity, specificity, and overall accuracy for exercise echocardiography from a pooled analysis of data in the literature were 86%, 81%, and 85%, respectively.[17] Presence of ischemia on exercise echocardiography is a good predictor of future cardiac events and, in a multivariate model, was the strongest independent predictor of cardiac death, myocardial infarction, or unstable angina.[18] In patients with good exercise capacity, extent and severity of exercise-induced LV dysfunction provided independent and incremental prognostic value.[19] Exercise echocardiography, like exercise SPECT, is particularly useful in patients with an intermediate-risk Duke Treadmill Score. The mortality rate is approximately 1% per annum in patients with normal exercise echocardiograms.[17]

Dobutamine echocardiography, with atropine administered for low heart rates, also provides prognostic value in patients with suspected or known CAD. Patients with a normal dobutamine–atropine stress echocardiogram have a low annual event rate of cardiac death or non-fatal infarction.[17] The rate of cardiac death or myocardial infarction in patients with new wall motion abnormalities or extensive resting wall motion abnormalities is increased.

Limitations of stress SPECT myocardial perfusion imaging and stress echocardiography

Radionuclide and echocardiographic stress testing are not without certain limitations.[20] Limitations of exercise or pharmacologic SPECT perfusion imaging include suboptimal specificity because of artifacts, long procedure time when rest and stress performed with ^{99m}Tc-labeled agents, no standardized correction for attenuation and scatter, poor quality images in obese patients, inability to quantitate absolute blood flow in mL min^{-1}g^{-1}, radiation exposure, and an underestimation of three-vessel disease in patients with diffusely abnormal flow reserve.

Limitations of exercise or pharmacologic stress echocardiography include decreased sensitivity for detection of one-vessel disease or mild stenosis with post-exercise imaging, inability to image all of the left ventricle in some patients, the technique is highly operator-dependent for image analysis, there is no standardized quantitative measurements for LVEF, and poor acoustic window in some patients. Myocardial contrast echocardiography, which enables the assessment of myocardial perfusion by ultrasound as well as regional function, may improve detection of CAD and permit a more accurate determination of disease extent.

Clinical decision-making

Exercise or pharmacologic SPECT myocardial perfusion imaging provides incremental diagnostic and prognostic value over clinical and exercise ECG test information, particularly in patients with an intermediate or intermediate-to-high pretest likelihood of CAD. Clearly, patients who exhibit normal myocardial perfusion and function on gated SPECT at high exercise heart rates or workloads have an excellent prognosis and should be referred for a non-cardiac evaluation for determining the etiology of presenting symptoms. Such patients should be intervened upon with respect to primary prevention and reduction of those CAD risk factors that are identified. Conversely, patients with high-risk scans may benefit from an early invasive strategy with a view towards revascularization, depending on coronary anatomic findings. A large number of patients will show mild ischemia without a multivessel disease scan pattern and absence of an extensive defect in the supply zone of the left anterior descending coronary artery. Such patients who also have good exercise tolerance may initially be treated medically with risk factor reduction and the administration of anti-ischemic drugs, such as beta-blockers and long-acting nitrates. An exception may be diabetics who, even with mild ischemia, may have extensive underlying CAD. Figure 9.7 shows a decision-making algorithm incorporating these concepts for patients presenting with undiagnosed chest pain.[21]

The future

For the future, the diagnostic and prognostic value of myocardial perfusion imaging will be enhanced with technologic advancements including attenuation-correction algorithms and the introduction of new perfusion tracers that are more linear with flow in the hyperemic range. Positron emission tomography (PET) imaging with rubidium-82 may prove cost-effective and more accurate than SPECT perfusion imaging for detection of CAD. PET–CT hybrid instruments may permit the simultaneous assessment of myocardial perfusion and coronary anatomy with non-invasive coronary angiography. CT scanners that can image at 64 slices per second have recently been introduced and have shown great feasibility for evaluating coronary anatomy. SPECT-CT hybrid imaging devices have also been introduced into the clinical setting. Currently, the CT scanning segment of the instrument is most often used for attenuation correction of the SPECT perfusion studies. Finally, molecular imaging technology is being explored, which ultimately may be useful in imaging inflamed vulnerable plaques as well as such biological phenomena as apoptosis and angiogenesis.

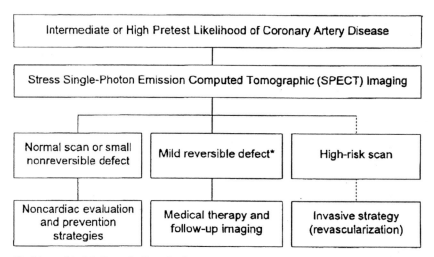

*A mild reversible defect is one that is confined to one coronary vascular region and does not include the entire risk zone of the left anterior descending coronary artery (apex, anterolateral wall, and septum).

Figure 9.7 Clinical decision-making algorithm for patients presenting with chest pain and an intermediate or high pretest likelihood of coronary artery disease (CAD). Patients who have normal or near-normal myocardial perfusion scans have an excellent prognosis and can undergo non-cardiac evaluation and prevention strategies. Patients with a high-risk scan would be candidates for an invasive strategy which could include revascularization. Patients with a mild reversible defect may be initially treated with aggressive medical therapy (Rx) with follow-up (F/U) imaging performed to assess efficacy of such therapy. *Defect that does not reflect a multivessel scan pattern or a defect pattern consistent with proximal left anterior descending CAD. (Reproduced with permission from Beller and Zaret [2000].[21])

Case Presentation (Continued)

The patient had a positive exercise ECG at peak stress characterized by less than 1.0 mm horizontal ST-segment depression. However, the myocardial perfusion scan was entirely within normal limits. This patient was placed on a non-steroidal anti-inflammatory agent for presumed musculoskeletal chest pain and, 1 week later, his symptoms disappeared. This case is an example of how myocardial perfusion imaging can be employed to distinguish between true and false-positive ST-segment depression on exercise testing. It should also be pointed out that, in this case, the ST-segment depression resolved within 1 min of recovery, which is a clue that it could be a false-positive response. Based on the data provided in this review, this patient's prognosis with a normal perfusion scan at a heart rate exceeding 85% of its maximum predicted heart rate is excellent.

References

1 Gianrossi R, Detrano R, Mulvihill D, *et al*. Exercise-induced ST depression in the diagnosis of coronary artery disease: a meta-analysis. *Circulation* 1989;**80**:87–98.

2 Gibbons RJ, Balady GJ, Bricker JT, *et al*. American College of Cardiology/American Heart Association (ACC/AHA) Task Force on Practice Guidelines 2002 guideline update for exercise testing: a report of the ACC/AHA Task Force on Practice Guidelines (Committee to Update the 1997 Exercise Testing Guidelines). *Circulation* 2002;**106**:1883–92. (Also available at: www.acc.org/clinical/guidelines/exercise/dir Index.htm)

3 Klocke FJ, Baird MG, Lorell BH, *et al*. American College of Cardiology/American Heart Association/American Society for Nuclear Cardiology (ACC/AHA/ASNC) guidelines for the clinical use of cardiac radionuclide imaging: a report of the ACC/AHA/ASNC Committee to Revise the 1995 Guidelines for the Clinical Use of Cardiac Radionuclide Imaging. *J Am Coll Cardiol* 2003;**42**:1318–33. (Also available at: http://www.acc.org/clinical/guidelines/radio/index.pdf)

4 Heller GV, Bateman TM, Johnson LL, *et al*. Clinical value of attenuation correction in stress-only Tc-99m sestamibi SPECT imaging. *J Nucl Cardiol* 2004;**11**:273–81.

5 Beller GA. First annual Mario S. Verani, MD, memorial lecture: clinical value of myocardial perfusion imaging in coronary artery disease. *J Nucl Cardiol* 2003;**10**:529–42.

6 Shaw LJ, Iskandrian AE. Prognostic value of gated myocardial perfusion SPECT. *J Nucl Cardiol* 2004;**11**:171–85.

7 Lima RS, Watson DD, Goode AR, *et al*. Incremental value of combined perfusion and function over perfusion alone by gated SPECT myocardial perfusion imaging for detection of severe three-vessel coronary artery disease. *J Am Coll Cardiol* 2003;**42**: 64–70.

8 Hachamovitch R, Berman DS, Shaw LJ, *et al*. Incremental prognostic value of myocardial perfusion single photon emission computed tomography for the prediction of cardiac death: differential stratification for risk of cardiac death and myocardial infarction. *Circulation* 1998;**97**:535–43. (Erratum in *Circulation* 1998;**98**:190.)

9 Hachamovitch R, Berman DS, Kiat H, *et al*. Exercise myocardial perfusion SPECT in patients without known coronary artery disease: incremental prognostic value and use in risk stratification. *Circulation* 1996;**93**:905–14.

10 Berman DS, Abidov A, Kang X, *et al*. Prognostic validation of a 17-segment score derived from a 20-segment score for myocardial perfusion SPECT interpretation. *J Nucl Cardiol* 2004;**11**:414–23.

11 Poornima IG, Miller TD, Christian TF, Hodge DO, Bailey KR, Gibbons RJ. Utility of myocardial perfusion imaging in patients with low-risk treadmill scores. *J Am Coll Cardiol* 2004;**43**:194–9.

12 Giri S, Shaw LJ, Murthy DR, *et al*. Impact of diabetes on the risk stratification using stress single-photon emission computed tomography myocardial perfusion imaging in patients with symptoms suggestive of coronary artery disease. *Circulation* 2002; **105**:32–40.

13 Hachamovitch R, Berman DS, Kiat H, *et al*. Incremental prognostic value of adenosine stress myocardial perfusion single-photon emission computed tomography and impact on subsequent management in patients with or suspected of having myocardial ischemia. *Am J Cardiol* 1997;**80**:426–33.

14 Thomas GS, Miyamoto MI, Morello AP III, *et al*. Technetium 99m sestamibi myocar-

dial perfusion imaging predicts clinical outcome in the community outpatient setting: the Nuclear Utility in the Community (NUC) Study. *J Am Coll Cardiol* 2004;**43**:213–23.

15 Hachamovitch R, Hayes SW, Friedman JD, Cohen I, Berman DS. Comparison of the short-term survival benefit associated with revascularization compared with medical therapy in patients with no prior coronary artery disease undergoing stress myocardial perfusion single photon emission computed tomography. *Circulation* 2003;**107**: 2900–7.

16 Hachamovitch R, Shaw LJ, Berman DS. The ongoing evolution of risk stratification using myocardial perfusion imaging in patients with known or suspected coronary artery disease. *ACC Curr J Rev* 1999;**8**:66–71.

17 Cheitlin MD, Armstrong WF, Aurigemma GP, *et al*. ACC/AHA/ASE 2003 guideline update for the clinical application of echocardiography: a report of the ACC/AHA task force on practice guidelines (ACC/AHA/ASE Committee to Update the 1997 Guidelines for the Clinical Application of Echocardiography). *Circulation* 2003;**108**: 1146–62.

18 Marwick TH, Mehta R, Arheart K, Lauer MS. Use of exercise echocardiography for prognostic evaluation of patients with known or suspected coronary artery disease. *J Am Coll Cardiol* 1997;**30**:83–90.

19 McCully RB, Roger VL, Mahoney DW, *et al*. Outcome after abnormal exercise echocardiography for patients with good exercise capacity: prognostic importance of the extent and severity of exercise-related left ventricular dysfunction. *J Am Coll Cardiol* 2002;**39**:1345–52.

20 Beller GA. Relative merits of cardiac diagnostic techniques. In: Zipes DP, Libby P, Bonow RO, Braunwald E, eds. *Braunwald's Heart Disease*, 7th edn. Saunders/Elsevier, Philadelphia, 2005: 373–94.

21 Beller GA, Zaret BL. Contributions of nuclear cardiology to diagnosis and prognosis of patients with coronary artery disease. *Circulation* 2000;**101**:1465–78.

CHAPTER 10

Peripheral vascular disease

Serge Kownator

Introduction

The importance of peripheral vascular disease is often underestimated in clinical cardiology. However, it is impotant to recognize and diagnose peripheral vascular lesions for two reasons. First, to perform an accurate evaluation of the patient's status and to determine the appropriate therapeutic strategy. Second, to stratify the level of risk in so far as peripheral vascular disease is an important marker and a strong predictor for cardiovascular events, in particular myocardial infarction and stroke.

The diagnosis of peripheral vascular disease relies extensively on the clinical evaluation, but in many circumstances the sensitivity of clinical examination appears rather poor. Therefore, imaging becomes a major step in the screening, diagnosis, and evaluation of vascular disease.

Techniques

Angiography

Since the 1920s angiography has been considered as the gold standard for vascular imaging. Even with the development of digital angiography it remains an invasive technique, with an overall risk of approximately 2–3% according to different studies.[1] Furthermore, angiography remains luminography without any reliable information on the vascular wall, and hemodynamic consequences. In addition, the costs of the technique may also be a limiting factor. Therefore, with the development of non-invasive imaging, it is now well accepted that digital angiography must not, in most cases, be used for the screening and diagnosis of peripheral vascular disease. However, it remains a major step in a number of cases before surgery and angioplasty.

Doppler ultrasound

Doppler ultrasound for vascular evaluation was introduced 40 years ago. In the beginning, only continuous wave Doppler was used for vascular applications in order to detect and quantify arterial stenosis using the Bernoulli equation. Severe stenoses were identified and quantified mainly by the peak systolic velocities. Today, Doppler ultrasound includes B-mode echography (for vascular wall evaluation), pulsed wave Doppler, color Doppler, and power Doppler. This full range of modalities is mandatory for a complete vascular evaluation. The technical advances allow high-resolution imaging resulting in enhanced performance of this technique. Doppler ultrasound is actually the most readily available and most commonly used technique for the screening and diagnosis of vascular lesions. Despite its dependence on the expertise of the operator, accuracy and reproducibility can be dramatically improved by education and experience.[2]

CT angiography

Introduced in 1998, multislice spiral CT allows a larger anatomic volume to be scanned, with a reduced contrast dose and a shorter acquisition time compared with single slice CT. Post-processing techniques improve the quality of reconstructed images such as multiplanar reconstructions, 3D, and maximum intensity projections. Very long segment areas can be imaged, enabling CT angiography (CTA) of the lower extremities and single acquisitions of the aorto-iliac or carotid systems. The combination of source images and post-processing allows comprehensive evaluation of the degree of stenosis, wall abnormalities such as soft or calcified plaques, aneurysmal dilatation, the presence of collaterals, and other incidental lesions. Although multislice CT has some impressive strengths, there are also some weaknesses. The ability to visualize calcium on CT is an advantage; however, it is also a disadvantage because calcifications can "bloom," and extensive vessel wall calcifications can make assessment of the vessel lumen and stenosis quantification virtually impossible. Renal insufficiency, iodine allergy, and radiation are also major limitations. Reconstruction algorithms need further validation for accurate stenosis quantification.[3] Despite its limitations, multislice CT is a major step forward in vascular imaging, with a good level of cost effectiveness and widespread availability.

Magnetic resonance angiography

Gadolinium-enhanced magnetic resonance angiography (MRA) has proven valuable for the non-invasive assessment of peripheral vascular disease. Furthermore, non-contrast methods are able to provide information about stenosis and the direction of flow. MRA can also analyze the vascular wall structure, plaque characterization, and tissue perfusion. Numerous studies have emphasized the accuracy of MRA compared with contrast angiography. Despite the extensive validation, discrepancies can be observed between MRA and conventional angiography. With MRA, there is sometimes an overestimation of the degree of stenosis. In addition, the inability to detect calcification of the arterial wall can be a problem. In some indications, a single breath-hold is not long enough for the acquisition. In general, however, MRA is relatively fast and easy to perform. For patients with renal failure or iodine allergy it appears to be the technique of choice (versus CTA or conventional angiography).[4] Although stents are not a contraindication for MRA, the presence of stents limits the interpretation of the images. Besides the usual contraindications such as pacemakers or claustrophobia, the main limitations for widespread use of this technique are its availability and cost.

Table 10.1 Imaging techniques: advantages and limitations.

Technique	Advantage	Limitation
Conventional angiography	Gold standard	Invasive
		Risk
		Cost
MRA	Non-invasive	Availability
		Cost
CTA	Non-invasive	Iodine injection
	Widely available	Validation
Ultrasound	Non-invasive	Operator dependent
	Widely used	
	Low cost	

CTA, computed tomography angiography; MRA, magnetic resonance imaging.

The strengths and limitations of the different imaging techniques are summarized in Table 10.1.

Clinical indications

The clinical indication depends on the patient's status and the availability and local expertise of the technique. We can differentiate risk stratification, screening of peripheral vascular lesions in high-risk patients, evaluation of clinical disorders such as vascular murmurs, and more severe situations such as transient ischemic attack (TIA), stroke, or leg ischemia. Risk stratification and screening are discussed in the following paragraphs, whereas evaluation of clinical disorders is illustrated in the case presentations.

Risk stratification

According to several recommendations, target organ damage is now part of the stratification of the risk in individuals. Of the different modalities, carotid ultrasound takes a major place in order to measure intima-media thickness (IMT) (Fig. 10.1). Validated by Pignoli in 1986, IMT has been correlated to risk factors associated with the development of atherosclerosis in all arterial beds including coronary and peripheral arteries and is also a predictor of cardiovascular events. In the Cardiovascular Health Study the risk for myocardial infarction or stroke is increased by a factor of 4 in the highest quintile of IMT, as compared with the lowest quintile.[5] In epidemiologic studies different protocols have been proposed. On the one hand, the measurement of different arterial areas allows the evaluation of a "mean maximum IMT," which includes diffuse thickness and plaques. This protocol is limited by the difficulty in assessing the different seg-

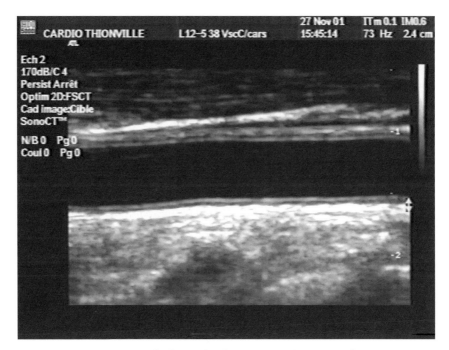

Figure 10.1 Common carotid echography showing normal intima media.

ments in all patients and requires a high level of skill. On the other hand, the measurement of the far wall of the common carotid artery is relatively easy to perform in all individuals but does not enable the evaluation of plaques, particularly at carotid bifurcation. A compromise protocol that includes the measurement of the far wall of the common carotid artery and the detection of plaques at the bifurcation could be suitable for daily practice. Another challenge lies in the determination of normal values for the different populations according to their age and gender because IMT is highly associated to these variables. In a French population normal values have been obtained, according to age and gender, but such data are not available in most countries; therefore the ESC/ESH guidelines for hypertension recommend a threshold of 0.9 mm. If IMT is very well assessed in epidemiologic and clinical studies, further data are necessary to recommend a wide utilization in daily practice.

Screening

Screening is a major concern in different clinical situations. Carotid stenosis, aortic aneurysms, and renal artery stenosis are often totally asymptomatic during much of their evolution. Therefore, a screening strategy can be useful in order to follow their evolution and to prevent complications.

Carotid stenosis

In high-risk patients, a one-time screening program of a population with a high prevalence of ≥60% asymptomatic carotid stenosis has been shown to be cost-effective.[6] This high-risk population includes, for example, patients with severe coronary disease or peripheral artery disease. Doppler ultrasound appears to be the most effective technique despite the fact that its accuracy can vary considerably between institutions. The low cost and large number of studies validating this technique support its widespread clinical use.

Abdominal aortic aneurysms

The MAAS and the ADAM[7] studies have emphasized the effectiveness of ultrasound screening for abdominal aneurysms in men over 65 years. Besides a dedicated program, it appears that measurement of the abdominal aorta should be routinely performed during echocardiography in exposed patients (Fig. 10.2).

Renal artery stenosis

Some groups have proposed angiographic screening for renal artery stenosis in all patients with high blood pressure during cardiac catheterization because incidental stenosis is found in 15–25% of these patients. Considering the high prevalence, non-invasive screening for renal artery stenosis can be also

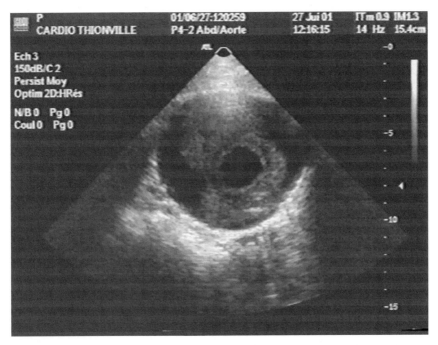

Figure 10.2 Abdominal aortic aneurysm: echography transverse view. Diameter 8 cm — heterogenic mural thrombus.

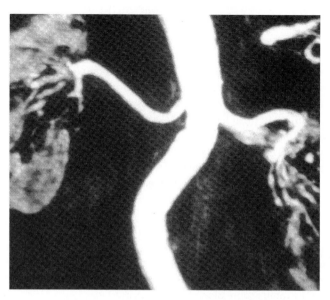

Figure 10.3 Magnetic resonance angiogram (MRA) of normal renal arteries.

proposed in hypertensive patients and individuals with multivascular disease. In these patients, Doppler ultrasound requires an experienced operator. This technique appears ideal for screening for this disorder, although MRA and multislice CT may also be suitable for this indication (Fig. 10.3).

Peripheral arterial disease

Although peripheral arterial disease is a predictor of poor outcome, it remains largely underestimated as shown by the PARTNERS program in the USA.[8] For one symptomatic patient at least one is asymptomatic. The systematic evaluation of Anckle Brachial Index (ABI) with continuous wave Doppler in exposed patients will increase the rate of awareness and will allow the identification of these very high-risk patients. An ABI under 0.9 allows the diagnosis of peripheral arterial disease. Under some circumstances, a stress test is mandatory to assess the diagnosis of peripheral artery disease. Doppler ultrasound allows an extensive evaluation of the aorta, the iliac, and the lower limb arteries; the technique provides both anatomic and hemodynamic information. More recently, MRA and multislice CT have been introduced to evaluate disease and provide even more precise imaging of the distal vessels. In view of the improvement of these non-invasive techniques, conventional angiography is no longer required for the assessment of peripheral arterial disease.

Case Presentation 1

A 69-year-old man was treated for hypertension and dyslipidemia. The patient had a history of coronary artery disease and underwent coronary artery bypass surgery in 1991. In 1999 he underwent surgery for abdominal aortic and iliac aneurysms. Prior to this surgical intervention, carotid Doppler ultrasound was performed and demonstrated bilateral, non-significant atheromatous lesions of the carotid bifurcations. In January 2004, a murmur over the right carotid artery was noted, in the absence of neurologic symptoms. Carotid Doppler ultrasound now showed a 60% (moderate) stenosis (peak systolic velocity [PSV] 220 cm/s) of the right internal carotid artery related to a hypoechoic atheromatous plaque. Considering the asymptomatic status of the patient, conservative medical therapy (with aspirin, angiotensin II antagonists, beta-blockers, and statins) appeared the treatment of choice.

In July 2004, carotid Doppler ultrasound showed progression of the stenosis, now being greater than 70%, with an increase in PSV to 440 cm/s (Fig. 10.4). CTA was performed and confirmed a severe stenosis (Fig. 10.5). Although the patient remained asymptomatic, he was referred to surgery for carotid endarterectomy, because of the rapid progression of the lesion.

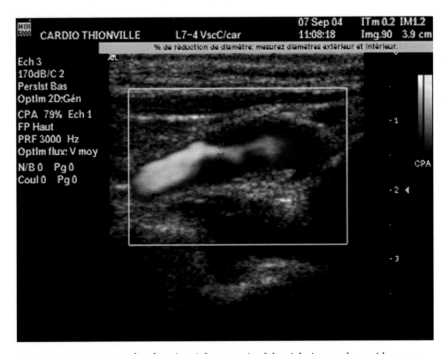

Figure 10.4 Power Doppler showing tight stenosis of the right internal carotid artery.

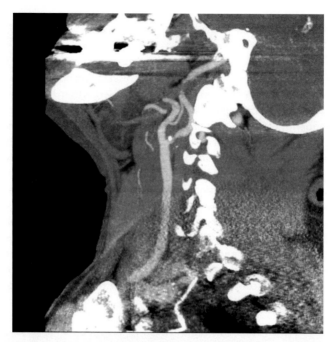

Figure 10.5 Multislice CT showing confirmation of the stenosis of the right internal carotid artery.

In this high-risk patient, the finding of a carotid murmur justified Doppler ultrasound as the first imaging technique. Considering a 60% stenosis with a PSV 220 cm/s, medical therapy and 6-month follow-up was selected based on previous publications.

However, considering the rapid progression of the stenosis in this asymptomatic patient, surgery appeared the most appropriate therapy. Confirmation of the echography by CTA was performed. In most institutions, there is no further indication for conventional angiography except if there are discrepancies between the findings on ultrasound and CTA or MRA.

Case Presentation 2

A 42-year-old woman presented with newly diagnosed hypertension in July 2003. She had no risk factors for cardiovascular disease and no family history of hypertension. Renal function and potassium level were within normal limits. Because of this new onset hypertension, renal artery stenosis was suspected. She was subsequently referred for a renal artery Doppler ultrasound examination. Bilateral renal artery fibromuscular dysplasia was detected (Fig. 10.6). The middle part of the right renal artery showed a tight stenosis with a PSV of 320 cm/s (Fig. 10.7). The left renal artery did not show significant stenosis. The arterial screening showed additional dysplasia of the iliac arteries with a right iliac artery stenosis. No dysplasia was detected in the carotid arteries.

Accordingly, right renal artery angioplasty was scheduled. Angiography confirmed the bilateral fibromuscular dysplasia (Fig. 10.8) and the stenosis of the right renal artery. Balloon angioplasty was successfully performed during the same session. At 1-year follow-up, the patient does not have restenosis. Her blood pressure is well-controlled without any medication, except for aspirin.

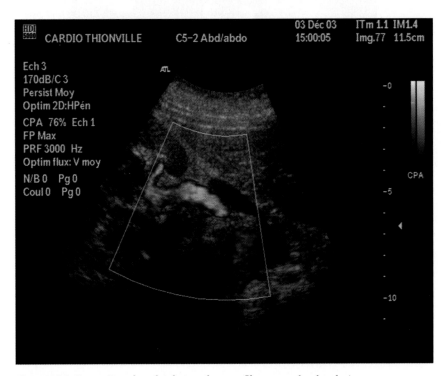

Figure 10.6 Power Doppler of right renal artery fibromuscular dysplasia.

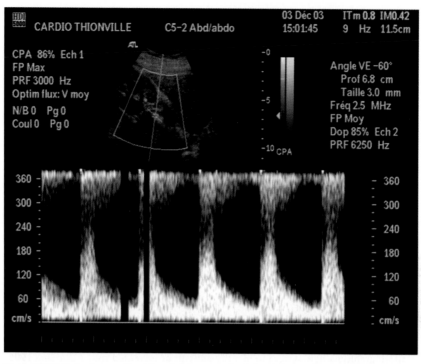

Figure 10.7 Pulsed wave Doppler of tight stenosis of the right renal artery. PSV > 300 cm/s.

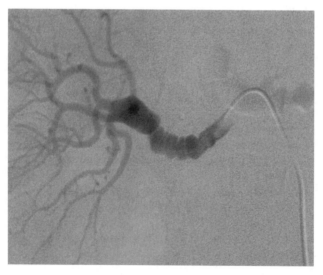

Figure 10.8 Angiography demonstrating confirmation of renal artery fibromuscular dysplasia.

In this case a renal artery stenosis was suspected based on the clinical history: new onset of hypertension in a young women without any risk factors. In an experienced vascular laboratory, Doppler ultrasound is the easiest imaging technique to assess the diagnosis. With a sensitivity and specificity of greater than 85%, this technique is an excellent first-line imaging modality.

Conclusions

The diagnosis of peripheral vascular disease relies greatly on imaging techniques, particularly in asymptomatic patients. As a result of technical improvements, non-invasive imaging is now preferred to angiography. If an experienced, validated vascular laboratory is available, Doppler ultrasound should be the first choice technique because of its low cost and high diagnostic accuracy. The use of MRA and/or CTA is increasing, but its use is dependent on local availability. It is clear that conventional angiography is no longer mandatory for the diagnosis but remains necessary in patients who need to undergo surgery or percutaneous interventions.

References

1 Egglin TK, O'Moore PV, Feinstein AR, Waltman AC. Complications of peripheral arteriography: a new system to identify patients at increased risk. *J Vasc Surg* 1995; **22**:787–94.
2 Strandness DE. *Duplex Scanning in Vascular Disorders*, 3rd edn. Philadelphia: Lippincott Williams & Wilkins, 2002.
3 Rubin GD. Data explosion: the challenge of multidetector-row CT. *Eur J Radiol* 2000;**36**:74–80.
4 Yucel EK, Anderson CM, Edelman RR, *et al.* AHA scientific statement. Magnetic resonance angiography: update on applications for extracranial arteries. *Circulation* 1999;**100**:2284–301.
5 O'Leary DH, Polak JF, Kronmal RA, Manolio TA, Burke GL, Wolfson SK. Carotid-artery intima and media thickness as a risk factor for myocardial infarction and stroke in older adults. Cardiovascular Health Study Collaborative Research Group. *N Engl J Med* 1999;**340**:14–22.
6 Derdeyn CP, Powers WJ. Cost-effectiveness of screening for asymptomatic carotid atherosclerotic disease. *Stroke* 1996;**27**:1944–50.
7 Lederle FA, Johnson GR, Wilson SE, *et al.* The aneurysm detection and management study screening program: validation cohort and final results. *Arch Intern Med* 2000;**160**:1425–30.
8 Hirsch AT, Criqui MH, Treat-Jacobson D, Regensteiner JG, *et al.* Peripheral arterial disease detection, awareness, and treatment in primary care. *JAMA* 2001;**286**: 1317–24.

CHAPTER 11

Risk stratification post-infarction

Frank M. Bengel

Introduction

After myocardial infarction with or without ST-segment elevation, assessment of the individual risk for further cardiac events such as reinfarction or death is important to guide decision-making.

Generally, acute coronary syndromes are occurring in a heterogeneous group of patients with different clinical presentations and differences in the underlying extent of atherosclerosis and functional alterations. Additionally, the success of an early reperfusion strategy may vary from one patient to another. Thus, in order to select the appropriate treatment and to prevent future cardiac events, precise characterization of the individual patient's disease status and the resulting prognosis is needed.

Clinical, laboratory, and ECG parameters are of value for rapid risk assessment at low cost, but non-invasive functional imaging techniques such as echocardiography and myocardial scintigraphy provide additional and incremental information. Important outcome-related parameters can be derived from these imaging techniques (Table 11.1), allowing for precise and reliable risk stratification in the in-hospital and pre-/post-discharge course.

Risk markers derived from rest imaging

Left ventricular ejection faction (LVEF) is stably and reproducibly determined by echocardiography, radionuclide angiography, ECG-gated myocardial perfusion scintigraphy, or cine magnetic resonance imaging, and is known to be one of the most powerful predictors of cardiovascular outcome.[1,2] In addition to LVEF, the aforementioned techniques allow for assessment of ventricular end-systolic volume as another prognostic parameter.

Resting myocardial perfusion imaging allows for semi-quantitative measurement of infarct size as another strong determinant of outcome. Using circumferential profile analysis of single photon emission computed tomography (SPECT) data sets in 274 patients after acute myocardial infarction, Miller *et al.*[3] found a significant association between infarct size and overall, as well as cardiac mortality at mid-term follow-up.

Table 11.1 Imaging markers of cardiovascular risk in post myocardial infarction patients.

Parameter	Technique
Resting LVEF and volumes	Echocardiography, gated SPECT, RNA, MRI
Stress LVEF and volumes	Stress echocardiography, RNA, MRI
Infarct size	Resting perfusion SPECT, late enhancement MRI
Myocardial salvage	Serial resting perfusion SPECT
Extent and severity of ischemia/ myocardium at risk	Stress perfusion SPECT, stress echocardiography
Myocardial viability	SPECT, PET, dobutamine echocardiography/MRI

LVEF, left ventricular ejection fraction; MI, myocardial infarction; MRI, magnetic resonance imaging; PET, positron emission tomography; RNA, radionuclide angiography; SPECT, single photon emission computed tomography.

Another attractive, but more laborious approach is to combine measurements of infarct size with an earlier performed SPECT study characterizing the initial area at risk prior to reperfusion. This allows for calculation of myocardial salvage as a surrogate endpoint of therapeutic efficacy. For assessment of the area at risk, the SPECT perfusion tracer is injected in the acute situation prior to treatment. Because tracers such as technetium-99m (^{99m}Tc) sestamibi or ^{99m}Tc tetrofosmin are retained by myocardium without significant redistribution, SPECT imaging can be performed within an interval of 8–10 h after reperfusion therapy and patient stabilization. Images then still reflect the initial extent of ischemic myocardium. Myocardial salvage is defined as the reduction of resting perfusion defect between area at risk study and a second scan several days after treatment. In a recent study in 765 patients with acute myocardial infarction treated by different approaches, SPECT-determined myocardial salvage was an independent predictor of mortality after 6 months.[4]

Magnetic resonance imaging (MRI) late after injection of gadolinium DTPA is a novel, attractive approach for measuring infarct size. Scar tissue shows a persisting accumulation of contrast agent, also known as "late enhancement," allowing for precise assessment of the transmurality and extent of an infarct. This sensitive technique detects smaller subendocardial infarcts even in patients with normal myocardial perfusion scans,[5] but the extent of scar early after an event may be slightly overestimated, probably as a result of peri-infarct edema. Despite the attractiveness of the approach, the clinical role or prognostic value of late enhancement MRI have not yet been established and need to be defined in larger scale clinical trials.

Risk markers derived from stress imaging

Stress testing provides information about the ischemic burden from underlying residual coronary artery disease. As such, it is another very important parameter for the definition of outcome. It has been demonstrated in various trials that results of functional testing are closer related to the prognosis of disease than its morphologic (i.e. angiographic) appearance.[6,7] Especially in post-infarct patients, exercise ECG is often difficult to interpret and inconclusive, thus emphasizing the need for an additional imaging technique. Both stress echocardiography and stress myocardial perfusion SPECT provide accurate information about risk after myocardial infarction.[8] In the early phase after an acute coronary event, however, physical exercise may not be desired. Under these conditions, pharmacologic stress imaging is of special interest. Brown *et al.*[9] were able to demonstrate that myocardial perfusion imaging under pharmacologic vasodilatation with dipyridamole is safely performed as early as 2–4 days after the infarct, and has better prognostic value than predischarge submaximal exercise SPECT imaging at 6–12 days.

The question of residual myocardial viability especially comes into play in patients with extensive left ventricular dysfunction, where the risk of revascularization is increased and where states of severely ischemically compromised myocardium are more frequent. Viability is linked to myocardial ischemia, as only viable myocardium can become ischemic under stress conditions. Ischemic episodes or constant hypoperfusion, however, may also be present at rest, causing repetitively stunned or hibernating myocardium. These states of jeopardized but viable myocardium are difficult to separate from scar tissue by conventional imaging techniques. Therefore, modified protocols such as SPECT imaging after reinjection of thallium-201, nitrate enhanced SPECT imaging, or low-dose dobutamine echocardiography have been developed and other specific techniques such as perfusion/metabolism positron emission tomography (PET) and late-enhancement MRI have been introduced. They all provide relatively high accuracy for prediction of functional recovery after revascularization,[10] but are limited to a few patients where the status of myocardial viability remains unclear from standard imaging techniques.

Risk-guided clinical decision-making

Because of the excellent capability for risk stratification, a non-invasive stress imaging test is recommended prior to discharge or after discharge in patients after myocardial infarction with and without ST-segment elevation, according to ESC task force reports.[1,2] The choice between echocardiography and perfusion scintigraphy in this situation is left open and should be dependent on local expertise and availability. Imaging provides a variety of prognostic parameters which then should be integrated to determine the overall risk of the patient for future events.

If non-invasive imaging suggests a high risk (e.g. LVEF less than 35% and/or extensive ischemia), then an early, invasive work-up with angiography and evaluation for revascularization is appropriate. If imaging is almost normal, thereby indicating low risk, patients can be managed by optimized medical therapy and clinical risk factor modification. A conservative strategy will be most cost-effective in such patients. Finally, if patients are in the border zone between low and high-risk according to imaging criteria, the choice between

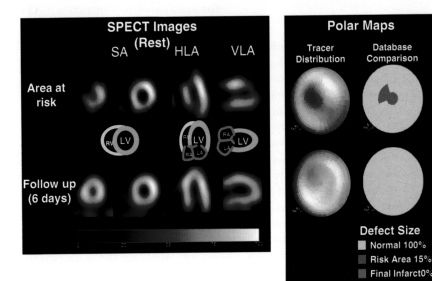

Figure 11.1 Resting myocardial perfusion SPECT for assessment of area at risk, myocardial salvage, and final infarct size. Area at risk is measured by ^{99m}Tc sestamibi injection in the acute situation prior to intervention and comprises 15% of left ventricle as determined from polar map analysis. Final infarct size and myocardial salvage are determined from rest images 6 days after intervention. No residual scar is evident in this case, demonstrating successful salvage by percutaneous transluminal coronary angioplasty (PTCA) and stenting.

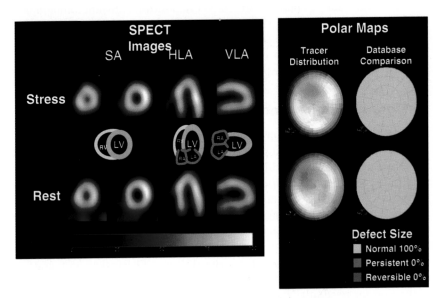

Figure 11.2 Predischarge myocardial perfusion SPECT at rest and during pharmacologic stress (dipyridamole). No stress-induced ischemia is observed, suggesting a low-risk situation.

invasive and conservative work-up can be based on their symptomatic status. Angiography is preferred in those with persistent angina and those with minimal symptoms are managed medically.

Case Presentation

A 63-year-old man with no prior history of cardiovascular disease was admitted to the emergency room with new onset, increasing retrosternal chest pain at rest. His resting ECG showed no persistent ST-elevations, but ST-segment depressions of 1.5 mm and inverted R-waves in leads V1-4. Troponin T was elevated at 1.3 ng/dL, creatine kinase (CK) was 168 U/L. Chest pain persisted after anti-anginal medication with clopidogrel, metoprolol, and nitrates, so that the decision for invasive angiography was taken.

Prior to angiography, 800 MBq ^{99m}Tc sestamibi was injected intravenously to allow for subsequent assessment of the myocardial area at risk. Perfusion SPECT imaging, performed after angiography, revealed resting ischemia in the distal anteroseptal and apical wall, comprising 15% of the left ventricle (Fig. 11.1).

Angiography showed subtotal occlusion of the mid portion of the left anterior descending coronary artery (LAD), which was identified as the culprit lesion and successfully treated by percutaneous transluminal coronary angioplasty (PTCA) and stenting, resulting in relief of symptoms. An additional 50% stenosis of the mid right coronary artery (RCA) was identified, but not treated interventionally.

The patient recovered and remained asymptomatic following intervention. He had an uncomplicated course during his hospital stay. Five days after the acute event, gated myocardial perfusion SPECT imaging at rest and during dipyridamole stress was performed for risk assessment and to determine hemodynamic relevance of the mild to moderate RCA stenosis. ^{99}Tc sestamibi 400 MBq was injected at rest, followed by pharmacologic stress with 0.56 mg/kg dipyridamole over 8 min and a second injection of 1000 MBq ^{99m}Tc sestamibi for stress imaging. No ECG abnormalities or symptoms were observed during dipyridamole testing. Comparison of resting images after intervention with the previous area at risk scan revealed a complete myocardial salvage with no significant residual perfusion defect, indicating the absence of larger scar (Fig. 11.1). Stress imaging ruled out myocardial ischemia in all vascular territories (Fig. 11.2). Gated SPECT revealed a normal LVEF of 52%. Only mild regional hypokinesia in distal anteroseptal wall was still present, consistent with post-ischemic stunning (Fig. 11.3; Video clips 8 and 9 ⊙). An additionally performed MRI late after injection of gadolinium revealed non-transmural late enhancement in distal anteroseptal wall, indicative of only small amounts of non-transmural residual scar tissue (Fig. 11.4).

Based on the results of non-invasive imaging, the risk of the patient for future cardiac events was considered to be low. He was therefore discharged on medication with clopidogrel, aspirin, metoprolol, and atorvastatin. Clinical follow-up examinations after 6 and 12 months were unremarkable. The patient remained symptom-free and did not have any complications.

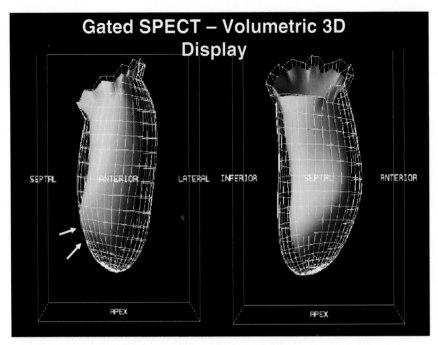

Figure 11.3 Volumetrical display of ECG-gated post-stress perfusion images in two different projections. Endocardial borders at end-diastole are depicted by the grid structure, endocardial borders at end-systole are marked by the colored shape. Regional hypokinesia in distal anteroseptal wall (arrows) is still present despite normal perfusion, indicating stunned myocardium. See also Video clips 8 and 9 ⬚.

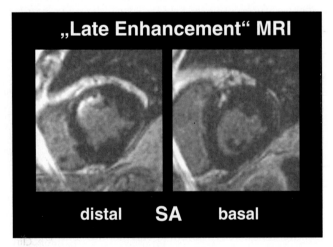

Figure 11.4 Contrast enhanced magnetic resonance studies late after injection of gadolinium-DTPA, performed prior to discharge. A small area of subendocardial contrast enhancement is observed in distal anteroseptal wall, indicating minor amounts of non-transmural scar tissue which are not identified at SPECT imaging.

References

1 Bertrand ME, Simoons ML, Fox KA, *et al.* Management of acute coronary syndromes in patients presenting without persistent ST-segment elevation. *Eur Heart J* 2002; **23**:1809–40.

2 Van de Werf F, Ardissino D, Betriu A, *et al.* Management of acute myocardial infarction in patients presenting with ST-segment elevation. The Task Force on the Management of Acute Myocardial Infarction of the European Society of Cardiology. *Eur Heart J* 2003;**24**:28–66.

3 Miller TD, Christian TF, Hopfenspirger MR, Hodge DO, Gersh BJ, Gibbons RJ. Infarct size after acute myocardial infarction measured by quantitative tomographic ^{99m}Tc sestamibi imaging predicts subsequent mortality. *Circulation* 1995;**92**:334–41.

4 Ndrepepa G, Mehilli J, Schwaiger M, *et al.* Prognostic value of myocardial salvage achieved by reperfusion therapy in patients with acute myocardial infarction. *J Nucl Med* 2004;**45**:725–9.

5 Wagner A, Mahrholdt H, Holly TA, *et al.* Contrast-enhanced MRI and routine single photon emission computed tomography (SPECT) perfusion imaging for detection of subendocardial myocardial infarcts: an imaging study. *Lancet* 2003;**361**:374–9.

6 Brown KA. Prognostic value of thallium-201 myocardial perfusion imaging: a diagnostic tool comes of age. *Circulation* 1991;**83**:363–81.

7 Picano E, Lattanzi F, Sicari R, *et al.* Role of stress echocardiography in risk stratification early after an acute myocardial infarction. EPIC (Echo Persantin International Cooperative) and EDIC (Echo Dobutamine International Cooperative) Study Groups. *Eur Heart J* 1997;**18**(Suppl D):78–85.

8 Zanco P, Zampiero A, Favero A, *et al.* Prognostic evaluation of patients after myocardial infarction: incremental value of sestamibi single-photon emission computed tomography and echocardiography. *J Nucl Cardiol* 1997;**4**:117–24.

9 Brown KA, Heller GV, Landin RS, *et al.* Early dipyridamole (99m)Tc-sestamibi single photon emission computed tomographic imaging 2 to 4 days after acute myocardial infarction predicts in-hospital and postdischarge cardiac events: comparison with submaximal exercise imaging. *Circulation* 1999;**100**:2060–6.

10 Bax JJ, Wijns W, Cornel JH, Visser FC, Boersma E, Fioretti PM. Accuracy of currently available techniques for prediction of functional recovery after revascularization in patients with left ventricular dysfunction due to chronic coronary artery disease: comparison of pooled data. *J Am Coll Cardiol* 1997;**30**:1451–60.

CHAPTER 12
Risk stratification before non-cardiac surgery

Miklos D. Kertai and Don Poldermans

Introduction

Cardiac complications are the major cause of perioperative morbidity and mortality in patients undergoing non-cardiac surgery.[1] It is estimated that approximately 1.5 million non-cardiac surgical procedures are performed annually in the Netherlands, of which 15,000 patients die during hospital stay and 30% of deaths are attributable to cardiac causes.[2] This high incidence of perioperative cardiac complications is particularly true for those patients with previous coronary artery disease (CAD) and those scheduled for high-risk surgery. Subsequently, a great deal of clinical research has focused on detection and modifying cardiac risk before non-cardiac surgery.[3]

Perioperative cardiac complications such as myocardial infarction are caused either by rupture of a coronary atherosclerotic plaque and thrombus formation similar to myocardial infarction occurring in a non-perioperative setting,[4] or by a mismatch between myocardial oxygen supply and demand. Factors that increase myocardial oxygen demand mainly result from surgical stress such as tachycardia, hypertension, pain, interruption of beta-blockers, or the use of sympathomimetic drugs. On the other hand, hypotension, vasospasm, anemia, hypoxia, or coronary artery plaque rupture with thrombosis may lead to decreased myocardium oxygen supply.[5]

The guidelines of the American College of Cardiology (ACC) and the American Heart Association (AHA) for perioperative cardiovascular evaluation for non-cardiac surgery provide recommendations for identifying low- and high-risk patients by perioperative clinical and non-invasive cardiac evaluation.[3]

The first step of this algorithm is to determine the urgency of the planned surgery. Patients needing acute procedures should proceed to surgery without the delay of additional cardiac evaluation. However, elective procedures allow a more thorough evaluation of cardiac risk to be carried out. With the help of these guidelines, minor, intermediate, and major clinical risk factors and degree of functional capacity can be determined as predictors of perioperative cardiac complications (Table 12.1). Accordingly, patients with only minor or intermediate clinical predictors and adequate functional capacity represent a low-risk

Table 12.1 Clinical predictors of increased perioperative cardiovascular risk.[3]

Major predictors
Unstable coronary syndromes
Decompensated congestive heart failure
Significant arrhythmias (high-grade atrioventricular block, ventricular arrhythmias)
Severe valvular disease

Intermediate predictors
Mild angina pectoris (Canadian class I and II)
Prior myocardial infarction
Compensated or prior congestive heart failure
Diabetes mellitus

Minor predictors
Advanced age
Abnormal electrocardiogram (left ventricular hypertrophy, left bundle branch block)
Rhythm other than sinus rhythm (e.g. atrial fibrillation)
Low functional capacity (less than four metabolic equivalents)
History of stroke
Uncontrolled systemic hypertension

---

population, irrespective of type of surgery, and further evaluation is unnecessary. However, if any of the clinical markers of cardiac risk present include history of myocardial infarction, diabetes mellitus, congestive heart failure, angina pectoris, and advanced age (age over 70 years) in patients scheduled for high-risk surgery, additional non-invasive evaluation should be considered. Several non-invasive tests have been described for evaluation of cardiac risk. In most ambulatory patients, the test of choice is exercise electrocardiography (ECG) testing, which can both provide an estimate of functional capacity and detect myocardial ischemia through changes in the ECG and hemodynamic response.[3] Nevertheless, patients with one or more intermediate predictors of cardiac risk often have important abnormalities on their resting ECG (e.g. left bundle-branch block, left ventricular hypertrophy with strain pattern), which may preclude reliable ST-segment analyses. Moreover, these patients more often have limited exercise capacity resulting from non-cardiac diseases such as peripheral artery disease, arthrosis, and chronic pulmonary disease. Therefore, other non-invasive and non-exercise-dependent techniques should be considered such as evaluation of left ventricular function and pharmacologic stress echocardiography or myocardial perfusion scintigraphy.

Imaging techniques to assess preoperative cardiac risk

Myocardial perfusion scintigraphy
Detection of CAD using myocardial perfusion scintigraphy is based on a differential blood flow distribution through the left ventricular myocardium, per-

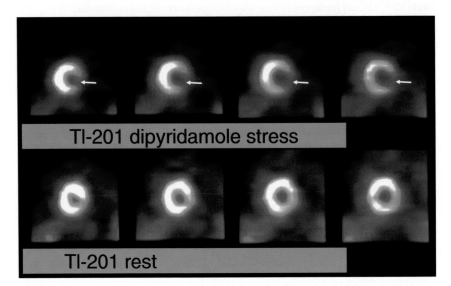

Figure 12.1 Dipyridamole thallium-201 (^{201}Tl) myocardial perfusion scintigraphy at rest (lower panel) and during dipyridamole stress (upper panel). The arrows indicate the presence of a reversible perfusion defect in the lateral wall, secondary to a stenosis in the left circumflex coronary artery. (Images courtesy Dr. JJ Bax, Department of Cardiology, Leiden University Medical Center, the Netherlands.)

fused by normal or stenotic coronary vessels.[6] A perfusion abnormality detected during the test may vary by size and reversibility (Fig. 12.1). Coronary artery stenoses involving the left anterior descending artery usually have larger perfusion defects than stenoses in the right or circumflex coronary arteries.[7] Patients with multivessel CAD may also have larger perfusion defects than patients with single-vessel disease.[8] The reversibility of thallium-201 (^{201}Tl) perfusion defects can be assessed by repeated imaging 3–4 h after obtaining the initial images. In clinical assessment, regions are semi-quantitatively scored as having normal tracer uptake, moderately decreased uptake, or severely reduced uptake.[9]

Myocardial perfusion scintigraphy is the most extensively studied non-invasive approach to cardiac risk stratification. Initial reports indicated that patients who exhibited myocardial perfusion defects following dipyridamole infusion that normalized within 3–4 h were at increased cardiac risk.[10,11] However, these results were later questioned by other investigators.[9,12] Indeed, a recent meta-analysis of 23 studies showed that despite the high sensitivity (83%) of the test, its specificity (49%) was too low for the prediction of cardiac death and myocardial infarction.[13] There are several possible explanations for these findings:

1 The test is more widely used in consecutive patients presenting for non-cardiac surgery than in selected patients with clinical risk factors.

2 Unblinded test results are available to clinicians, thus influencing perioperative care.

3 Repeat imaging 3–4 h after ^{201}Tl injection may not allow sufficient time for thallium redistribution.

4 ^{201}Tl uptake may be uniformly restricted in patients with severe and diffuse coronary artery disease.

Semi-quantitative analysis of the data, taking into account the defect severity and extent, has been demonstrated to increase the predictive value of the test.[14]

Dobutamine stress echocardiography

Pharmacologic stress echocardiography with dobutamine (DSE) has been described as a useful tool for preoperative cardiac risk stratification in patients undergoing non-cardiac surgery.[15,16] Dobutamine infusion increases myocardial oxygen demand through positive chronotropic and inotropic effects and impairs myocardial oxygen supply by shortening diastole.[15,17] These effects result in myocardial ischemia and systolic contractile dysfunction in regions supplied by critically stenotic coronary arteries.[18] If the chronotropic response is inadequate (i.e. the age-corrected target heart rate is not achieved), atropine in 0.25-mg increments up to 2.0 mg may be administered. During the dobutamine stress test, the 12-lead ECG is continuously monitored and recorded at 1-min intervals (Fig. 12.2a,b). Images are obtained at rest and during dobutamine-induced stress and are analyzed off-line according to the 17-segment model of the American Society of Echocardiography (Fig. 12.2c,d; Video clips 10 and 11), and wall motion is scored in each segment on a 5-point scale.[19] The test results are considered positive when wall motion in any segment deteriorates by one grade or more (Fig. 12.2d).

The role of DSE in cardiac risk stratification has been studied extensively in recent reports.[15,20] Data combined from a recent meta-analysis showed that the sensitivity and specificity of DSE for perioperative cardiac death and myocardial infarction are high (85% and 70%, respectively).[13] A combination of cardiac risk assessment with DSE was also shown to be useful for further risk stratification of patients at intermediate to high risk for cardiac complications.[15] DSE can be performed safely with reasonable patient tolerance (incidence of cardiac arrhythmias and hypotension 8% and 3%, respectively) and may provide additional diagnostic information about valvular dysfunction.[21] The test has some limitations: it should not be used in patients with severe arrhythmias, significant hypertension, or hypotension.

Comparison of non-invasive tests used for preoperative risk stratification

There have been few comparisons of the various non-invasive diagnostic tests used for preoperative cardiac risk assessment. In a meta-analysis of 20 studies, Mantha et al.[22] compared the predictive value of dipyridamole myocardial perfusion scintigraphy, radionuclide ventriculography, ambulatory electrocardiography and DSE for perioperative cardiac death and myocardial infarction. The

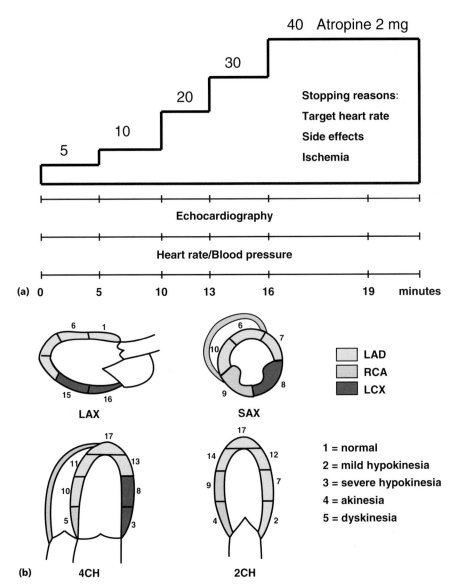

Figure 12.2 (a) The study protocol of dobutamine stress echocardiography. (b) The 17-segment model as defined by the American Society of Echocardiography. LAD, left anterior descending coronary artery; LAX, long-axis view; LCX, left circumflex coronary artery; RCA, right coronary artery; SAX, short-axis view; 2 CH, two-chamber view; 4 CH, four-chamber view. *Continued on facing page.*

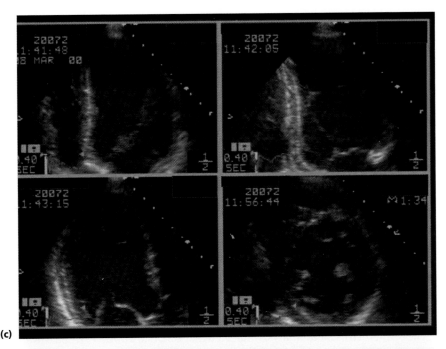

(c)

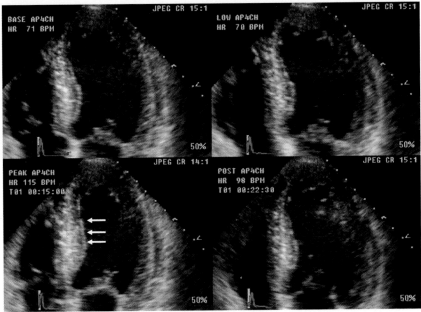

(d)

Figure 12.2 *Continued.* (c) Quad-screen of a normal echocardiography at rest. Panels are apical four-chamber view (left upper), apical two-chamber view (right upper), apical three-chamber view (left lower), and short axis view (right lower). See also Video clip 10 ⬤. (d) Dobutamine stress-induced myocardial ischemia. The images show left ventricular hypertrophy, and myocardial ischemia developed at peak stress (lower left panel) in the posterior septum (indicated by arrows). See also Video clip 11 ⬤.

results showed that with the exception of DSE, each of the tests demonstrated a bias for a better predictive value in the earlier studies. Although DSE appeared to be the best among these tests and ambulatory electrocardiography to have the least predictive value, the available data analyzed were not sufficient to determine which test is optimal. Results of a similar meta-analysis by Shaw *et al.*[23] comparing the predictive value of dipyridamole ^{201}Tl scintigraphy and DSE for risk stratification before vascular surgery, showed that the prognostic value of both non-invasive stress tests had similar predictive accuracy but the summed odds ratios for cardiac death and myocardial infarction were greater for DSE than for dipyridamole perfusion scintigraphy. Recently, Kertai *et al.*[24] compared the predictive value of dobutamine and dipyridamole stress echocardiography and dipyridamole ^{201}Tl scintigraphy in 2204 patients undergoing major vascular surgery. Of these 2204 consecutive patients, 1093 underwent DSE, 394 patients had dipyridamole stress echocardiography, and 717 patients had dipyridamole ^{201}Tl scintigraphy before major vascular surgery. There was no statistically significant difference in the predictive value of a positive test result for dipyridamole stress echocardiography and DSE but a positive test result for dipyridamole ^{201}Tl scintigraphy had a significantly lower prognostic value. Finally, using a novel meta-analytic approach, the predictive values of six non-invasive tests used for preoperative cardiac risk assessment were compared.[13] The results of this meta-analysis indicated that DSE had a positive trend towards a better diagnostic performance for the prediction of perioperative cardiac complications for vascular surgery compared with the other tests (ambulatory electrocardiography, exercise electrocardiography, radionuclide ventriculography, myocardial perfusion scintigraphy, and dipyridamole stress echocardiography), but only a significant difference in the comparison with myocardial perfusion scintigraphy was demonstrated.

In summary, the results of these studies indicate that DSE provides additional prognostic information comparable with other tests, and may be the preferred test if additional questions about valvular and left ventricular dysfunction exist. The physician's choice of the method of preoperative cardiac testing, however, should also take into account factors such as local expertise and experience, availability, and costs.

Cardiac magnetic resonance for the detection of myocardial ischemia

Cardiac magnetic resonance (CMR) has been shown to have high accuracy and reproducibility for the evaluation of cardiac structure and ventricular function.[25,26] The use of dipyridamole-induced hyperemia or dobutamine-induced wall motion abnormalities have been described as possible diagnostic tools for the detection of myocardial ischemia.[27,28] Compared with dipyridamole, administration of dobutamine infusion is well tolerated and appears to be a more appropriate agent for provoking myocardial ischemia.[29] Similarly to DSE, cine images are obtained at baseline and then repeated every 5 min during gradual increases of dobutamine infusion. Additional recovery images are also recorded 10 min after the test. The assessment of left ventricular wall motion abnormalities is similar to with DSE, and segments are scored as normal, hypokinetic, akinetic, or dyskinetic (Fig. 12.3a; Video clips 12–15 👁). In Fig. 12.3(a) dobutamine-stress cardiac magnetic resonance imaging are shown at rest, at low-dose and at peak dobutamine stress. At peak dobutamine stress, as indicated by arrows in Fig. 12.3, a stress induced wall-motion abnormality has developed. Studies have shown that dobutamine-stress CMR has a sensitivity of 91% and specificity of 80% for the identification of wall-motion abnormalities; the sensitivities for the detection of one-, two- and three-vessel disease were 88%, 91% and 100%, respectively.[30] In general, DSE and dobutamine-stress CMR have similar accuracy, but CMR may offer an alternative approach when the DSE images are not optimal (e.g. because of a suboptimal acoustic window).[31]

Dobutamine-stress CMR has also been investigated for the assessment of myocardial ischemia and preoperative cardiac risk assessment.[32] Preliminary data suggest that dobutamine CMR-induced myocardial ischemia in patients at intermediate risk for cardiac complications was associated with an increased risk of perioperative cardiac events.[32] Of the 102 non-cardiac surgery patients studied, 26 (25%) had dobutamine CMR-induced myocardial ischemia, of whom 20% developed cardiac events. The test had a sensitivity of 84% with a specificity of 78% for the prediction of perioperative cardiac complications. Although these findings will require additional studies to assess the utility of dobutamine-stress CMR for preoperative risk assessment, this non-invasive stress test could be an alternative to DSE in patients with an intermediate risk who are unable to undergo DSE.

Perioperative cardioprotective medical therapy

Several studies have suggested that perioperative use of beta-blockers may reduce the incidence of postoperative myocardial ischemia, myocardial infarction, and cardiac mortality.[33–35] A randomized study by Mangano et al.[36] showed no difference in perioperative mortality of 200 patients randomized to atenolol or placebo, but mortality was significantly lower at 6 months following discharge (0% versus 8%, $P < 0.001$), over the first year (3% versus 14%, $P = 0.005$), and over 2 year follow-up (10% versus 21%, $P = 0.02$) in patients receiving atenolol compared with patients receiving placebo. A more recent study by Poldermans et al.[37] demonstrated the cardioprotective effect of beta-blocker use in 112 high-risk vascular patients randomized to perioperative bisoprolol use or standard care. This study showed a significant reduction in the incidence of perioperative cardiac death and myocardial infarction in patients receiving bisoprolol compared with patients receiving standard care (3.3% versus 34%). In patients with contraindications to beta-blockers, α_2-adrenergic agonists (clonidine, mivazerol) as alternative treatment for the reduction of perioperative cardiac complications may be considered. In a large-scale, randomized, controlled trial of intravenous use of the α_2-adrenergic agonist mivazerol,

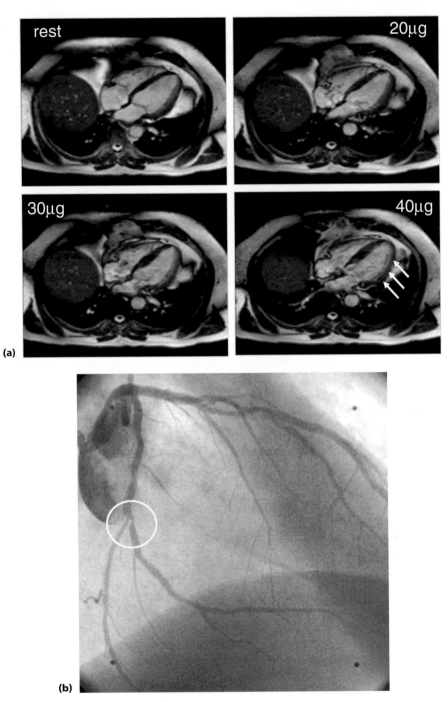

Figure 12.3 (a) Dobutamine-stress cardiac magnetic resonance imaging. Arrows indicate dobutamine-stress-induced wall-motion abnormality. (Images courtesy Dr. I Paetsch, Department of Internal Medicine/Cardiology, German Heart Institute, Berlin, Germany.) See also Video clips 12 (rest), 13 (20 μg), 14 (30 μg), 15 (40 μg) . (b) Corresponding coronary angiography of the patient, showing a critical stenosis (indicated by the circle) in the left circumflex coronary artery.

Oliver *et al.*[38] also found no significant effect for the reduction of perioperative cardiac complication in patients undergoing non-cardiac surgery, although a significant reduction of cardiac complications and mortality was observed in a subset of patients undergoing major vascular surgery. Similarly, results from recent meta-analyses also showed that α_2-adrenergic agonist use was associated with a significantly reduced incidence of myocardial ischemia and may also have effects on perioperative cardiovascular complications especially in high-risk patients.[39,40] Thus, the intraoperative use of α_2-adrenergic agonists may indeed reduce perioperative cardiac events, especially in patients undergoing major vascular surgery.

Despite the beneficial effect of beta-blockers for the reduction of perioperative cardiac complications, some patients identified by clinical risk factors and DSE as being at high risk often still have a considerable perioperative cardiac complication rate.[20] For these patients, additional therapy aiming at prevention (e.g. statin therapy) may further optimize risk reduction. A case–control study by Poldermans *et al.*[41] showed that vascular patients who were on statin therapy had a fourfold reduction in all-cause mortality compared with patients without statin use. This observation was consistent in subgroups of patients according to the type of vascular surgery, cardiac risk factors, and beta-blocker use. Similarly, Durazzo *et al.*[42] reported a significantly reduced incidence of cardiovascular events within 6 months after vascular surgery in patients who were randomly assigned to atorvastatin compared with placebo (atorvastatin versus placebo, 8.3% vs. 26.0%). Finally, Lindenauer *et al.*[43] demonstrated a 28% relative risk reduction of in-hospital mortality in statin users compared with non-users in 780,591 patients undergoing major non-cardiac surgery. Although these initial results are promising, prospective, large-scale studies are needed to confirm the beneficial effect and safety of perioperative statin therapy.

Clinical management of patients with a negative test result

Intermediate- or high-risk patients with a normal test, no stress-induced myocardial ischemia, could be scheduled for non-cardiac surgery at relatively low risk. Although there are no prospective randomized trials available evaluating the cardioprotective effect of beta-blockers and statins in this population, these patients may benefit from perioperative beta-blocker therapy in a similar way to patients with a history of CAD.[44]

Clinical management of patients with a positive test result

If the result of a non-invasive test is abnormal perioperative management is complex. The decision whether to perform surgery with cardioprotective medical therapy or to perform additional cardiac catheterization and, if possible, coronary revascularization should be based on the extent and severity of

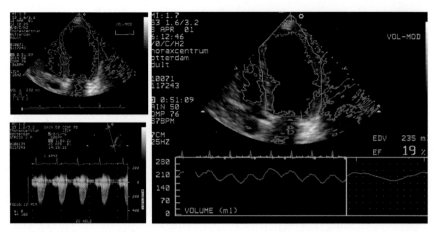

Figure 12.4 Echocardiography and low-dose dobutamine stress echocardiography in a patient with reduced left ventricular function and aortic valve stenosis. Measurement of left ventricular function at rest (upper left); continuous wave Doppler of aortic valve stenosis at rest (lower left); left ventricular function during low-dose dobutamine stress echocardiography (right). See also Video clip 16 ⬬.

stress-induced myocardial ischemia.[45] In patients with limited stress-induced myocardial ischemia, suggesting one- or two-vessel disease, a combination of beta-blocker and statin use with intensive perioperative monitoring may prevent the occurrence of perioperative cardiac complications.[20,41] After surgery these patients should be regularly followed up and undergo repetitive late cardiac non-invasive testing to re-evaluate the progression of coronary artery disease.[46] In patients with extensive myocardial ischemia, suggesting left main or severe three-vessel disease, coronary artery bypass surgery should be considered.[47]

Clinical Presentation

A 72-year-old man was referred to the vascular surgery outpatient clinic because of progressive intermittent claudication of the left leg. His medical history revealed hypertension, hypercholesterolemia, and smoking. He has smoked for over 50 years and is still a smoker. There were no symptoms of angina pectoris or previous myocardial infarction. The general physician had already started angiotensin-converting enzyme (ACE) inhibitor and statin therapy. Physical examination revealed blood pressure 125/75 mmHg and pulse rate 82 b min^{-1}. Auscultation of the heart revealed an early to mid systolic murmur with a systolic thrill in the aortic area (grade III of VI), radiating to the neck. There was a soft diastolic murmur. No other cardiac abnormalities were observed during physical examination. Arterial pulsations over the left dorsalis pedis and tibialis posterior arteries were absent. Twelve-lead electrocardiography showed a sinus rhythm, normal conduction, and left ventricular hypertrophy. Laboratory examination showed no abnormalities in renal and liver function. The total cholesterol was 4.2 mmol/L. Two-dimensional echocardiography revealed thickened and calcified aortic leaflets with reduced leaflet motion, and concentric left ventricular hypertrophy. The left ventricular ejection fraction was 19%, and Doppler echocardiography showed a mean transvalvular pressure gradient of 40 mmHg.

This 72-year-old vascular patient showed typical physical and echocardiographic signs of moderate aortic valve stenosis. However, given the presence of a reduced left ventricular function, the severity of the aortic stenosis is likely to be underestimated. In these patients, stress echocardiography with low-dose dobutamine is recommended to assess whether the aortic stenosis is fixed or dynamic (i.e. flow-dependent).[48] As shown in Fig. 12.4 and Video Clip 16 👁, the mean aortic valve gradient increased to 80 mmHg during low-dose dobutamine. In these patients, the risk of perioperative mortality is five times higher compared with patients without aortic valve stenosis.[49] Therefore, this patient was referred for aortic valve replacement prior to vascular surgery.

References

1 Mangano DT. Perioperative cardiac morbidity. *Anesthesiology* 1990;**72**:153–84.

2 Landelijke Medische Registratie, years 1991–2000. Prismant, 2004. Utrecht. Electronic data file. Accessed 30 August 2004. www.prismant.nl.

3 Eagle KA, Berger PB, Calkins H, *et al*. Committee to Update the 1996 Guidelines on Perioperative Cardiovascular Evaluation for Non-cardiac Surgery. ACC/AHA guideline update for perioperative cardiovascular evaluation for non-cardiac surgery: executive summary a report of the American College of Cardiology/American Heart Association Task Force on Practice Guidelines. *Circulation* 2002;**105**:1257–67.

4 Dawood MM, Gupta DK, Southern J, *et al*. Pathology of fatal perioperative myocardial infarction: implications regarding pathophysiology and prevention. *Int J Cardiol* 1996;**57**:37–44.

5 Warltier DC, Pagel PS, Kersten JR. Approaches to the prevention of perioperative myocardial ischemia. *Anesthesiology* 2000;**92**:253–9.

6 Iskandrian AE, Verani MS. Nuclear imaging techniques. In: Topol EJ, ed. *Textbook of Cardiovascular Medicine*. Philadelphia: Lippincott Williams & Wilkins, 2002:1191–212.

7 Gallik DM, Obermueller SD, Swarna US, *et al.* Simultaneous assessment of myocardial perfusion and left ventricular function during transient coronary occlusion. *J Am Coll Cardiol* 1995;**25**:1529–38.

8 Mahmarian JJ, Boyce TM, Goldberg RK, *et al.* Quantitative exercise thallium-201 single photon emission computed tomography for the enhanced diagnosis of ischemic heart disease. *J Am Coll Cardiol* 1990;**15**:318–29.

9 Baron JF, Mundler O, Bertrand M, *et al.* Dipyridamole-thallium scintigraphy and gated radionuclide angiography to assess cardiac risk before abdominal aortic surgery. *N Engl J Med* 1994;**330**:663–9.

10 Boucher CA, Brewster DC, Darling RC, *et al.* Determination of cardiac risk by dipyridamole-thallium imaging before peripheral vascular surgery. *N Engl J Med* 1985; **312**:389–94.

11 Cutler BS, Leppo JA. Dipyridamole thallium 201 scintigraphy to detect coronary artery disease before abdominal aortic surgery. *J Vasc Surg* 1987;**5**:91–100.

12 Mangano DT, London MJ, Tubau JF, *et al.* Study of Perioperative Ischemia Research Group. Dipyridamole thallium-201 scintigraphy as a preoperative screening test: a re-examination of its predictive potential. *Circulation* 1991;**84**:493–502.

13 Kertai MD, Boersma E, Bax JJ, *et al.* A meta-analysis comparing the prognostic accuracy of six diagnostic tests for predicting perioperative cardiac risk in patients undergoing major vascular surgery. *Heart* 2003;**89**:1327–34.

14 Eagle KA, Coley CM, Newell JB, *et al.* Combining clinical and thallium data optimizes preoperative assessment of cardiac risk before major vascular surgery. *Ann Intern Med* 1989;**110**:859–66.

15 Poldermans D, Arnese M, Fioretti PM, *et al.* Improved cardiac risk stratification in major vascular surgery with dobutamine-atropine stress echocardiography. *J Am Coll Cardiol* 1995;**26**:648–53.

16 Das MK, Pellikka PA, Mahoney DW, *et al.* Assessment of cardiac risk before non-vascular surgery: dobutamine stress echocardiography in 530 patients. *J Am Coll Cardiol* 2000;**35**:1647–53.

17 Fung AY, Gallagher KP, Buda AJ. The physiologic basis of dobutamine as compared with dipyridamole stress interventions in the assessment of critical coronary stenosis. *Circulation* 1987;**76**:943–51.

18 Poldermans D, Bax JJ, Thomson IR, *et al.* Role of dobutamine stress echocardiography for preoperative cardiac risk assessment before major vascular surgery: a diagnostic tool comes of age. *Echocardiography* 2000;**17**:79–91.

19 Schiller NB, Shah PM, Crawford M, *et al.* American Society of Echocardiography Committee on Standards, Subcommittee on Quantitation of Two-Dimensional Echocardiograms. Recommendations for quantitation of the left ventricle by two-dimensional echocardiography. *J Am Soc Echocardiogr* 1989;**2**:358–67.

20 Boersma E, Poldermans D, Bax JJ, *et al.* Predictors of cardiac events after major vascular surgery: role of clinical characteristics, dobutamine echocardiography, and beta-blocker therapy. *JAMA* 2001;**285**:1865–73.

21 Poldermans D, Rambaldi R, Bax JJ, *et al.* Safety and utility of atropine addition during dobutamine stress echocardiography for the assessment of viable myocardium in patients with severe left ventricular dysfunction. *Eur Heart J* 1998;**19**:1712–8.

22 Mantha S, Roizen MF, Barnard J, *et al*. Relative effectiveness of four preoperative tests for predicting adverse cardiac outcomes after vascular surgery: a meta-analysis. *Anesth Analg* 1994;**79**:422–33.

23 Shaw LJ, Eagle KA, Gersh BJ, Miller DD. Meta-analysis of intravenous dipyridamole-thallium-201 imaging (1985–1994) and dobutamine echocardiography (1991–1994) for risk stratification before vascular surgery. *J Am Coll Cardiol* 1996;**27**:787–98.

24 Kertai MD, Boersma E, Sicari R, *et al*. Which stress test is superior for perioperative cardiac risk stratification in patients undergoing major vascular surgery? *Eur J Vasc Endovasc Surg* 2002;**24**:222–9.

25 Viswamitra S, Higgins CB, Meacham DF, Mehta JL. Magnetic resonance imaging in myocardial ischemia. *Curr Opin Cardiol* 2004;**19**:510–6.

26 Laddis T, Manning WJ, Danias PG. Cardiac MRI for assessment of myocardial perfusion: current status and future perspectives. *J Nucl Cardiol* 2001;**8**:207–14.

27 Miller DD, Holmvang G, Gill JB, *et al*. MRI detection of myocardial perfusion changes by gadolinium-DTPA infusion during dipyridamole hyperemia. *Magn Reson Med* 1989;**10**:246–55.

28 Pennell DJ, Underwood SR, Manzara CC, *et al*. Magnetic resonance imaging during dobutamine stress in coronary artery disease. *Am J Cardiol* 1992;**70**:34–40.

29 Schvartzman PR, White RD. Magnetic resonance imaging. In: Topol EJ, ed. *Textbook of Cardiovascular Medicine*. Lippincott Williams & Wilkins, 2002: 1213–56.

30 van Rugge FP, van der Wall EE, Spanjersberg SJ, *et al*. Magnetic resonance imaging during dobutamine stress for detection and localization of coronary artery disease: quantitative wall motion analysis using a modification of the centerline method. *Circulation* 1994;**90**:127–38.

31 Baer FM, Theissen P, Crnac J, *et al*. Head to head comparison of dobutamine-transoesophageal echocardiography and dobutamine-magnetic resonance imaging for the prediction of left ventricular functional recovery in patients with chronic coronary artery disease. *Eur Heart J* 2000;**21**:981–91.

32 Rerkpattanapipat P, Morgan TM, Neagle CM, *et al*. Assessment of preoperative cardiac risk with magnetic resonance imaging. *Am J Cardiol* 2002;**90**:416–9.

33 Stone JG, Foex P, Sear JW, *et al*. Myocardial ischemia in untreated hypertensive patients: effect of a single small oral dose of a beta-adrenergic blocking agent. *Anesthesiology* 1988;**68**:495–500.

34 Raby KE, Brull SJ, Timimi F, *et al*. The effect of heart rate control on myocardial ischemia among high-risk patients after vascular surgery. *Anesth Analg* 1999;**88**:477–82.

35 Urban MK, Markowitz SM, Gordon MA, *et al*. Postoperative prophylactic administration of beta-adrenergic blockers in patients at risk for myocardial ischemia. *Anesth Analg* 2000;**90**:1257–61.

36 Mangano DT, Layug EL, Wallace A, Tateo I. Multicenter Study of Perioperative Ischemia Research Group. Effect of atenolol on mortality and cardiovascular morbidity after non-cardiac surgery. *N Engl J Med* 1996;**335**:1713–20.

37 Poldermans D, Boersma E, Bax JJ, *et al*. Dutch Echocardiographic Cardiac Risk Evaluation Applying Stress Echocardiography Study Group. The effect of bisoprolol on perioperative mortality and myocardial infarction in high-risk patients undergoing vascular surgery. *N Engl J Med* 1999;**341**:1789–94.

38 Oliver MF, Goldman L, Julian DG, Holme I. Effect of mivazerol on perioperative cardiac complications during non-cardiac surgery in patients with coronary heart disease: the European Mivazerol Trial (EMIT). *Anesthesiology* 1999;**91**:951–61.

39 Wijeysundera DN, Naik JS, Scott Beattie W. α_2-Adrenergic agonists to prevent perioperative cardiovascular complications: a meta-analysis. *Am J Med* 2003;**114**:742–52.

40 Stevens RD, Burri H, Tramer MR. Pharmacologic myocardial protection in patients undergoing non-cardiac surgery: a quantitative systematic review. *Anesth Analg* 2003;**97**:623–33.

41 Poldermans D, Bax JJ, Kertai MD, *et al*. Statins are associated with a reduced incidence of perioperative mortality in patients undergoing major non-cardiac vascular surgery. *Circulation* 2003;**107**:1848–51.

42 Durazzo AES, Machado FS, Ikeoka DT, *et al*. Reduction in cardiovascular events after vascular surgery with atorvastatin: a randomized trial. *J Vasc Surg* 2004;**39**:967–75.

43 Lindenauer PK, Pekow P, Wang K, *et al*. Lipid-lowering therapy and in-hospital mortality following major non-cardiac surgery. *JAMA* 2004;**291**:2092–9.

44 Smith SC, Blair SN, Bonow RO, *et al*. AHA/ACC guidelines for preventing heart attack and death with atherosclerotic cardiovascular disease: 2001 update. A statement for healthcare professionals from the American Heart Association and the American College of Cardiology. *Circulation* 2001;**104**:1577–9.

45 Gibbons RJ, Abrams J, Chatterjee K, *et al*. Committee on the Management of Patients With Chronic Stable Angina. ACC/AHA 2002 Guideline Update for the Management of Patients With Chronic Stable Angina: summary article: A report of the American College of Cardiology/American Heart Association Task Force on Practice Guidelines. *Circulation* 2003;**107**:149–58.

46 Kertai MD, Boersma E, Bax JJ, *et al*. Optimizing long-term cardiac management after major vascular surgery: role of beta-blocker therapy, clinical characteristics, and dobutamine stress echocardiography to optimize long-term cardiac management after major vascular surgery. *Arch Intern Med* 2003;**163**:2230–5.

47 Eagle KA, Guyton RA, Davidoff R, *et al*. Committee to Revise the 1991 Guidelines for Coronary Artery Bypass Graft Surgery. ACC/AHA Guidelines for Coronary Artery Bypass Graft Surgery: Executive Summary and Recommendations: A report of the American College of Cardiology/American Heart Association Task Force on Practice Guidelines. *Circulation* 1999;**100**:1464–80.

48 Bountioukos M, Kertai MD, Schinkel AF, *et al*. Safety of dobutamine stress echocardiography in patients with aortic stenosis. *J Heart Valve Dis* 2003;**12**:441–6.

49 Kertai MD, Bountioukos M, Boersma E, *et al*. Aortic stenosis: an underestimated risk factor for perioperative complications in patients undergoing non-cardiac surgery. *Am J Med* 2004;**116**:8–13.

Section three
Heart failure

CHAPTER 13

Acute dyspnea (diastolic, systolic LV dysfunction, and pulmonary embolism)

Michael V. McConnell and Brett E. Fenster

Introduction

There are a myriad of evanescent processes that cause acute dyspnea (Table 13.1). Many of these disease states can be diagnosed using non-invasive imaging techniques. A successful diagnostic strategy requires consideration of the relative advantages and disadvantages of available imaging modalities, including performance, convenience, procedure time, invasiveness, risk, availability, and cost. This chapter discusses the ability of a number of non-invasive modalities to assess systolic and diastolic dysfunction, myocardial ischemia and infarction, valvular dysfunction, and pulmonary embolism.

Systolic and diastolic left ventricular dysfunction

Evaluation of the patient with acute dyspnea necessitates consideration of both myocardial systolic and diastolic dysfunction as an etiology. While heart failure is ultimately a clinical diagnosis, the limitations of physical examination, chest X-ray radiography, and biomarkers often require additional non-invasive imaging to assure accurate diagnosis and effective treatment.

Echocardiography

Because of its well-established performance, instantaneous processing, inexpensiveness, and comprehensiveness, echocardiography remains the initial study of choice in assessing systolic dysfunction. Global systolic function can be determined both quantitatively by Simpson's rule (method of disk) and wall motion index, and qualitatively by visual assessment of endocardial thickening. In the 10% of cases in which poor visualization limits the determination of contractility, perfluten microsphere contrast agents or transesophageal echocardiography can improve functional assessment. Suspected ventricular septal defects can be evaluated by surveying myocardial septal integrity with color Doppler and intravascular contrast techniques.

Echocardiography remains the gold standard for identifying diastolic dys-

Table 13.1 Important etiologies of acute dyspnea in non-invasive imaging.

Ventricular dysfunction
Systolic dysfunction
  Myocardial ischemia or infarction
  Myocarditis
  Acute-on-chronic systolic dysfunction
  Congenital heart disease
  Arrhythmia

Diastolic dysfunction
  Myocardial ischemia or infarction
  Pericardial disease (tamponade, constriction)
  Acute-on-chronic diastolic dysfunction (including restriction)

Mechanical complications from myocardial infarction
Ventricular septal defect
Left ventricular free wall rupture

Valvular dysfunction
Acute MR resulting from papillary muscle or chordal rupture, ischemia, or endocarditis
Acute aortic regurgitation resulting from dissection or endocarditis
Prosthetic valve dysfunction resulting from acute thrombosis or dehiscence
Congenital heart disease

Pulmonary embolism

---

function through the assessment of pulsed wave Doppler mitral valve and pulmonary vein inflow patterns, deceleration times, interventricular relaxation times, and tissue Doppler patterns. Diminished mitral valve inflow association with inspiration and/or right-sided chamber collapse in the presence of significant pericardial effusion remains the reference standard for the non-invasive diagnosis of pericardial tamponade. Similar inflow patterns in the absence of effusion suggest constriction.

A considerable advantage of echocardiography over other imaging modalities is its portability. Unstable patients who require critical care monitoring may be unsuitable for transport to scanner facilities. Furthermore, dyspneic patients who cannot tolerate the supine position necessary for other modalities can be imaged in the upright position by echocardiography. However, echocardiography can be limited by the poor acoustic windows associated with obesity, severe pulmonary disease, or unusual body habitus. In addition, echocardiography cannot adequately characterize myocardial tissue, limiting its ability to visualize myocardial infiltrative processes or scarring.

Cardiac magnetic resonance imaging
Unlike echocardiographically determined calculations of cardiac function, which rely upon two-dimensional data sets that assume a uniform myocardial

geometry, cardiac magnetic resonance imaging (CMR) utilizes three-dimensional data sets to generate an exquisitely accurate assessment of ventricular volumes, output, and contractility. Accordingly, CMR is viewed to be the reference standard for determining cardiac function and mass. CMR is particularly useful when echocardiographic examinations are limited by poor acoustic windows. Compared with echocardiography, CMR has superior visualization of the right ventricle, which can be of particular use in evaluating isolated right ventricular myopathies. With its superior delineation of myocardial anatomy, CMR can assess for specific etiologies of systolic dysfunction including infarction (Fig. 13.1), arrythmogenic right ventricular dysplasia, and myocarditis.

CMR can check for diastolic dysfunction through evaluation of relaxation abnormalities using tissue tagging and left ventricle (LV) three-dimensional diastolic motion techniques. However, limited data exist to validate this methodology with clinical findings. CMR is particularly useful in the diagnosis

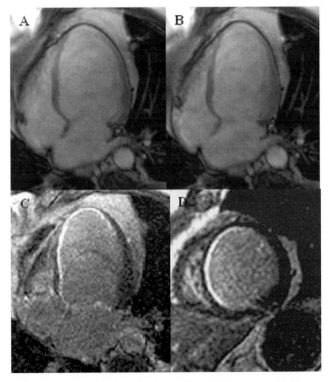

Figure 13.1 Cardiac magnetic resonance imaging (CMR) steady-state free precession (SSFP) imaging in the four-chamber view: (A) end-diastole; (B) end-systole. There is left ventricular enlargement with severe systolic dysfunction and apical dyskinesis. Delayed enhancement imaging in (C) the four-chamber and (D) short-axis views shows a large septal and apical infarct.

of pericardial disease through characterization of pericardial anatomy and detection of restricted motion at the pericardial–myocardial interface using tagging techniques.

Despite the broad range of applications of CMR, numerous factors currently limit its use. CMR is contraindicated in patients with pacemakers or implantable defibrillators and ferromagnetic cerebral aneurysm clips. Irregular rhythms that often accompany acute heart failure can result in inadequate cardiac gating and suboptimal examinations, although more rapid imaging and real-time acquisitions can obviate this potential limitation. Adequate respiratory gating requires patients to be supine while performing breath-holds, limiting feasibility in some patients with acute dyspnea. Limited availability outside of most major medical centers remains a significant impediment to routine use of CMR as does the increased cost compared with echocardiography. Although most CMR image acquisition and processing are instantaneous, volumetric quantitation requires additional post-processing time. Finally, the small confines of scanners can provoke claustrophobia in patients, requiring patient sedation or premature study termination.

Nuclear studies

Gated single photon emission computed tomography (SPECT) permits simultaneous evaluation of regional and global ventricular function as well as perfusion. However, severe perfusion abnormalities can preclude accurate assessment of left ventricular function and volume, resulting in an underestimation of ejection fraction.[1] Techniques such as peak filling rate, time to peak filling, and filling fraction can assess for diastolic dysfunction but will require improved temporal resolution and a reliable diastolic filling phase for results that rival echocardiography. Although multiple gated blood pool acquisition (MUGA) produces highly accurate ejection fraction measurements, peak filling rate assessments of diastolic dysfunction can have considerable beat-to-beat variation. Furthermore, many centers are not staffed to perform emergent MUGA or SPECT studies, limiting availability.

Myocardial ischemia and infarction

In the absence of ST-segment elevation infarction that would necessitate emergent X-ray angiography, a variety of non-invasive methodologies exist to evaluate for acute myocardial ischemia, stenotic coronary artery disease, or both.

Single positron emission computed tomography

Acute rest myocardial perfusion imaging (ARMPI) for the detection of perfusion defects and associated wall motion abnormalities is an accurate method of detecting acute ischemia. ARMPI during chest pain episodes has a sensitivity of 96% and a specificity of 79% for detecting coronary artery disease (CAD).[2] However, this technique is insensitive in the pain-free state, making it less efficacious in patients with acute dyspnea without angina. Moreover, ARMPI protocols have not been incorporated into routine use at most centers.

Echocardiography

In the acute setting where ischemia is suspected, resting echocardiography can be used to assess for the presence of a new regional wall motion abnormality or LV dysfunction. Echocardiography performed within 4 h of presentation has a sensitivity of 96% and a specificity of 75% in predicting cardiac events.[3]

Cardiac magnetic resonance imaging

CMR offers the potential to serve as a comprehensive modality for evaluating ischemic heart disease in the acute setting. Resting myocardial perfusion, wall motion, and viability assessment in patients with acute chest pain has a superior sensitivity (85%) to ECG, troponin I, and thrombolysis in myocardial infarction (TIMI) risk score for the detection of acute coronary syndrome.[4] Real-time CMR can detect regional ischemia via wall motion abnormalities as well as myocardial tagging techniques.

CMR is unique in its ability to evaluate multiple myocardial parameters during a single study, including subendocardial ischemia, myocardial viability and, most intriguingly, coronary anatomy via angiography (CMRA) (Fig. 13.2). In contrast to computed tomography (CT), CMRA requires no nephrotoxic contrast agents or radiation. However, the small size of coronary arteries, complex course, and perpetual motion pose significant obstacles to achieving ideal resolution. Furthermore, contemporary coronary stents create "black hole" artifacts that preclude angiographic visualization. Despite these limitations, CMRA is effective in diagnosing left main disease, proximal three-vessel CAD, coronary artery bypass graft patency, and anomalous coronary arteries.[5]

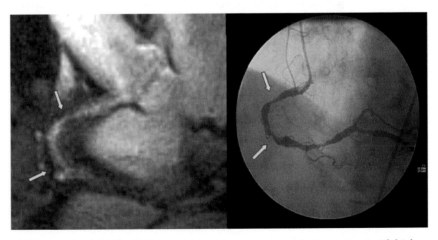

Figure 13.2 CMR (left) and X-ray (right) coronary angiography in a patient with high-grade proximal and mid right coronary artery stenoses (arrows). (Courtesy of Dr. Phillip Yang, Stanford University.)

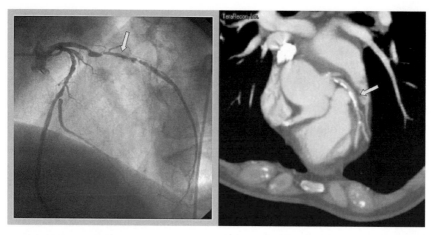

Figure 13.3 16-row MDCT (right) and X-ray coronary angiography (left) in a 74-year-old man showing the left anterior descending coronary artery (arrows) with sequential high-grade calcific stenoses. (Courtesy of Dr. Frandics Chan, Stanford University.)

Computed tomography

ECG-gated multi-detector computed tomography (MDCT) is emerging as a sensitive (95%) and specific (86%) method for detecting CAD (Fig. 13.3).[6] However, significant coronary calcification can cause scatter artifacts that obscure adequate lumen visualization. CT is limited by number of factors, including the use of nephrotoxic contrast agents and significant radiation exposure. Furthermore, CT is currently unable to reliably assess myocardial wall motion and perfusion abnormalities. Finally, adequate temporal resolution necessitates relatively low heart rates, often requiring pharmacologic measures for rate control.

Valvular disease

Acute dyspnea can herald underlying valvular dysfunction in the form of stenotic disease or regurgitation resulting from ischemia, endocarditits, or aortic dissection. Dyspnea in patients with prosthetic valves raises the possibility of valvular thrombosis, dehiscence, endocarditis, or perivalvular leak.

Echocardiography

Echocardiography is the mainstay in valvular dysfunction assessment in both native and prosthetic valves. Echocardiography is superior in its ability to directly assess valvular morphology, vegetations, and subvalvular structures. Color Doppler is the non-invasive gold standard for characterization of regurgitant and flow acceleration jets (Fig. 13.4). Valvular gradients may be quantitated with Doppler techniques, which closely approximate invasive measurements. The inherent limitations of transthoracic echocardiography in

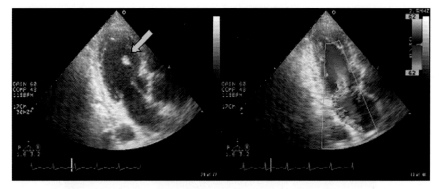

Figure 13.4 Apical three-chamber transthoracic echocardiogram in an 83-year-old man with acute pulmonary edema 2 days after acute anterior myocardial infarction demonstrating anterior papillary muscle rupture (arrow) and flail anterior mitral valve leaflet. Color Doppler revealed severe eccentric mitral regurgitation.

interrogating metallic prosthetic valve dysfunction or ascending aortic dissection can be overcome with transesophageal echocardiography. Additionally, echocardiography provides concomitant information about ventricular function and chamber size relevant for valvular disease management decisions.

Cardiac magnetic resonance imaging

CMR techniques such as volume measurements, signal-void phenomena, and velocity mapping can be used for an integrated evaluation of valvular disease. Velocity-encoded mapping can generate an accurate measurement of both regurgitant volume and fraction as well as stenotic peak flow velocity, but does require post-processing. It is also well-validated in evaluating aortic dissection. Temporal resolution is less optimal than echocardiography, and there is limited valvular morphologic characterization. Non-ferromagnetic prosthetic valves can be safely imaged but often create a localized signal defect which impairs adequate visualization.

Acute pulmonary embolism

Acute pulmonary embolism (PE) is a vexing clinical entity with protean manifestations which requires timely diagnosis and treatment. Although plasma biomarkers have been used successfully to risk-stratify patients, the ultimate diagnosis frequently necessitates non-invasive imaging.

Computed tomography

Spiral CT has supplanted ventilation–perfusion (V/Q) scanning as the first-line imaging modality for diagnosis of PE. In contrast to V/Q scans, CT offers the distinct advantage of direct thrombus visualization and determination of the lung parenchymal and mediastinal abnormalities, leading to alternative diagnoses

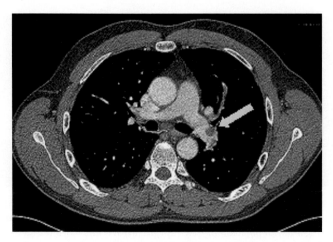

Figure 13.5 Chest CT angiogram in a 48-year-old man with dyspnea with a non-occlusive filling defect (arrow) in the left pulmonary artery indicative of pulmonary embolus.

for dyspnea (Fig. 13.5). Furthermore, CT venography of the lower extremity venous system can be performed simultaneously to assess for concurrent deep venous thrombosis.

Compared with single-row detector CT, MDCT has increased the sensitivity of PE diagnosis from 70% to 90%.[7] However, this improved sensitivity has resulted in the frequent finding of previously undiagnosed, small (2–3 mm) peripheral emboli, often in patients with minimal symptoms. Such a situation creates a quandary because the clinical significance of these small PEs is unclear.

Ventilation–perfusion scintigraphy

V/Q scans remain an important alternative to CT in patients with renal insufficiency, contrast allergy, motion artifact, or poor right ventricular function resulting in inadequate opacification of the pulmonary vascular bed. Tempering the utility of V/Q scans is the fact that the vast majority of lung scans (73%) are read as intermediate probability, necessitating the use of additional imaging or simple empiric therapy.[8] Furthermore, wide interobserver variability exists with scan interpretations.

Magnetic resonance angiography

Although gadolinium-enhanced magnetic resonance pulmonary angiography (MRPA) allows for excellent tissue characterization, it is infrequently utilized because of its lower spatial and temporal resolution compared with CT.

Echocardiography

Because 50% of patients with angiographically proven PE have normal echocardiograms, echocardiography is not recommended for the primary diagnosis of PE.[9] However, echocardiography is a rapid and practical test that can

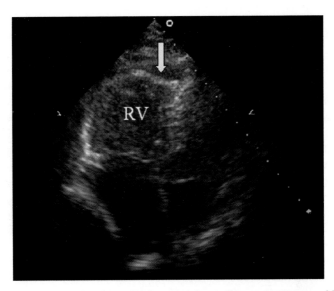

Figure 13.6 Apical four-chamber transthoracic echocardiogram in 79-year-old woman with acute dyspnea 10 days after a left knee arthroplasty demonstrating a right ventricular (RV) dilatation and dysfunction with preserved apical contractility (arrow) consistent with acute pulmonary embolism. Ventilation–perfusion scanning revealed bilateral basal and apical perfusion abnormalities. Following anticoagulation therapy, the right ventricular function normalized.

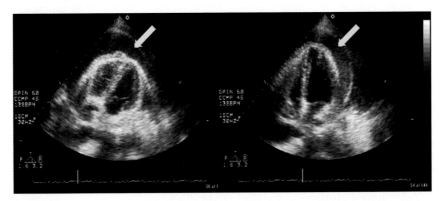

Figure 13.7 Apical four-chamber transthoracic echocardiogram demonstrating large, circumferential, pericardial effusion (arrows) and cardiac "swinging" within the pericardium over one cardiac cycle (left to right frames), indicative of tamponade.

risk stratify and prognosticate acute PE patients. Echocardiographic findings suggestive of a large PE include right ventricle (RV) dilatation and regional RV dysfunction (Fig. 13.6), interventricular septal flattening and paradoxical motion, and tricuspid regurgitation. Patients with high-risk echocardiographic findings warrant consideration of thrombolysis or embolectomy.

Case Presentation

A 58-year-old woman with Stage IV breast cancer complicated by bilateral malignant pleural effusions was admitted to the oncology service with protracted emesis, dehydration, and tachycardia presumed to be secondary to a recently completed chemotherapy. During the placement of an indwelling subclavian catheter, a normal saline bolus was administered intravenously resulting in sudden onset of respiratory distress. A bedside transthoracic echocardiogram revealed a large circumferential pericardial effusion with interventricular dependence and diminished tricuspid valve inflow patterns (Fig. 13.7). Urgent pericardiocentesis yielded 260 mL bloody exudative fluid with an opening pericardial pressure of 20 mmHg. Following the pericardiocentesis, the patient had a modest improvement in hypoxemia but remained tachycardic. Repeat echocardiography showed a small residual effusion but new evidence of right ventricular hypokinesis suggestive of PE. Chest CT angiography demonstrated bilateral segmental and subsegmental branch PE. An inferior vena cava filter was placed and the patient was started on unfractionated heparin and warfarin, resulting in significant clinical improvement.

Conclusions

Multiple non-invasive imaging modalities exist to facilitate the accurate detection of the myriad disease processes that manifest as acute dyspnea. Ultimately, no single imaging modality is superior in evaluating all potential diagnoses. Rather, the current spectrum of imaging techniques are complementary and their effective use requires an appreciation of each modality's strengths and weaknesses. While echocardiography remains a vital modality for the rapid evaluation of multiple clinical scenarios, emerging technologies such as CMR and MDCT will likely continue to have a larger role in imaging patients with acute dyspnea.

References

1 Manrique A, Faraggi M, Vera P, *et al.* [201]Ti and ^{99m}Tc-MIBI gated SPECT in patient with large perfusion defects and left ventricular dysfunction: comparison with equilibrium radionuclide angiography. *J Nucl Med* 1999;**40**:805–9.

2 Bilodeau L, Theroux P, Gregoire J, *et al.* Technetium-99m sestamibi tomography in patients with chest pain: correlations with clinical, electrocardiographic, and angiographic findings. *J Am Coll Cardiol* 1991;**18**:1684–91.

3 Kontos MC, Arrowood JA, Paulsen WH, *et al.* Early echocardiography can predict cardiac events in emergency department patients with chest pain. *Ann Emerg Med* 1998;**31**:550–7.

4 Kwong RY, Schussheim AE, Rekhraj S, *et al.* Detecting acute coronary syndrome in the emergency department with cardiac magnetic resonance imaging. *Circulation* 2003;**107**:531–7.

5 Kim WY, Danias PG, Stuber G, *et al*. Coronary magnetic resonance angiography for the detection of coronary stenoses. *N Engl J Med* 2001;**345**:1863–69.

6 Nieman K, Cademartiri F, Lemos PA, *et al*. Reliable non-invasive coronary angiography with fast submillimeter multislice spiral computed tomography. *Circulation* 2002;**106**: 2051–4.

7 Qanadh SD, Hajjarn ME, Mesurolle B, *et al*. Pulmonary embolism detection: prospective evaluation of dual-section helical CT versus selective angiography in 157 patients. *Radiology* 2000;**217**:447–55.

8 The PIOPED investigators. Value of the ventilation/perfusion scan in acute pulmonary embolism: results of the Prospective Investigation of Pulmonary Embolism Diagnosis (PIOPED). *JAMA* 1990;**263**:2753–9.

9 Goldhaber SZ. Echocardiography in the management of pulmonary embolism. *Ann Intern Med* 2002;**136**:691–700.

CHAPTER 14

Echocardiographic evaluation of patients with chronic dyspnea

Jong-Won Ha and Jae K. Oh

Introduction

Dyspnea is defined as an abnormally uncomfortable awareness of breathing that occurs whenever the work of breathing is excessive. The mechanisms responsible for dyspnea vary in different conditions. Although cardiac and pulmonary diseases can cause pathologic dyspnea, other systemic conditions such as anemia, obesity, neuromuscular diseases, and metabolic acidosis should be suspected as a possible cause of this symptom. Cardiac causes of dyspnea include systolic dysfunction, myocardial ischemia, valvular diseases, cardiomyopathies, pericardial diseases, congenital heart disease, cardiac masses, and primary diastolic dysfunction. Most of these conditions are easily detected by a comprehensive echocardiography examination. Because valvular heart diseases and cardiomyopathies are discussed in other chapters, this chapter primarily reviews evaluation of diastolic function and other less common but important causes of chronic dyspnea that can be reliably identified by echocardiography.

The common hemodynamic event responsible for cardiac dyspnea is increased diastolic filling pressure resulting from various causes. Therefore it is essential that diastolic filling pressures as well as underlying structural and functional abnormality are evaluated by echocardiography in patients with dyspnea.

Evaluation of left ventricular systolic function

The most readily detectable cardiac condition responsible for dyspnea is reduced systolic function from previous myocardial infarction, severe myocardial ischemia, or dilated cardiomyopathy. The most popular systolic parameters measured by echocardiography are fractional shortening and ejection fraction. Fractional shortening, which is a percentage change in left ventricular cavity dimension with systolic contraction, is not used clinically. Ejection fraction represents stroke volume as a percentage of left ventricular end-diastolic volume, hence its determination requires left ventricular volume measurement. The American Society of Echocardiography recommends the simplified Simpson's method to estimate ventricular volume from two orthogonal apical views. However, the detection of systolic dysfunction or reduced ejection fraction does not automatically indicate that dyspnea is caused by systolic dysfunction. We need to demonstrate increased filling pressure and/or pulmonary systolic pressure.

One of most important reasons for dyspnea is myocardial ischemia resulting from severe coronary artery disease. Regional wall motion abnormalities at rest or with stress (exercise or dobutamine infusion) usually, although not always, indicate the presence of coronary artery disease. Left ventricular regional wall motion analysis is usually based upon grading of contractility of individual myocardial segments. For the purpose of standardized analysis, the left ventricle is divided into three levels (basal, mid, apical) and 16 segments. Basal and mid (papillary muscle) level is subdivided into six segments, and the apical level into four segments. All 16 segments can be visualized from multiple tomographic planes of surface echocardiography.

It has recently been shown that among patients referred for exercise echocardiography, those with the primary symptom of dyspnea were at high risk of having coronary artery disease.[1] Among patients with dyspnea but no chest pain, 42% had echocardiographic evidence of ischemia and 59% had an abnormal exercise echocardiogram. During 3.1 ± 1.8 years' follow-up, myocardial infarction, coronary revascularization, or death occurred in 23% of these patients. Therefore, patients with dyspnea have a high likelihood of ischemia and a high incidence of cardiac events during follow-up. Exercise echocardiography permits combined assessment of exercise capacity, left ventricular systolic function, and exercise-induced ischemia. It also provides independent information for identifying patients at risk of cardiac events.

Evaluation of diastolic function

In patients with heart failure, the increase in left ventricular filling pressures is the primary mechanism responsible for dyspnea, irrespective of the presence or severity of systolic dysfunction. Therefore, the assessment of left atrial pressure or left ventricular filling pressures is crucial to determine the etiology of the dyspnea. Left ventricular filling pressure can be estimated by mitral inflow deceleration time (especially when there is left ventricular systolic dysfunction), pulmonary vein flow velocity analysis, comparison of flow duration (mitral A wave versus pulmonary venous atrial flow reversal), and transmitral flow early diastolic velocity to mitral annular early diastolic velocity ratio (E/E'). Currently, E/E' is the most practical and reliable parameter to estimate left ventricle (LV) filling pressure, regardless of underlying systolic function.[2,3]

Mitral flow

Assessment of transmitral blood flow velocities serves as the backbone of diastolic functional evaluation by Doppler echocardiography. The velocity curve is influenced by several parameters including preload, afterload, contractile state, heart rate, myocardial relaxation, and left ventricular compliance. Theoretical models, computer simulation, and experimental animal models have shown that left atrial pressure, rate of isovolumic ventricular relaxation (τ), end-systolic volume and left ventricular minimal pressure are major determinants of transmitral Doppler filling. Impairment of left ventricular relaxation, which is the earliest manifestation of diastolic dysfunction, results in a prolongation of the isovolumic relaxation time and a reduction in the early transmitral flow velocity (E) with prolongation of the E-wave deceleration time and augment A velocity. In contrast, increasing filling pressures result in shortening of the iso-volumic relaxation time, increased early transmitral gradient and consequently a high early transmitral flow (E) velocity, shortening of the deceleration time and reduction in atrial flow (A) velocity. Because the mitral flow Doppler profile depends on both of the above parameters, progressive elevation of left atrial pressure in ventricles with reduced isovolumic relaxation will reverse the classic pattern of impaired myocardial relaxation towards a "normal" appearing profile, the so-called pseudonormal pattern.

Transmitral flow velocity curves show characteristic patterns as diastolic dysfunction advances (Fig. 14.1). In a normal middle-aged subject, the mitral flow velocity curve consists of an E/A ratio slightly greater than 1.0 and a deceleration time of approximately 200 ms. In the early stages of diastolic dysfunction, referred to as mild diastolic dysfunction (grade 1 diastolic dysfunction), impaired (delayed) relaxation of the left ventricle predominates, resulting in a typical mitral flow velocity profile. At this stage there is little if any increase in rest left ventricular diastolic pressure or mean left atrial pressure. Increased filling pressure may develop with exercise because of shortening of the diastolic filling period which blunts the diastolic filling because of atrial contraction. With progression of diastolic dysfunction the filling pressures start to increase at rest, thus increasing the driving pressure gradient across the mitral valve. This has the effect of normalizing mitral inflow velocity with normal E/A ratio and DT. This phase represents moderate diastolic dysfunction (grade 2 diastolic dysfunction). In more advanced stage of diastolic dysfunction, effective operative compliance decreases, the left atrial pressure becomes even higher producing a restrictive filling pattern characterized by a tall E velocity, shortened DT, and small A velocity (grade 3–4 diastolic dysfunction). In patients with left ventricular systolic dysfunction, a restriction to filling pattern has been associated with a worse functional class and exercise intolerance. A short deceleration time (less than 140 ms) is indicative of a poor prognosis, independent of the degree of systolic dysfunction. On the basis of this progression of disease patterns, a grading system for the severity of diastolic dysfunction as assessed by Doppler echocardiography has been proposed (Fig. 14.1).[4] In a patient with grade 3 diastolic dysfunction, the velocity profile may revert to grade 2 or even grade 1 diastolic dysfunction indicative of good prognosis. On the other hand, some patients with severe abnormalities of ventricular compliance and end-stage heart dis-

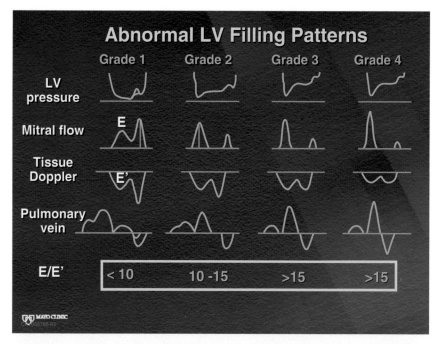

Figure 14.1 Grading of left ventricle (LV) diastolic filling abnormalities (see text for details).

ease maintain a severe restrictive pattern even after optimal medical therapy. These are the patients with the poorest prognosis and they are classified as grade 4 (irreversible) diastolic dysfunction.[5]

Because of the opposing effects on these variables by relaxation and filling pressures, it is often difficult to evaluate the relaxation properties of the left ventricle when the left atrial pressure is unknown. Moreover, the relationships between deceleration time or E/A ratio and filling pressures are not as strong in patients with normal systolic function. Therefore, it is desirable to have additional variables to complement mitral inflow velocity in the evaluation of diastolic function. Recording of mitral annulus velocity by tissue Doppler echocardiography provides the information regarding myocardial relaxation and is most helpful in estimating LV filling pressure in conjunction with mitral inflow velocity.

Tissue Doppler imaging

Tissue Doppler imaging (TDI) is a recent, pulsed wave Doppler application that allows direct measurement of myocardial tissue velocities. TDI is the easiest and most reproducible method to evaluate myocardial relaxation by measuring mitral annulus velocity during diastole. The mitral annulus velocity reflects shortening and lengthening of the left ventricular myocardial fibers along a longitudinal plane (base to apex plane). With prolonged myocardial relaxation, early diastolic annulus motion is reduced. It has been shown that the early diastolic mitral annulus velocity (E') as determined by TDI is relatively pre-load independent (Fig. 14.1),[6] especially in patients with reduced myocardial relaxation.[7] As left ventricular filling pressure increases, mitral E velocity becomes progressively higher whereas E' velocity remains reduced. Nagueh *et al.*[3] have recently shown that when the mitral E velocity was corrected for the influence of myocardial relaxation (i.e. the E/E' ratio), it was found to correlate well with the mean pulmonary capillary wedge pressure (PCWP). Ommen *et al.*[2] have assessed the association between E' (septal annulus) and left ventricular filling pressures in 100 consecutive patients referred for cardiac catheterization and found that E/E' ratio greater than 15 identified increased left ventricular filling pressure (Fig. 14.2). Nagueh *et al.*[7] also showed that E' remained unchanged with increased transmitral gradient in subjects with diastolic dysfunction whereas it increases in subjects with normal τ.

Although E/E' ratio accurately predicts elevated filling pressures in myocardial disease, an exception is constrictive pericarditis. In constrictive pericarditis,

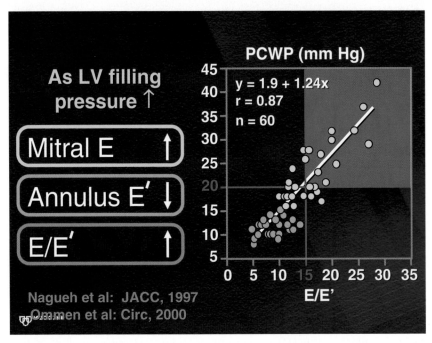

Figure 14.2 Relationship between E/E' and pulmonary capillary wedge pressure (PCWP). As left ventricular filling pressure increase mitral E velocity becomes progressively higher, whereas E' velocity remains reduced. Therefore, when the mitral E velocity was corrected for the influence of myocardial relaxation (i.e. the E/E' ratio), it correlates well with the mean PCWP. (Adapted from Nagueh *et al.*[3])

E' is usually well preserved or even accentuated despite increased filling pressures, and the finding of preserved E' has been proven to be useful for distinguishing constrictive pericarditis from restrictive cardiomyopathy.

Diastolic stress echocardiography

Primary diastolic dysfunction is responsible for up to 50% of congestive heart failure, whose hemodynamic correlate is elevated diastolic filling pressures even at rest. More commonly, patients' symptoms of primary diastolic dysfunction occur only during exertion because diastolic filling pressure is normal at rest and increases only with exertion.[8] Many elderly subjects and patients with hypertension or left ventricular hypertrophy have Doppler echocardiographic evidence of impaired diastolic function, but do not have symptoms of heart failure or dyspnea at rest. In most patients with chronic congestive heart failure, symptoms are not present at rest but develop with exertion. Because patients with significant heart disease may have entirely normal hemodynamics in the resting state and cardiac symptoms may be precipitated only by exertion or some other stresses, it may be important to assess hemodynamic status during some form of stress such as exercise. Therefore exercise hemodynamic responses, rather than evaluation of diastolic function at rest alone, should provide additional physiologic and diagnostic information in these patients. Recently, assessment of diastolic function during exercise has been shown to be feasible[9,10] and may be beneficial in dyspneic patients. *Diastolic stress echocardiography*, a novel, non-invasive, diagnostic test using supine, bicycle exercise, and Doppler echocardiography, provides valid additional information that may help to identify individuals with primary diastolic dysfunction and heart failure. In patients with normal diastolic function E/E' remains less than 10 with exercise, whereas it increases in patients with exercise-induced high filling pressures (Fig. 14.3). Patients without evidence of exercise-induced deterioration of diastolic function may not benefit from conventional heart failure treatment. Conversely, subjects who show exercise-induced diastolic dysfunction and symptoms of exertional dyspnea may have clinical improvement after proper treatment based on their hemodynamic profiles with exercise. This test is potentially an excellent way to distinguish cardiac from non-cardiac dyspnea in patients with multiple coexisting conditions that can cause exertional dyspnea. Normal values of diastolic parameters at baseline and exercise are shown in Table 14.1.

Dyspnea associated with hypoxia

Pulmonary hypertension
Shortness of breath is a characteristic feature of pulmonary hypertension caused by pulmonary vascular disease. Echocardiography allows measurement of the thickness of the right ventricular wall and can show enlargement of the right ventricular cavity in relation to that of the left. The interventricular

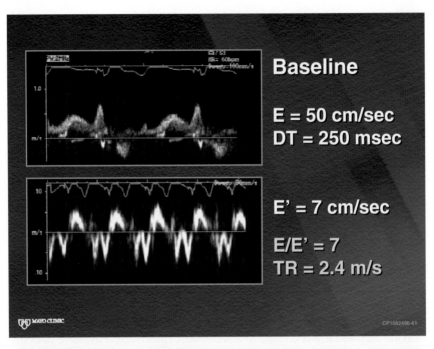

Baseline

E = 50 cm/sec
DT = 250 msec

E' = 7 cm/sec

E/E' = 7
TR = 2.4 m/s

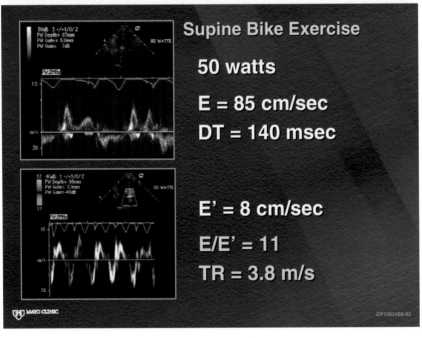

Supine Bike Exercise

50 watts

E = 85 cm/sec
DT = 140 msec

E' = 8 cm/sec

E/E' = 11
TR = 3.8 m/s

Table 14.1 Diastolic stress test normal values.

	Baseline	Exercise
E (cm s^{-1})	73 ± 19	90 ± 25
A (cm s^{-1})	69 ± 17	87 ± 22
DT (ms)	192 ± 40	176 ± 42
E' (cm s^{-1})	12 ± 4	15 ± 5
E/E'	6.7 ± 2.2	6.6 ± 2.5

septum may be displaced leftward and thus shows characteristic D-shaped left ventricular cavity. It may be difficult to distinguish acute cor pulmonale (pulmonary embolism) from chronic obstructive lung disease. Right ventricular hypertrophy is common in chronic form. In both forms, the right-side chambers are dilated and there is two-dimensional Doppler evidence of right ventricular pressure overload as described above. The left ventricular cavity is relatively small and hyperdynamic unless there is left-side cardiac pathology also present. Although certain two-dimensional echocardiographic features suggest pulmonary hypertension, Doppler echocardiography is the primary means to determine actual pulmonary pressures by tricuspid regurgitation velocity.

Platypnea-orthodeoxia

Platypnea-orthodeoxia is a rare syndrome that is often associated with interatrial shunting through a patent foramen ovale (PFO) or atrial septal defect. Patients with this abnormality usually have progressive dyspnea and hypoxia when standing, which is relieved by assuming the recumbent position. After detection of a PFO by transesophageal echocardiography, the diagnosis is confirmed by transthoracic echocardiography using saline contrast injection while

Figure 14.3 Mitral inflow and mitral annulus velocity at baseline (top) and with supine bicycle exercise (bottom) were obtained from a 50-year-old woman with poorly controlled hypertension and diabetes who presented with a chief complaint of exertional dyspnea. At baseline, diastolic filling pattern showed grade 1 diastolic dysfunction (E/A velocity ratio less than 1, prolonged deceleration time, and E/E' 7) indicating relatively normal filling pressure despite impaired myocardial relaxation. Diastolic function assessment showed grade 3 diastolic filling pattern (shorter deceleration time, higher E/A velocity ratio, and E/E' increased to 11) with moderate exercise indicating moderate elevation of filling pressure. Normal pulmonary artery systolic pressure at baseline also increased markedly with exercise. The patient's blood pressure was 180/68 mmHg at rest and 180/96 mmHg after 5 min exercise on supine bicycle achieving 4.9 MET. Heart rate increased from 50 to 72 b min^{-1} with exercise. She was treated with an angiotensin-receptor blocker and her exertional dyspnea improved as well as her blood pressure control.

lying supine and standing upright. This maneuver demonstrates a large right-to-left shunt through a PFO while the patient is in an upright position and no significant shunt while in a recumbent position.

Uncommon cardiac conditions associated with dyspnea

Pulmonary vein stenosis

Atrial fibrillation is a common arrhythmia that is found in 1% of persons older than 60 years and it is a predictor of stroke. Pulmonary vein ablation offers the potential to cure patients with atrial fibrillation. However, the risk of significant pulmonary vein stenosis or occlusion after radiofrequency catheter ablation of refractory atrial fibrillation has been reported. The clinical manifestations of pulmonary vein stenosis are variable, including chest pain, cough, hemoptysis, recurrent lung infection, pulmonary hypertension, and dyspnea. In patients with dyspnea and a history of radiofrequency catheter ablation for atrial fibrillation, pulmonary vein stenosis should be suspected. In echocardiographic examination, two-dimensional echocardiography alone is not sufficient to detect this anomaly. Color Doppler imaging can easily demonstrate turbulent flow from the entry point of the pulmonary vein and thus suggest obstruction. Transesophageal echocardiography is well suited to examination of the pulmonary veins and to diagnosis of pulmonary venous obstruction. Frequency aliasing observed by transthoracic color Doppler imaging is also an important clue in the diagnosis of pulmonary vein stenosis. Doppler echocardiography can be used in the quantitative analysis of severity of functional abnormality. However, in some instances of increased angle to flow, the actual pressure gradient produced by the obstruction may be underestimated.

Constrictive pericarditis

Constrictive pericarditis is a form of diastolic heart failure as a fibrotic, thickened, and adherent pericardium restricts diastolic filling of the heart. The symmetrical constricting effect of the pericardium results in elevation and equilibrium of diastolic pressures in all four cardiac chambers. In patients with dyspnea and other symptoms and signs of right heart failure, constriction should be included as a possible diagnosis. Hatle et al.[11] described the unique feature of respiratory variation in mitral inflow and hepatic vein velocities in patients with constrictive pericarditis, and this substantially improved the accuracy for diagnosis. However, a subset of patients with constrictive pericarditis do not demonstrate such respiratory variation in Doppler velocities, and mitral inflow velocities may be indistinguishable from those of other causes of heart failure.

Recently, it was shown that E' measured by TDI is reduced in patients with restrictive cardiomyopathy, whereas it is relatively normal or even accentuated in constrictive pericarditis.[12,13] Recording of E' by TDI is another useful means of diagnosing constrictive pericarditis when mitral inflow velocity reveals a restrictive filling pattern without sufficient respiratory variation. Therefore, the recording of E' by TDE should be an essential part of echocardiographic Doppler evaluation of all patients with heart failure, especially when constrictive pericarditis is suspected. Most patients with constrictive pericarditis show characteristic two-dimensional echocardiographic abnormalities. These include abnormal ventricular septal motion with prominent respiratory septal "bounce," calcified or thickened pericardium, and dilated inferior vena cava. These abnormal two-dimensional echocardiographic findings should raise the diagnostic possibility of constrictive pericarditis. Further demonstration of characteristic Doppler findings such as respiratory variation in mitral inflow velocity and a normal to increased E' will confirm a diagnosis of constrictive pericarditis.

Conclusions

Chronic dyspnea is often challenging to evaluate because there are many causes for this non-specific symptom. Echocardiography is an ideal imaging tool to evaluate cardiac function, structure, and hemodynamics comprehensively in patients with dyspnea. The capability to assess diastolic function and filling pressures at rest and with exercise by echocardiography enhances our diagnostic ability and allows better management of patients with chronic dyspnea.

References

1 Bergeron S, Ommen S, Bailey K, Oh J, McCully R, Pellikka P. Exercise echocardiographic findings and outcome of patients referred for evaluation of dyspnea. *J Am Coll Cardiol* 2004;**43**:2242–6.

2 Ommen S, Nishimura R, Appleton C, *et al*. Clinical utility of Doppler echocardiography and tissue Doppler imaging in the estimation of left ventricular filling pressures: a comparative simultaneous Doppler–catheterization study. *Circulation* 2000; **102**:1788–94.

3 Nagueh S, Middleton K, Koplen H, Zoghbi W, Quinones M. Doppler tissue imaging: a non-invasive technique for evaluation of left ventricular relaxation and estimation of filling pressures. *J Am Coll Cardiol* 1997;**30**:1527–33.

4 Nishimura R, Tajik A. Evaluation of diastolic filling of left ventricle in health and disease: Doppler echocardiography is the clinician's Rosetta Stone. *J Am Coll Cardiol* 1997;**30**:8–18.

5 Pinamonti B, Zecchin M, Di Lenarda A, Gregori D, Sinagra G, Camerini F. Persistence of restrictive left ventricular filling pattern in dilated cardiomyopathy: an ominous prognostic sign. *J Am Coll Cardiol* 1997;**29**:604–12.

6 Sohn D, Chai I, Lee D, *et al*. Assessment of mitral annulus velocity by Doppler tissue imaging in the evaluation of left ventricular diastolic function. *J Am Coll Cardiol* 1997;**30**:474–80.

7 Nagueh S, Sun H, Kopelen H, Middleton K, Khoury D. Hemodynamic determinants of the mitral annulus diastolic velocities by tissue Doppler. *J Am Coll Cardiol* 2001;**37**:278–85.

8 Kitzman D, Higginbotham M, Cobb F, Sheikh K, Sullivan M. Exercise intolerance in

patients with heart failure and preserved left ventricular systolic function: failure of the Frank–Starling mechanism. *J Am Coll Cardiol* 1991;**17**:1065–72.

9 Ha J, Lulic F, Bailey K, *et al*. Effects of treadmill exercise on mitral inflow and annular velocities in healthy adults. *Am J Cardiol* 2003;**91**:114–5.

10 Ha J, Oh J, Pellikka P, *et al*. Diastolic stress echocardiography: a novel non-invasive diagnostic test for diastolic dysfunction using supine bicycle exercise Doppler echocardiography. *J Am Soc Echocardiogr* In press.

11 Hatle L, Appleton C, Popp R. Differentiation of constrictive pericarditis and restrictive cardiomyopathy by Doppler echocardiography. *Circulation* 1989;**79**:357–70.

12 Garcia M, Rodriguez L, Ares M, Griffin B, Thomas J, Klein A. Differentiation of constrictive pericarditis from restrictive cardiomyopathy: assessment of left ventricular diastolic velocities in longitudinal axis by Doppler tissue imaging. *J Am Coll Cardiol* 1996;**27**:108–14.

13 Ha J, Ommen S, Tajik A, *et al*. Differentiation of constrictive pericarditis from restrictive cardiomyopathy using mitral annular velocity by tissue Doppler echocardiography. *Am J Cardiol* 2004;**94**:316–9.

CHAPTER 15
Resynchronization therapy

Ole-A. Breithardt

Introduction

Cardiac resynchronization therapy (CRT) aims to normalize the disturbed electrical activation sequence that is frequently observed in patients with systolic dysfunction and left ventricular (LV) dilatation in order to improve cardiac hemodynamics. This ambitious goal is typically achieved by the implantation of a LV pacing lead through the coronary sinus tributaries to allow for advanced stimulation of the delayed activated posterolateral wall of the LV. Several prospective trials demonstrated that this strategy is likely to be successful in terms of symptomatic and hemodynamic improvement in the majority of patients with heart failure and left bundle branch block (LBBB).

However, not all heart failure patients respond to therapy. The therapeutic efficacy of a CRT device depends on several factors, including the LV pacing site, device programing (atrioventricular [AV] delay, right–left interventricular [VV] delay), the extent of myocardial scars in ischemic cardiomyopathies, the presence of valvular disease, and the individual degree of dyssynchrony. Most of these factors can be evaluated and monitored at the bedside by transthoracic echocardiography. Other imaging techniques may also be suited to answer some of these issues, such as cardiac magnetic resonance imaging for the identification of scars and radionuclide angiography for the measurement of ejection fraction and quantification of interventricular dyssynchrony, but are technically more demanding and less widely available.

Pathophysiology of cardiac dyssynchrony in LBBB

The physiologic AV contraction sequence with a short PQ interval (less than 150–200 ms) is optimal to allow for complete ventricular emptying and filling. Within the ventricles the electrical activation wavefront spreads rapidly through the His bundle and the Purkinje fibers with a short time delay between the earliest and latest activated myocardial segment of less than 40–50 ms.[1] Left ventricular pre-ejection pressure is slightly higher than in the right ventricle and septal motion is normal.[2] This well-coordinated contraction sequence optimizes the myocardial energy expenditure and its hemodynamic performance.

In the failing heart, myocardial contractility is depressed and highly dependent on pre- and afterload. The presence of an electrical conduction delay—most frequently a LBBB and a prolonged PQ interval more than 150–200 ms — further impairs myocardial energy consumption and the hemodynamic performance of the heart. The LV is activated slowly through the septum from the right side and the LV endocardial activation time may exceed 100 ms.[3] Left ventricular pre-ejection pressure is lower than in the right ventricle and septal motion is abnormal. This results in an uncoordinated contraction sequence and delays LV ejection at the expense of diastolic filling.[4]

Echocardiography in CRT candidates

A careful echocardiographic evaluation is one of the most important steps to select good clinical responders before implantation. Information on the presence and extent of mechanical cardiac dyssynchrony can be derived from conventional echocardiographic parameters during every routine examination. Newer techniques such as tissue Doppler imaging (TDI) and three-dimensional (3D) echocardiography help to characterize the disturbed contraction patterns more precisely, but are technically more demanding.

Data from several small, single-center studies suggest that such echocardiographic information about mechanical asynchrony and its impact on hemodynamics is a better predictor for CRT success than baseline QRS width alone. It is frequently observed that CRT does not decrease QRS width, but nevertheless reduces mechanical dyssynchrony and improves hemodynamics.

Conventional echocardiographic parameters

Table 15.1 provides an overview on the available conventional parameters that are valuable for the assessment of dyssynchrony before CRT implantation and for follow-up.

Parasternal M-mode

Beyond the measurement of ventricular dimensions, the classic parasternal M-mode provides information about the intraventricular septal to posterior wall motion delay (SPWMD). In a small trial on 20 patients, the baseline SPWMD predicted the CRT-related LV reverse remodeling effect better than preimplant QRS width.[5] The SPWMD is measured between the first peak of systolic posterior motion of the septum and the peak anterior motion of the posterior wall. Alternatively, the onset of septal and posterior wall thickening can be compared. A preimplant SPWMD of more than 130–140 ms is seen in good long-term responders. During successful CRT, the SPWMD should be reduced significantly below the cut-off value of 130 ms; frequently it will be close to zero (Fig. 15.1).

Pre-ejection interval by Doppler

The time interval between the onset of electrical activation and the onset of ventricular outflow is defined as the ventricular pre-ejection delay (PEI). It is

Table 15.1 Parameters valuable in the assessment of dyssynchrony.

Method	Measure	Objective	Comment
Parasternal long-axis M-mode	SPWMD >130–140 ms	Intraventricular dyssynchrony (septum–posterior wall)	Often difficult to acquire, limited prospective data
2D apical four- and two-chamber view	Biplane ejection fraction and volumes	Document presence of systolic HF and baseline volumes for FU	Not a marker for dyssynchrony
CW Doppler of pulmonary and aortic outflow	RV–LV pre-ejection interval (ΔPEI) >40 ms	Interventricular dyssynchrony (RV vs. LV)	Robust and reproducible, affected by afterload
PW Doppler of mitral inflow	Diastolic filling time <40–45% of cycle length	Hemodynamic impact of dyssynchrony on diastole	Robust, reproducible; only indirect measure, affected by heart rate
CW Doppler of mitral regurgitation jet (if present)	Slope of regurgitant jet for estimation of LV peak + dP/dt	Non-invasive estimate of LV peak + dP/dt	Tends to underestimate invasive peak + dP/dt, only indirect measure

CW, continuous wave; FU, follow-up; HF, heart failure; LV, left ventricle; peak + dP/dt, peak positive rate of pressure rise; PEI, pre-ejection interval; PW, pulsed wave; RV, right ventricle; SPWMD, septal posterior wall motion delay.

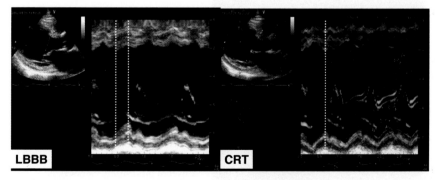

Figure 15.1 Parasternal anatomic M-mode (post-processed M-mode from 2D data set) in left bundle branch block (LBBB, left) and during cardiac resynchronization therapy (CRT, right). In LBBB, biphasic septal motion with early inward motion is present. Inward motion of the posterior wall is delayed by approximately 240 ms. During successful CRT both walls show simultaneous inward motion (right).

measured by Doppler echocardiography from the onset of the QRS to the opening click of the pulmonary valve (RV-PEI) and to the opening click of the aortic valve (LV-PEI). Typical values in LBBB patients are 100 ms for the RV-PEI and 150 ms for the LV-PEI. However, these values may differ substantially between measurements and patients, depending on the applied Doppler technique (pulsed wave [PW] or continuous wave [CW]) and on the reference point on the ECG tracing (onset of QRS). Thus, it is most important to use the same Doppler modality and reference points when calculating the "interventricular mechanical delay" (IVMD), as the difference between the LV-PEI and the RV-PEI:

IVMD = LV-PEI – RV-PEI

The IVMD by Doppler echocardiography is typically prolonged (more than 40 ms) in heart failure patients with LBBB resulting from the delayed ejection of the LV (Fig. 15.2). CRT normalizes the IVMD to values below 20–30 ms by synchronizing both ventricles.

Diastolic filling time
In the normal heart, more than 60% of the cycle length at rest is reserved for

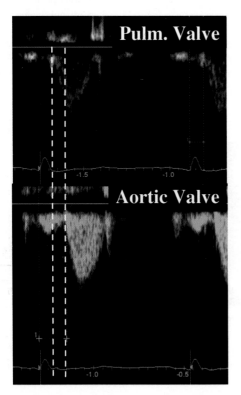

Figure 15.2 Continuous wave Doppler across the pulmonary (above) and aortic valve (below). The pulmonary pre-ejection interval, measured from the onset of the QRS complex as the reference point to the onset of pulmonary ejection, is significantly shorter than the aortic pre-ejection interval. The resulting calculated interventricular mechanical delay is approximately 60 ms.

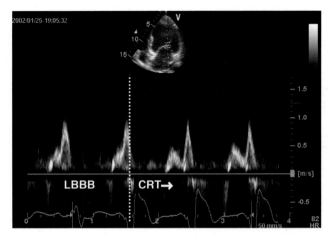

Figure 15.3 Effect of CRT on the mitral inflow profile. During LBBB, the early and late diastolic filling waves are fused and the diastolic filling time is markedly reduced to less than 40% of the corresponding cycle length (left, first two beats). Immediately with the onset of CRT, the diastolic filling time increases above 50% of cycle and the inflow profile normalizes with clear separation of the early and late diastolic filling wave.

diastolic filling. A long PR interval and the delayed activation in LBBB go at the expense of the diastolic filling time (dFT), which can be measured by PW Doppler between the opening and closure of the mitral valve as the total duration of the E-wave and the A-wave. In patients with marked dyssynchrony, the dFT lies below 40–45% of the corresponding cycle length and frequently the early and late diastolic filling waves are fused. CRT and proper AV delay optimization may improve the dFT by more than 15–20% of its baseline value and restore a normal inflow pattern with a separated E- and A-wave.[6,7] These changes can be easily followed online while reprograming the pacemaker (Fig. 15.3; see also p.184).

Functional mitral regurgitation and LV systolic performance

A characteristic feature of delayed AV conduction in heart failure is the presence of presystolic mitral regurgitation (Fig. 15.4, left). The delayed onset of the LV pressure rise after termination of active atrial filling leads to incomplete mitral valve closure with presystolic regurgitation. Presystolic mitral regurgitation should be eliminated by AV delay optimization (Fig. 15.4, right).

Additional important information on LV systolic function can be obtained from the regurgitation jet. The slope of the regurgitant jet by CW Doppler allows estimation of the LV rate of pressure rise (LV peak + dP/dt)[8] and is an indicator for hemodynamic improvement by CRT (Fig. 15.4). Quantification of LV peak + dP/dt at baseline may enable later comparison during follow-up and allows the identification of hemodynamic responders.[6,9]

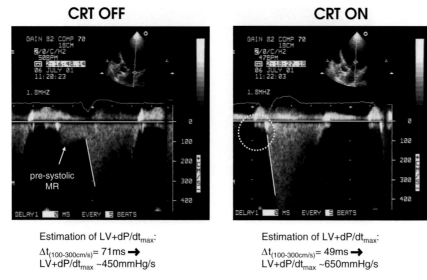

Estimation of LV+dP/dt$_{max}$:
$\Delta t_{(100-300cm/s)} = 71ms$ ➡
LV+dP/dt$_{max}$ ~450mmHg/s

Estimation of LV+dP/dt$_{max}$:
$\Delta t_{(100-300cm/s)} = 49ms$ ➡
LV+dP/dt$_{max}$ ~650mmHg/s

Figure 15.4 Continuous wave Doppler of functional mitral regurgitation in a patient with LBBB and a prolonged PQ interval of more than 300 ms (left). Presystolic mitral regurgitation is present and left ventricular systolic function is poor, as estimated by the slow increase of the regurgitant velocity (LV peak dP/dt). During CRT and successful AV delay optimization, the presystolic component of the regurgitant signal is eliminated and systolic function is improved (right).

Aortic stroke volume

Invasive and non-invasive studies demonstrated that successful CRT acutely increases aortic stroke volume by 10–15%.[7] This effect can be accurately measured by PW Doppler and has been evaluated in several trials. However, calculation of stroke volume is relatively time-consuming, because it requires careful positioning of the PW Doppler sample volume at the level of the LV outflow tract, measurement of the LV outflow tract diameter, and averaging of several beats, which makes it less attractive in daily practice. Alternatively, in patients with a stable heart rate, the velocity time integral ("stroke distance") by aortic CW Doppler can be used to compare the acute changes with CRT.

In summary, conventional echocardiographic parameters provide helpful information about the funtional status of possible CRT candidates and on the impact of asynchrony on LV function. During follow-up these measurements help to verify CRT efficacy and can be used to optimize the pacemaker settings. The analysis can be performed online on every standard echocardiographic scanner and requires no specific expertise. However, a complete analysis is time-consuming and most of the described parameters provide only indirect information about mechanical synchrony.

Tissue Doppler imaging

Tissue Doppler imaging (TDI) measures the velocity of myocardial motion with a high temporal resolution and therefore seems ideally suited to identify LV dyssynchrony and to quantify the resynchronization effect. Unlike conventional Doppler, the high-frequency, low-amplitude signals of myocardial blood flow are filtered out and myocardial tissue velocities are displayed as a spectral Doppler waveform (PW-TDI) or in a color-coded manner similar to color flow Doppler. Today, the temporal resolution of both TDI techniques is high enough to resolve the short-lived cardiac events. Frame-rates above $100–120 \, s^{-1}$ are required to identify reliably the isovolumic events and the onset of regional motion.

Several strategies have been tested to identify synchrony of myocardial motion based on the myocardial velocity profile. Some investigators identified dyssynchrony by the presence and extent of post-systolic shortening (delayed longitudinal contraction, DLC) in the basal segments and demonstrated that CRT reduces the extent of DLC.[10] However, most investigators followed a more quantitative approach and concentrated either on the timing of the onset of systolic myocardial motion or on the timing of peak systolic velocity.[6,11–15]

In the normal heart, the onset of systolic motion occurs briefly after the isovolumic velocity spike and almost simultaneously in all myocardial segments. Earliest onset of systolic motion is typically observed in the posterobasal segment with a short delay of the other walls, resulting in synchronous longitudinal contraction and a negligible inter- and intraventricular delay. In contrast, most patients with heart failure and a conduction delay frequently show a significantly increased inter- and intraventricular delay of more than $50–100 \, ms$.[16] The prevalence of inter- and intraventricular dyssynchrony is generally higher in patients with LBBB and wide QRS prolongation; however, the correlation between the QRS width and the degree of dyssynchrony is poor. In particular, in patients with normal (less than 120 ms) or relatively narrow QRS (less than 150 ms), the intraventricular delay cannot be reliably predicted by the QRS duration alone. Thus, in this subgroup echocardiography is of particular value to identify patients with correctable inter- and intraventricular dyssynchrony.[11,16]

A similar comparison was performed by Bleeker *et al.*[17] who focused on septal and lateral peak systolic motion in the basal segments obtained by color-coded TDI (Fig. 15.5). The authors found a poor overall correlation between QRS duration and the septal–lateral peak systolic delay (SL-delay). Up to 40% of patients with a QRS width above 120 ms showed no dyssynchrony by TDI (SL-delay less than 60 ms) and almost 30% of patients with normal QRS width (less than 120 ms) presented with clear signs of dyssynchrony, defined as a SL-delay more than 60 ms. In two other publications, the same group demonstrated that the SL-delay with a cut-off value of 60–65 ms is a good predictor for identifying clinical CRT responders,[13] that the degree of baseline dyssynchrony predicts the extent of reverse remodeling during follow-up,[18] and that the im-

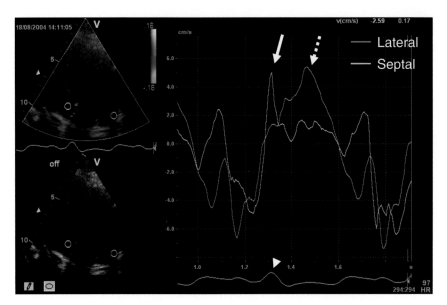

Figure 15.5 Color-coded tissue Doppler imaging in a patient with LBBB. The post-processed velocity curves from the basal septum (yellow) and the basal lateral wall (green) clearly indicate asynchronous longitudinal motion. Peak apical velocity of motion of the septum (arrow) occurs clearly before the lateral wall (dashed arrow). Arrowhead = QRS complex.

provement in ejection fraction is directly correlated to the reduction in the SL-delay.[13]

A third approach was tested by Yu *et al.*[6,14,19] who also measured the timing of regional peak systolic velocity but extended the analysis to the basal and mid segments in three apical views. From this 12-segment model they calculated the average delay from the onset of the QRS to the regional peak systolic velocity (Ts), the average of Ts from all segments, and the standard deviation of Ts (Ts-SD) as a marker for dyssynchrony. They were able to show that Ts-SD is significantly elevated in patients with heart failure and LBBB and that CRT reduces Ts-SD significantly.[6] In another series, the authors demonstrated that their dyssynchrony index Ts-SD was a good predictor for LV reverse remodeling, segregating responders (cut-off of more than 32 ms) from non-responders. Furthermore, they also confirmed that heart failure patients with normal QRS width can present with significant dyssynchrony: systolic dyssynchrony defined as a Ts-SD of more than 32 ms was found in 43% of patients with normal QRS duration and in 64% of patients with prolonged QRS of more than 120 ms.[19]

A clear disadvantage of the approach by Yu *et al.* is the time-consuming measurement of Ts in 12 different segments if the analysis is performed manually. However, new software algorithms promise a semi-automated online measure-

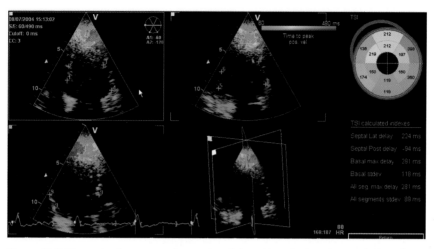

Figure 15.6 Example of a new semi-automated tissue Doppler imaging analysis tool (triplane tissue synchronization imaging, TSI). Three 2D imaging planes, corresponding to the conventional apical four-chamber, two-chamber, and long-axis views, are acquired simultaneously with a 3D matrix array transducer. Time to peak systolic velocity is automatically measured and displayed in a color-coded fashion (green, early systolic peak; yellow/red, late systolic peak). Six basal and six mid LV segments are analyzed and the calculated indices are displayed on the right side, indicating a significant delay within the left ventricle.

ment of Ts-SD from the complete LV. In combination with new matrix array transducers, a quick measurement of Ts-SD from three simultaneously acquired apical views becomes possible (Fig. 15.6).

Three-dimensional echocardiography

In an early, small study, Breithardt *et al.*[20] analyzed the effects of LBBB and CRT on LV dyssynchrony in 34 patients with heart failure and ventricular conduction delay from the Path-CHF study. A semi-automatic method for endocardial border delineation was applied to quantify the degree of LV dyssynchrony in two-dimensional (2D) echocardiographic sequences from the apical four-chamber view, thus focusing on the septal–lateral relationship. Regional wall movement curves were compared by a mathematical phase analysis, based on Fourier transformation. The resulting septal–lateral phase angle difference, a quantitative measure for intraventricular synchrony, was significantly elevated if compared with normal controls. CRT reduced the septal–lateral phase angle difference significantly and the degree of dyssynchrony before implantation of the CRT system predicted the acute hemodynamic response to optimized resynchronization therapy. An obvious limitation of this approach is the restriction to a single imaging plane. Any dyssynchrony in other walls will be overlooked and thus the precise extent of dyssynchrony cannot be measured adequately.

These limitations may be overcome by 3D echocardiography. With the introduction of real-time 3D echocardiography it is now possible to acquire 3D information more rapidly and without the necessity for time-consuming offline reconstruction. New matrix array transducers allow scanning of the complete LV within a few cardiac cycles. The acquired digital 3D data set can then be transferred to a separate workstation for offline analysis. Regional wall motion patterns can be visualized and quantified after segmentation of the LV chamber with semi-automatic contour tracing algorithms. Preliminary reports suggest that this approach enables a comprehensive analysis of LV wall motion before and during CRT with a direct comparison of endocardial wall motion between all LV segments. Segmental wall motion over time is measured in relation to a center point and can be quantitatively expressed as a regional stroke volume or ejection fraction. Preliminary experience has been reported;[21,22] however, the clinical feasibility of real-time 3D echocardiography still has to be proven.

Optimization of the atrio-ventricular delay

Atrio-ventricular synchronization is as important as resynchronizing the ventricles. In most patients a sensed AV delay in the range 100–150 ms is associated with the best hemodynamic performance. However, in some patients (approximately 25%) shorter or longer AV delays may yield better results. Thus, it is mandatory to verify that the programed AV delay (often the standard settings of the pacemaker) is beneficial and to optimize it further if necessary. Ritter *et al.*[23] proposed an algorithm for the optimization of the AV delay in patients with conventional DDD pacemakers, which requires the pacemaker to be programed to two different AV delays (short and long) and the transmitral inflow profile to be recorded at every stage. The principle is widely accepted and has been validated in small trials.[24] However, it has not been systematically validated in patients with advanced heart failure and LV-based pacing.

Most centers today use a simplified, iterative approach for AV delay optimization. The transmitral inflow is recorded at a long AV delay with complete ventricular capture, then shorter AV delays are tested until the A-wave is prematurely terminated. Finally, the shortest AV delay that produces the longest diastolic filling time without premature truncation of the A-wave is programed.

Optimization of the interventricular pacing interval (VV delay)

Modern CRT devices allow the pacing of both ventricles independently with a programable offset between RV and LV stimulation, the so-called VV-delay. This important option allows further optimization in many patients, in particular those who do not seem to benefit clinically and hemodynamically from "classic" simultaneous biventricular stimulation. Invasive hemodynamic studies have demonstrated that such a sequential stimulation protocol with individual optimization of the VV delay is associated with an approximately 10% additional absolute improvement in systolic function as measured by LV peak + dP/dt[25,26] and in improved resynchronization of wall motion.[27] In most patients, optimal resynchronization is achieved either by simultaneous stimulation (VV delay = 0) or by moderate LV pre-excitation of 20–30 ms before the RV is stimulated. In patients with an ischemic cardiomyopathy more extreme offsets of up to 60–70 ms LV pre-excitation may be required[26] and in some individuals even RV pre-excitation is superior. It should be noted, however, that the responses to sequential CRT may vary widely and depend on the presence of non-viable tissue and the individual lead position.

Echocardiographic-guided optimization of the VV delay involves the same variables that have been discussed for the assessment of dyssynchrony and for verification of CRT efficacy during follow-up. For practical purposes, a limited number of LV–RV offsets should be tested and compared, e.g. simultaneous stimulation and pre-excitation of 20, 40 and 60 ms of either ventricle. Depending on the experience of the operator and equipment, the effects can be followed either by conventional Doppler variables[25] or by TDI modalities.[27]

Conclusions

Echocardiography offers a variety of parameters that help to identify dyssynchrony, its hemodynamic impact, and the effects of resynchronization therapy. Important information can be obtained from every routine examination, but newer techniques such as TDI and — in the near future — 3D echocardiography will help to localize and quantify the degree of dyssynchrony more precisely.[28]

It is yet unclear whether a single echocardiographic parameter will be able to serve all needs in daily clinical practice: to identify the ideal candidate, to verify CRT efficacy, and to optimize CRT settings during follow-up. However, there is certainly enough firm evidence already to select a good CRT candidate and to verify CRT efficacy if all the available echocardiographic information on hemodynamics and mechanics is combined and correctly interpreted.

References

1 Cassidy DM, Vassallo JA, Marchlinski FE, Buxton AE, Untereker WJ, Josephson ME. Endocardial mapping in humans in sinus rhythm with normal left ventricles: activation patterns and characteristics of electrograms. *Circulation* 1984;**70**:37–42.

2 Little WC, Reeves RC, Arciniegas J, Katholi RE, Rogers EW. Mechanism of abnormal interventricular septal motion during delayed left ventricular activation. *Circulation* 1982;**65**:1486–91.

3 Vassallo JA, Cassidy DM, Marchlinski FE, *et al*. Endocardial activation of left bundle branch block. *Circulation* 1984;**69**:914–23.

4 Grines CL, Bashore TM, Boudoulas H, Olson S, Shafer P, Wooley CF. Functional abnormalities in isolated left bundle branch block: the effect of interventricular asynchrony. *Circulation* 1989;**79**:845–53.

5 Pitzalis MV, Iacoviello M, Romito R, *et al*. Cardiac resynchronization therapy tailored

by echocardiographic evaluation of ventricular asynchrony. *J Am Coll Cardiol* 2002; **40**:1615–22.

6 Yu CM, Chau E, Sanderson JE, *et al*. Tissue Doppler echocardiographic evidence of reverse remodeling and improved synchronicity by simultaneously delaying regional contraction after biventricular pacing therapy in heart failure. *Circulation* 2002;**105**: 438–45.

7 Breithardt OA, Stellbrink C, Franke A, *et al*. Acute effects of cardiac resynchronization therapy on left ventricular Doppler indices in patients with congestive heart failure. *Am Heart J* 2002;**143**:34–44.

8 Bargiggia GS, Bertucci C, Recusani F, *et al*. A new method for estimating left ventricular dP/dt by continuous wave Doppler echocardiography: validation studies at cardiac catheterization. *Circulation* 1989;**80**:1287–92.

9 Oguz E, Dagdeviren B, Bilsel T, *et al*. Echocardiographic prediction of long-term response to biventricular pacemaker in severe heart failure. *Eur J Heart Fail* 2002;**4**: 83–90.

10 Sogaard P, Egeblad H, Kim W, *et al*. Tissue Doppler imaging predicts improved systolic performance and reversed left ventricular remodeling during long-term cardiac resynchronization therapy. *J Am Coll Cardiol* 2002;**40**:723–30.

11 Faber L, Lamp B, Hering D, *et al*. Analyse der inter- und intraventrikulären Asynchronie mittels Fluss- und Gewebe-Dopplerechokardiographie [Analysis of inter- and intraventricular asynchrony by tissue Doppler echocardiography]. *Z Kardiol* 2003;**92**:994–1002.

12 Bax JJ, Molhoek SG, van Erven L, *et al*. Usefulness of myocardial tissue Doppler echocardiography to evaluate left ventricular dyssynchrony before and after biventricular pacing in patients with idiopathic dilated cardiomyopathy. *Am J Cardiol* 2003;**91**:94–7.

13 Bax JJ, Marwick TH, Molhoek SG, *et al*. Left ventricular dyssynchrony predicts benefit of cardiac resynchronization therapy in patients with end-stage heart failure before pacemaker implantation. *Am J Cardiol* 2003;**92**:1238–40.

14 Yu CM, Fung WH, Lin H, Zhang Q, Sanderson JE, Lau CP. Predictors of left ventricular reverse remodeling after cardiac resynchronization therapy for heart failure secondary to idiopathic dilated or ischemic cardiomyopathy. *Am J Cardiol* 2002;**91**: 684–8.

15 Schuster P, Faerestrand S, Ohm OJ. Colour tissue velocity imaging can show resynchronization of longitudinal left ventricular contraction pattern by biventricular pacing in patients with severe heart failure. *Heart* 2003;**89**:859–64.

16 Rouleau F, Merheb M, Geffroy S, *et al*. Echocardiographic assessment of the interventricular delay of activation and correlation to the QRS width in dilated cardiomyopathy. *Pacing Clin Electrophysiol* 2001;**24**:1500–6.

17 Bleeker GB, Schalij MJ, Molhoek SG, *et al*. Relationship between QRS duration and left ventricular dyssynchrony in patients with end-stage heart failure. *J Cardiovasc Electrophysiol* 2004;**15**:544–9.

18 Bax JJ, Bleeker GB, Marwick TH, *et al*. Left ventricular dyssynchrony predicts response and prognosis after cardiac resynchronization therapy. *J Am Coll Cardiol* 2004;**44**:1834–40.

19 Yu CM, Lin H, Zhang Q, Sanderson JE. High prevalence of left ventricular systolic and diastolic asynchrony in patients with congestive heart failure and normal QRS duration. *Heart* 2003;**89**:54–60.

20 Breithardt OA, Stellbrink C, Kramer AP, *et al*. Echocardiographic quantification of left

ventricular asynchrony predicts an acute hemodynamic benefit of cardiac resynchronization therapy. *J Am Coll Cardiol* 2002;**40**:536–45.

21 Kapetanakis S, Cooklin M, Monaghan MJ. Mechanical resynchronization in biventricular pacing illustrated by real-time transthoracic three-dimensional echocardiography. *Heart* 2004;**90**:482.

22 Franke A, Breithardt OA, Rulands D, Sinha AM, Kuhl HP, Stellbrink C. Quantitative
analysis of regional left ventricular wall motion patterns in patients with cardiac resynchronization therapy using real-time 3D echocardiography [Abstract]. *Circulation*
2003;**108**(Suppl S):2231.

23 Ritter P, Dib JC, Mahaux V, *et al*. New method for determing the optimal atrioventricular delay in patients paced in DDD mode for complete atrioventricular block [Ab-
stract]. *PACE* 1995;**18**:855.

24 Kindermann M, Fröhlig G, Doerr T, Schieffer H. Optimizing the AV delay in DDD
pacemaker patients with high degree AV block: mitral valve Doppler versus imped-
ance cardiography. *PACE* 1997;**20**:2453–62.

25 van Gelder BM, Bracke FA, Meijer A, Lakerveld LJ, Pijls NH. Effect of optimizing the
VV interval on left ventricular contractility in cardiac resynchronization therapy. *Am
J Cardiol* 2004;**93**:1500–3.

26 Perego GB, Chianca R, Facchini M, *et al*. Simultaneous vs. sequential biventricular
pacing in dilated cardiomyopathy: an acute hemodynamic study. *Eur J Heart Fail*
2003;**5**:305–13.

27 Sogaard P, Egeblad H, Pedersen AK, *et al*. Sequential versus simultaneous biventricular resynchronization for severe heart failure: evaluation by tissue Doppler imaging.
Circulation 2002;**106**:2078–84.

28 Bax JJ, Ansalone G, Breithardt OA, *et al*. Echocardiographic evaluation of cardiac resynchronization therapy: ready for routine clinical use? A critical appraisal. *J Am Coll
Cardiol* 2004;**44**:1–9.

CHAPTER 16

Hypertrophic cardiomyopathy

Petros Nihoyannopoulos

Introduction

Definitions

Cardiomyopathies are heart muscle conditions of no apparent cause. Cardiomyopathies are typically divided in four categories depending on morphologic and functional characteristics:

1 Hypertrophic
2 Dilated
3 Restrictive
4 Arhythmogenic right ventricular

However, this classification is based on the morphologic and functional characterization of genetically defined disease and patients often present with a combination of appearances. It is therefore possible that a patient with hypertrophic cardiomyopathy (HCM) may deteriorate in the long term and become dilated or even restrictive.

HCM is currently defined as an inherited, primary disease of the heart muscle characterized by ventricular hypertrophy, impaired diastolic function, and vigorous ventricular contraction in the absence of a cardiac or systemic cause.[1–3] There are several genes and hundreds of mutations that have been identified, involving primarily the sarcomeric proteins of the heart. This makes the condition genetically heterogeneous so it could include several disease entities.

Pathophysiology

Functional abnormalities include a forceful, ventricular contraction often with complete emptying, achieving an ejection fraction of 80–100%. The powerful contraction and complete emptying of the ventricle often occurs in association with intraventricular pressure gradients. When the gradient is subaortic, it occurs in association with a systolic anterior movement of the mitral valve (SAM). Gradients may be persistent at rest, labile (spontaneously variable), or appear only on provocation, and do not correlate with prognosis. Although initially HCM was thought to be mainly a disorder of left ventricular systolic function, it is now recognized that the main problem lies in diastole with impaired ventricular relaxation.

It has become progressively more difficult to define diagnostic limits of patients with "unexplained left ventricular hypertrophy," mainly because of the inability to exclude the disease unless a genetic screen is performed. The result has been that the clinical spectrum of HCM has widened with great heterogeneity of age, clinical presentation and natural history, and underscores the need to define the molecular basis of the condition. Until then, idiopathic hypertrophy represents the cornerstone of clinical diagnosis.

Diagnosis

The diagnosis of HCM is based upon the demonstration of unexplained, left ventricular hypertrophy producing a small, non-compliant, vigorously contracting left ventricle. The clinical findings of dyspnea, chest pain, dizziness, or syncope are the most frequent symptoms that lead to a discovery of HCM but they are present in only half of patients. In the remainder, particularly in children and adolescents, the diagnosis is made as a result of family screening or following the discovery of a murmur, or the electrocardiographic evidence of left ventricular hypertrophy. The wide use of echocardiography has brought to light many instances of HCM in patients thought to have had innocent murmurs, mitral valve prolapse, coronary artery disease, or normal hearts. The most dreaded symptom is sudden cardiac death. In a large study, Maron *et al.*[4] showed that 46% of patients who died suddenly were entirely asymptomatic and sudden death was the first manifestation of the disease.

The role of echocardiography

The diagnosis of HCM is made on the basis of the echocardiographic appearance of left ventricular hypertrophy in the absence of an underlying cause. However, echocardiography should have a supportive role in the clinical diagnosis of HCM, as the diagnosis of the condition is clinical and requires the exclusion of other causes of left ventricular hypertrophy.

The original M-mode recording techniques were invaluable in describing the early diagnostic criteria for HCM:

1 The presence of asymmetric hypertrophy of the ventricular septum (ASH), defined as the ratio of septal and posterior left ventricular wall thickness at end-diastole of ≥1.3 cm[5]

2 The systolic anterior motion of the mitral valve (SAM)

3 The premature, mid-systolic closure of the aortic valve in the presence of a small and vigorously contracting left ventricle (Fig. 16.1)

An inherent disadvantage of M-mode echocardiography, however, is that only a small section of the left ventricle can be examined with a single ultrasound beam, usually passing through the anterior septum and posterior walls. Patients with HCM may show a wide distribution of ventricular hypertrophy.

Two-dimensional echocardiography produces whole anatomic sections of the heart so that the true size and shape of the valves and cavities may be appreciated. The presence of ASH is not a prerequisite for the diagnosis of HCM. Other conditions such as systemic hypertension, athlete's heart, or even aortic steno-

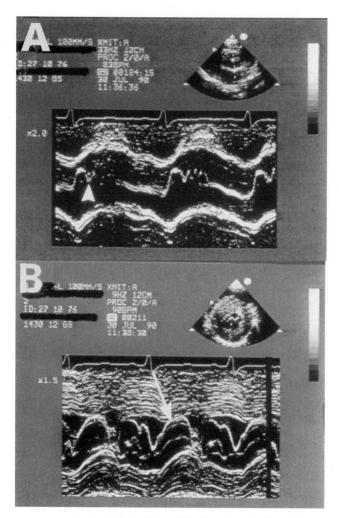

Figure 16.1 A representative M-mode echocardiogram from a patient with hypertrophic cardiomyopathy (HCM) highlighting the four main echocardiographic features of the condition. (A) Mid-systolic closure of the aortic valve (arrowhead). (B) Systolic anterior motion of the mitral valve (arrow) and asymmetric left ventricular hypertrophy together with a small, vigorously contracting left ventricle.

sis can cause the ventricular septum to appear thicker than the left ventricular free wall and, conversely, in many patients with HCM the septum and the free wall may be of similar thickness (concentric hypertrophy). The recent recognition of a group of patients with HCM but without left ventricular hypertrophy[5] has demolished the last cornerstone of a firm echocardiographic diagnosis of the condition.

The parasternal long-axis view is important in the visualization of the ventricular septum, left ventricular outflow tract, together with the mitral appara-

Figure 16.2 Two-dimensional echocardiogram of the parasternal long-axis view of the left ventricle in diastole showing marked ventricular septal hypertrophy, small end-diastolic dimensions (41 mm). Note that the mitral valve is impinging the ventricular septum (arrow). At the point of contact with the ventricular septum the anterior mitral leaflet and the endocardial surface of the septum are more echogenic, implying fibrosis.

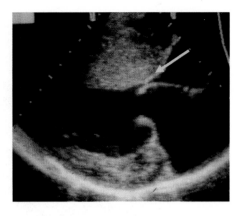

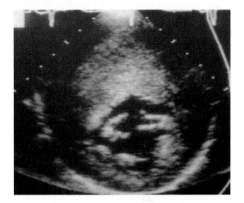

Figure 16.3 Short-axis parasternal view of a HCM patient with marked septal hypertrophy and normal posterior wall at mid-ventricular level.

tus (Fig. 16.2). It is the view of choice for the visualization of SAM of the mitral valve and mid-systolic closure of the aortic valve. While M-mode provides a better temporal resolution, two-dimensional echocardiography provides better spatial resolution. High-frequency phenomena, such as SAM and mid-systolic closure of the aortic valve, can thus be better appreciated using M-mode tracings.

Parasternal short-axis view is useful to localize and describe the extent of ventricular hypertrophy (Fig. 16.3). Serial parasternal short-axis views are crucial for the definition of the extent and shape of left ventricular hypertrophy. They provide the opportunity to determine whether segmental hypertrophy exists in other areas of the left ventricle, such as the posterior septum, anterolateral free wall, and posterolateral free wall. From these serial short-axis views the left ventricle can be divided into four segments at mitral and papillary muscle level and two at the apex, so that the anterior, lateral inferior, and posterior septal walls can be measured (Fig. 16.4). Thus, by combining the parasternal long- and short-axis views, the left ventricular walls can be examined comprehensibly and the localization and extent of ventricular hypertrophy can be fully

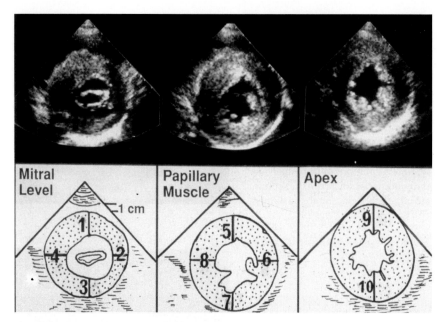

Figure 16.4 Serial short-axis, cross-sectional views of the left ventricle at mitral valve, papillary muscles level and apex, demonstrating the segments of myocardial wall measured routinely in patients with hypertrophic cardiomyopathy.

described. Occasionally, members of the same families with HCM may manifest a similar pattern of ventricular hypertrophy. Echocardiographic imaging of the right ventricle is also important, as approximately one-third of patients with HCM may have right ventricular hypertrophy.[6]

Echocardiographically, HCM is a condition characterized by:

1 Hypertrophy of all (concentric) or a portion of the left ventricular walls, that is, ventricular septum (asymmetric), or apex (distal)
2 Dilated left atrium
3 Small, non-dilated ventricles
4 Absence of any other cardiac or systemic condition producing hypertrophy (aortic stenosis—valvular, subvalvular, supravalvular, coarctation, systemic hypertension, renal failure, amyloidosis)
5 Normal or super-normal (vigorous) ventricular contraction in the absence of other hyperdynamic states (fever, pregnancy, hyperthyroidism)

Associated findings such as SAM or mid-systolic closure of the aortic valve should not be considered diagnostic. When all the echocardiographic features are present, together with the suggestive clinical picture, a firm diagnosis of HCM can be made. When only a number of these findings is present, the diagnosis can only be made after exclusion of other causes of ventricular hypertrophy.

Patterns of ventricular hypertrophy

Asymmetric septal hypertrophy (ASH) is the most frequent form of left ventricular hypertrophy and has been regarded as the hallmark of HCM. Although this hypertrophy usually involves the basal anterior septum to a variable extent and severity, it may also involve the apical, mid, or posterior septum in isolation.[7] ASH may be confined to the most proximal septum as a discrete "tumor-like" swelling in an otherwise normal ventricular septum. Variations in ventricular hypertrophy in HCM emphasize the need to obtain serial parasternal short-axis views at multiple levels along the left ventricle, so that the complete distribution of the ventricular hypertrophy can be ascertained.

Concentric or symmetrical left ventricular hypertrophy is also frequently seen in patients with HCM and when this occurs the echocardiographic differentiation from secondary causes of left ventricular hypertrophy such as systemic hypertension, cardiac amyloidosis, or "athlete's heart," may be difficult (Fig. 16.5).

Predominantly distal (apical) distribution of left ventricular hypertrophy is also found in a substantial number of patients (Fig. 16.6). Japanese authors indicate that patients with giant, negative T-waves have hypertrophy confined to the left ventricular apex, mild symptoms, and few adverse prognostic features.[8] This distribution of hypertrophy characteristically creates a spade-like deformity of the left ventricular cavity during diastole and this is well seen by two-dimensional echocardiography from the apical four-chamber projection.

HCM is seen with increasing frequency in the elderly. However, few patients have the "classic" clinical and echocardiographic features with left ventricular outflow tract gradient. Others are discovered incidentally while undergoing investigations of coronary artery disease and yet others have been discovered during investigation of hypertension. An association of elderly patients with HCM and mitral annular calcification has also been reported.[9] These patients also tend to have an angulated ventricular septum. The prognosis of these patients is

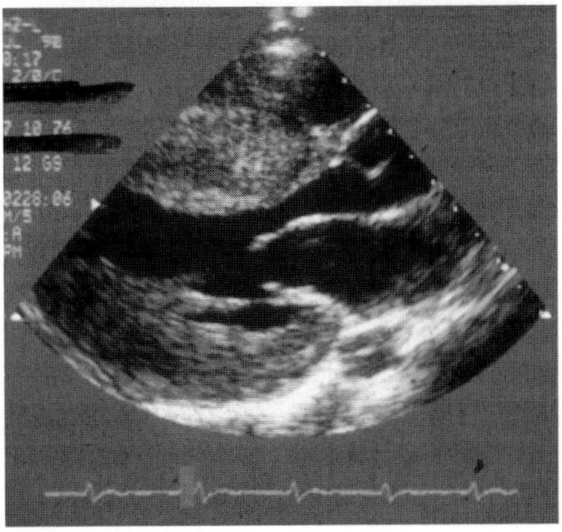

Figure 16.5 Parasternal long-axis view from a patient with HCM of the concentric type. Note that both the septum and the posterior wall are of similar thickness.

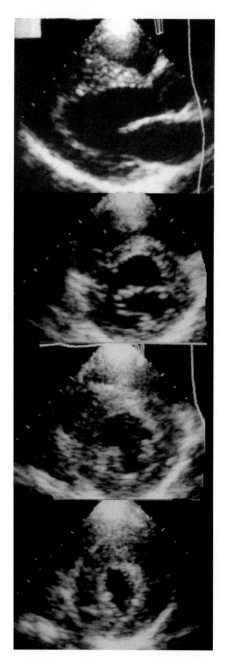

Figure 16.6 Parasternal long-axis and serial parasternal short-axis views of the left ventricle from a patient with hypertrophic cardiomyopathy of the apical type. Note that the wall thickness is normal at the base (upper panel), marginally thickened (13 mm) at papillary muscle level (middle panel) and clearly hypertrophied (22 mm) at the apex.

good, because they have survived the test of time, and it can be argued whether this patient group really represents the same disease.

Diagnostic difficulties

Patients with HCM present great phenotypic and genotypic heterogeneity. It is therefore reasonable to consider that no single diagnostic technique is currently sufficient to cover the entire spectrum of the disease and many clinical, electrocardiographic, and echocardiographic skills are needed to diagnose HCM.

It is important to investigate suspected cases of HCM in order to exclude the diagnosis, particularly in high-risk families. Although the absence of ventricular hypertrophy can, in most instances, be sufficient to exclude the diagnosis of HCM, in some cases showing mild, perhaps localized hypertrophy and good ventricular function it may be very difficult to exclude the diagnosis.

Although two-dimensional echocardiography is the diagnostic tool of choice, other entities that simulate HCM must be recognized. These include misinterpretations of normal variants of left ventricular shape, or can be caused by oblique longitudinal sections of the left ventricle (off-axis views) and the presence of other causes leading to ventricular hypertrophy. ASH may be a sensitive marker for HCM, but it is not specific for this condition.

One should be aware of the possible false diagnosis of asymmetrical septal hypertrophy when acute angulation of the ventricular septum occurs (sigmoid septum) (Fig. 16.7). In the elderly population the ventricular septum tends to continue from the anterior aortic wall in an acute angle, so that it easily gives the false impression of a localized subaortic septal thickening when viewed from left parasternal projections. Such angulation appears to form a localized septal thickening at the proximal portion of the anterior septum, particularly when the M-mode beam transects the septum at this level and can easily be misinterpreted as ASH and thus HCM. Left ventricular wall thickening, small outflow

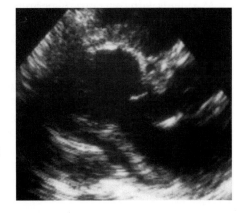

Figure 16.7 Parasternal long-axis view from an 81-year-old patient with a markedly angulated ventricular septum. Note that the very proximal portion of the septum is sharply angled towards the left ventricle outflow which risks being misinterpreted as hypertrophic cardiomyopathy.

tract dimensions, and a small incomplete SAM may complete the illusion of HCM.

ASH is relatively common in infants with congenital heart disease. The overall prevalence of disproportionate septal hypertrophy in one study was 10% and exceeded 20% in patients with pulmonary stenosis or pulmonary hypertension.

ASH may occur in conditions causing thinning or thickening of the left ventricular posterior wall relative to the septum. This abnormal septum to posterior wall thickness ratio is commonly encountered in patients with coronary artery disease either because of segmental hypertrophy of the septum (i.e. secondary to systemic hypertension) or, more commonly, as a result of transmural myocardial infarction of the posterior wall, causing thinning that produces an abnormal ratio even in the presence of normal septal thickness.

Concentric hypertrophy is the predominant pattern in secondary left ventricular hypertrophy. Patients with hypertensive heart disease, aortic stenosis, cardiac amyloidosis, and chronic renal failure show predominant concentric hypertrophy and may have echocardiograms with an appearance mimicking that of HCM with or without a gradient. The vigorous left ventricular systolic contraction, however, seen in HCM should, in the majority of cases, differentiate patients with HCM from those with cardiac infiltration where ventricular contraction is depressed. There is a subset of patients with small left ventricular cavity, moderate left ventricular hypertrophy, and hyperdynamic systolic function secondary to long-standing systemic hypertension. These patients are usually elderly and may exhibit a systolic anterior motion of the mitral valve, an outflow tract gradient, and impaired diastolic function. In practice, the diagnosis of HCM should not be made in these patients because the hypertrophy is secondary to a known aetiology. It is conceivable, however, to have a common disease such as systemic hypertension in association with a rare cardiac condition such as hypertrophic cardiomyopathy, in which case the differential diagnosis is extremely difficult clinically and should be avoided. Future genetic markers may perhaps be able to differentiate the two conditions.

Cardiac amyloidosis may occasionally prove difficult to differentiate from HCM patients with concentric hypertrophy, particularly at an early stage of the disease. Both may show a similar degree of concentric left and right ventricular hypertrophy and the described "sparkling" myocardial texture lacks specificity for cardiac amyloidosis. The depressed systolic function in cardiac amyloidosis usually contrasts well with the usual vigorous ventricular contraction seen in HCM. The thickened valves and atrial septum (with amyloid infiltration) may on occasion be of some help in the differential diagnosis. A low-voltage electrocardiogram in patients with cardiac amyloidosis will add to the differential diagnosis but cardiac biopsy will conclusively differentiate the two conditions.

Another major diagnostic difficulty occurs in some athletes who present with symmetric or even asymmetric left ventricular hypertrophy involving the septum more than the free wall. Ventricular hypertrophy may represent either a physiologic adaptation with more hypertrophy than usual or abnormal hypertrophy because of underlying HCM, putting the patient at risk for sudden death.

Regular intake of anabolic steroids, combined with intense isometric exercise, may lead to a further increase in left ventricular wall thickness in relation to internal ventricular dimensions[10] overshadowing an underlying primary myocardial disorder. The discrimination between HCM and physiologic adaptation often lies in the cavity dimensions rather than in the wall thickness, whether asymmetric or not. In HCM, the cavity dimensions tend to be at the lower end of the normal limits, particularly at end-systole, whereas the athlete is vagotonic with resting bradycardia and the ventricular dimensions are at the upper normal limits. Recent echocardiographic modalities using tissue Doppler and myocardial velocity gradients may more easily discriminate physiologic hypertrophy from pathologic hypertrophy of the heart.

The mitral apparatus

The mitral apparatus is visualized in its integrity from parasternal and apical long-axis as well as parasternal short-axis projections and these represent the optimal views for the visualization and assessment of SAM.

There are three hypotheses evoking the mechanisms of SAM:
1 Venturi effect, resulting in the mitral valve cusp being aspirated into the relatively low pressure chamber by the high velocity of blood flow through the left ventricular outflow tract
2 Abnormal mitral valve cusp apposition at the onset of systole in association with a small left ventricular cavity
3 Abnormal positioning of the papillary muscles, which are displaced forward and medially during systole in association with a small left ventricular cavity

Whatever the mechanism of SAM might be, its presence is not pathognomonic of HCM. This motion of the mitral valve can also occur whenever there is a small, hypertrophied left ventricle in association with a hyperdynamic ejection. SAM is also common in elderly patients with an angled septum or hypertensive heart, especially when preload and afterload have been reduced by diuretics. Similarly, the absence of SAM does not preclude the diagnosis of HCM.

The aortic valve

Early closure of the aortic valve is thought to occur when the left ventricular outflow tract gradient peaks in mid-to-late systole. Like SAM, mid-systolic closure of the aortic valve is non-specific and may be seen in other conditions such as discrete subaortic stenosis as well as in any hyperdynamic left ventricle.

Rarely, patients with HCM have aortic incompetence. This may be the result of annular distortion or of wear and tear of the cusps leading to aortic regurgitation. This valvular degeneration may become the site of vegetations should bacteremia be produced and therefore prevention should be instituted. The murmur of aortic regurgitation is usually soft and short and the regurgitation is only mild.

Doppler echocardiography

The addition of Doppler modalities to two-dimensional echocardiography has provided comprehensive hemodynamic assessment of HCM patients. Pulsed wave Doppler is particularly useful in the assessment of left ventricular filling. Systolic events are predominantly characterized by the presence of increased intraventricular velocities and the presence or absence of gradient. Continuous wave Doppler is a reliable method for measuring the peak systolic pressure drop (gradient) across the left ventricular outflow tract using the simplified Bernoulli equation ($\Delta P = 4V^2$). Color flow imaging complements the anatomic information obtained by two-dimensional echocardiography and facilitates further understanding of the underlying pathophysiologic changes occurring in HCM.

Diastolic events

The basic functional disorder in HCM occurs during diastole with impaired relaxation, filling, and compliance of the ventricles. Far from being uniform, myocardial dysfunction is patchy and irregular, depending upon the extent and distribution of the myofibrillar lesions.

Diastolic velocity waveforms are recorded with pulsed wave Doppler by positioning the sample volume at the tips of the mitral valve during diastole. Appleton et al.[11] demonstrated several patterns of left ventricular diastolic filling in a variety of different cardiac diseases dependent upon the interrelation of left ventricular relaxation, left atrial pressure, and intrinsic left ventricular chamber stiffness. In HCM, the period during which the heart is isovolumic is often prolonged, left ventricular filling is slow, and the proportion of filling volume resulting from atrial systole may be increased. These pathophysiologic changes are reflected in the pulsed wave Doppler recording of the transmitral waveform. Impaired ventricular relaxation results in prolonged isovolumic relaxation time, slower early ventricular filling (E wave), and a compensatory exaggerated atrial systolic filling (A wave), in patients with normal left atrial pressure, so that the ratio E/A is reduced (Fig. 16.8).

In more severe cases, with increased left atrial pressure (more than 15 mmHg), the extent of rapid filling is increased, with a consequent reduction of the atrial contribution, giving the wrong impression of "normalization" of left ventricular filling (pseudonormalized). More advanced still, with decreased compliance and high left ventricular filling pressures, there is accelerated rapid early filling and normal or reduced late filling similar to patients with restrictive physiology.

These Doppler diastolic parameters are sensitive but lack specificity because they may be influenced by multiple factors, including the intrinsic properties of the cardiac muscle and loading conditions of the heart as well as heart rate and the patient's age. Although heart rate and arterial pressure have important influences on left ventricular diastolic filling, it is the interplay between left atrial pressure at mitral valve opening, mitral regurgitation, left ventricular relaxation, and chamber stiffness that determine the rate and extent of early and late diastolic filling.

Color flow imaging can distinguish the high presystolic inflow velocity (A wave) from the lower velocity of the early diastolic filling flow (E wave) by the

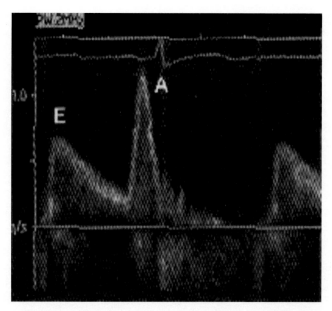

Figure 16.8 A typical transmitral velocity profile from a patient with HCM. Note the reduced E-wave velocity with prolonged deceleration time and a compensatory increase of the A-wave (impaired relaxation). This is the earliest diastolic abnormality that occurs in such patients and may not be associated with breathlessness.

increased brightness of the red–orange color occurring in late diastole, which also often aliases. Because patients with HCM usually have small left ventricular cavity dimensions, the higher velocity in late diastole may be seen into the left ventricular cavity and even on occasions reach the cardiac apex.

Systolic events

The systolic events may be categorized into two groups: those occurring in the left ventricular cavity and outflow tract in which the highlight is the gradient; and in the presence of mitral regurgitation.

Intraventricular flow velocity

Doppler echocardiography has been used to measure pressure gradients across stenotic valves. This has also be proven to be valid for calculating the dynamic gradient across the left ventricular outflow tract in patients with HCM. In contrast to fixed obstruction, the flow velocity profile in patients with HCM gradually increases and only reaches maximal velocity in late systole (Fig. 16.9). If there is no high velocity in the left ventricular outflow tract at rest, the late-peaking velocity contour may be brought out in some patients with provocative maneuvers following amyl nitrate inhalation, or during a Valsalva maneuver. The velocity contour reflects both the timing and the magnitude of the pressure drop across the left ventricular outflow tract.

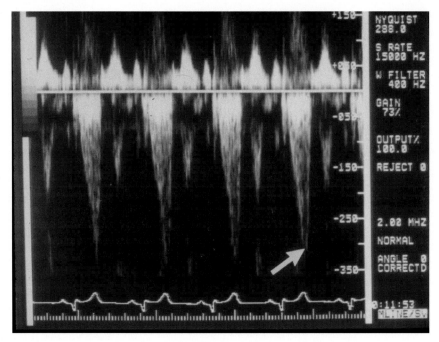

Figure 16.9 Continuous wave Doppler directed across the left ventricular outflow tract showing the characteristic delayed systolic peak (arrow) of the velocity waveform. In this patient the peak velocity was 3.2 m s^{-1} reflecting a pressure gradient of 42 mmHg.

Color flow imaging can identify the uniformity or the non-uniformity of the intraventricular flow. In patients with HCM, the intraventricular color flow map during systole is characterized by a non-homogeneous blue color with a lighter hue compared with normals and typically aliases at mid-ventricular level, at the level of the hypertrophied papillary muscles or at the level of the mitral valve. When SAM occurs, the systolic flow at this level becomes turbulent with a "mosaic" color pattern (Fig. 16.10). When the flow crosses the aortic valve into the ascending aorta it becomes laminar again with homogeneous red color, as seen from the suprasternal window (flow moving towards the transducer).

Mitral regurgitation

Mitral regurgitation is a well-recognized component of the complex pathophysiology encountered in patients with HCM. Its association with SAM of the mitral valve and the magnitude of the intraventricular gradient has also been well documented.[12] Patients who do not present with SAM of the mitral valve rarely present with mitral regurgitation.

Color flow imaging can detect the presence of mitral regurgitation with high sensitivity and specificity. When the jet is directed anteriorly it may be confused

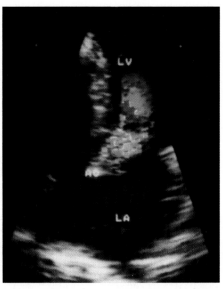

Figure 16.10 Color flow Doppler in a representative hypertrophic cardiomyopathy patient. From the apex, high-velocity systolic flow is apparent away from the transducer (light blue), passing from the middle of the left ventricle where it aliases into red color. When blood flow reaches the subaortic area, it becomes turbulent (green–yellow color) suggesting the presence of an outflow gradient.

with the turbulent jet of the left ventricular outflow tract. With continuous wave Doppler alone it can be very difficult to separate these two high velocity jets and a great deal of expertise is required in both the recording and the interpretation. The shape of the two systolic profiles is typically different, with the outflow tract velocity having a "scimitar" or "dagger" shaped late-peaking contour, as opposed to the more symmetrical velocity curve of mitral regurgitation. With color flow imaging the left ventricular outflow tract flow velocity and mitral regurgitant jet can readily be distinguished and allow for a better lining-up of the continuous wave Doppler beam and outflow tract velocity.

Predictors of prognosis

There is now evidence that the overall outcome of HCM is not that malignant but predictors of a good versus a bad outcome are not clear.

Diastolic left ventricular dysfunction, as assessed by Doppler, is particularly common in HCM patients but again these abnormalities may not be related to the patient's symptoms nor are they related to the presence of intracardiac gradients.[13] Perhaps one positive echocardiographic finding in relation to severe breathlessness would be the detection of severe mitral regurgitation.

During longitudinal studies on some patients with HCM, the development of progressive congestive heart failure can be associated with ventricular dilatation and impairment of a previously vigorous left ventricular contraction. This may also result in a progressive decrease in the ventricular gradient. Serial echocardiographic and Doppler studies could illustrate the turning point towards progressive deterioration in this subgroup of patients by demonstrating a gradual decrease in intraventricular systolic flow velocity.

Conclusions

While it is convenient to classify cardiomyopathies into four major groups, there is an overlap between the anatomic and functional characteristics in many instances. As the genetic demystification of the cardiomyopathies continues, the boundaries of the various types of cardiomyopathies may be better determined. Until that time, we should continue categorizing our patients in these four groups. HCM has a familial nature and it is important to screen family members, as often the diagnosis may be more revealing once family screening has been completed. As the causes and pathophysiology of HCM are better understood, it could be argued that the term idiopathic may no longer be sustainable.

References

1 Goodwin JF, Oakley CM. The cardiomyopathies. *Br Heart J* 1972;**34**: 545.
2 Maron BJ, Epstein SE. Hypertrophic cardiomyopathy: a discussion of the nomenclature. *Am J Cardiol* 1979;**43**:1242–4.
3 Report of the WHO/ISFC task force on the definition and classification of cardiomyopathies. *Br Heart J* 1980;**44**:672–3.
4 Maron BJ, Roberts WC, Epstein SE. Sudden death in hypertrophic cardiomyopathy: a profile of 78 patients. *Circulation* 1982;**65**:1388–94.
5 McKenna WJ, Nihoyannopoulos P, Davies MJ. Hypertrophic cardiomyopathy without hypertrophy: a description of two families with premature cardiac death and myocardial disarray in the absence of increased muscle mass. *Br Heart J* 1989;**61**:75.
6 McKenna WJ, Kleinebenne A, Nihoyannopoulos P, Foale R. Echocardiographic measurement of right ventricular wall thickness in hypertrophic cardiomyopathy: relation to clinical and prognostic features. *J Am Coll Cardiol* 1988;**11**:351–8.
7 Maron BJ, Gottdiener JS, Epstein SE. Patterns and significance of distribution of left ventricular hypertrophy in hypertrophic cardiomyopathy: a wide angle, two-dimensional echocardiographic study of 125 patients. *Am J Cardiol* 1981;**48**:418–28.
8 Yamaguchi H, Ishimura T, Nishiyama S, *et al.* Hypertrophic non-obstructive cardiomyopathy with giant, negative T-waves (apical hypertrophy); ventricular and echocardiographic features in 30 patients. *Am J Cardiol* 1979;**44**:401–12.
9 Kronzon I, Glassman E. Mitral ring calcification in idiopathic hypertrophic subaortic stenosis. *Am J Cardiol* 1978;**42**:60–6.
10 Urhausen A, Holpes R, Kindermann W. One and two dimensional echocardiography in bodybuilders using anabolic steroids. *Eur J Appl Physiol* 1989;**58**:633–40.
11 Appleton CP, Hatle LK, Popp RL. Relation of transmitral flow velocity patterns to left ventricular function: new insights from a combined hemodynamic and Doppler echocardiographic study. *J Am Coll Cardiol* 1988;**12**:426–40.
12 Yonezawa Y, Nihoyannopoulos P, McKenna WJ, Doi YL, Ozawa T. Mitral regurgitation in hypertrophic cardiomyopathy: a color Doppler echocardiographic study. *Am J Noninvasive Cardiol* 1988;**2**:195–8.
13 Maron BJ, Bonow RO, Canon RO III, Leon MD, Epstein SE. Hypertrophic cardiomyopathy: interrelation of clinical manifestations, pathophysiology and therapy. *N Engl J Med* 1987;**316**:780–9.

CHAPTER 17

Viability in ischemic cardiomyopathy

Gabe B. Bleeker, Jeroen J. Bax, and Ernst E. van der Wall

Case Presentation

A 62-year-old male patient experienced a gradual decline in exercise capacity over the last 2 years, and presented with heart failure symptoms according to New York Heart Association Class III without angina, and a 6-min walking distance of 220 m. The patient had a history of an antero-septal and an inferior infarction, 11 and 12 years before the current presentation. Seven years before presentation this patient had undergone coronary artery bypass grafting with a LIMA-graft to the left anterior descending artery and a venous jump-graft to an intermediate branch, the obtuse marginal branch and the right posterior descending artery. The ECG showed a wide QRS complex (238 ms) with left bundle branch block. How should this patient be further evaluated?

Introduction

Over the past decades the number of patients with chronic heart failure has increased dramatically. This condition is still associated with high morbidity and mortality despite advances in medical therapy. Coronary artery disease (CAD) is in large part responsible for the increased incidence of heart failure, being the cause of heart failure in at least 70% of cases. Initially, it was thought that ischemia-induced regional and/or global left ventricular (LV) dysfunction was the result of irreversible damage of cardiac myocytes whereby improvement of myocardial dysfunction was considered impossible.

However, observational studies showed that several patients with ischemia-induced LV dysfunction exhibited improvement in regional and global LV function following coronary revascularization.[1] Since then, many studies have confirmed that LV dysfunction in CAD patients is not necessarily an irreversible process. Both regional contraction and global LV function (LV ejection fraction) may markedly improve following revascularization.

In patients with ischemic heart failure, the severity of LV dysfunction is directly related to long-term survival and it was shown that improvement in LV function following revascularization was associated with a better prognosis compared with pharmacologic treatment alone. However, despite these promising results, not all patients improved in regional and/or global contractile function. The percentage improvement in contractile function following revascularization varies widely among studies, and has been reported at between 24% and 82% of all dysfunctional segments.[2] Further analysis of these patients showed that myocardial segments with improved contractility following revascularization contain cardiac myocytes that are still viable. To describe this phenomenon, the concept of "viability" was introduced.[3] Dysfunctional, but viable myocardium has the potential to regain contractile function following revascularization. On the other hand, revascularization of non-viable or scar tissue will not result in improvement of function. Moreover, it was shown that an improvement in contractile function following revascularization was associated with an increased annual survival rate. These findings have important diagnostic and therapeutic implications. Because coronary revascularization has the potential to improve LV function and increase patient survival, revascularization should be considered in every heart failure patient. However, revascularization is associated with substantial morbidity and mortality, especially in patients with impaired LV function. Therefore, it is of critical importance to select those patients who are most likely to benefit from revascularization in order to justify the procedural risks.

This chapter describes the pathophysiologic mechanisms responsible for LV dysfunction in patients with CAD and the most commonly used non-invasive imaging techniques for assessment of myocardial viability.

Stunning and hibernation

Myocardial ischemia can result in impaired myocardial function through several mechanisms. Dysfunctional but viable myocardium should be distinguished from non-viable myocardium or scar tissue. Prolonged severe ischemia of the myocardium often results in necrosis of cardiac myocytes, leading to irreversible damage of the myocardium, referred to as scar tissue.

However, ischemia does not always result in myocardial cell death. The two mechanisms responsible for reversible myocardial dysfunction in the presence of CAD are stunning and hibernation, during which the myocardium remains viable.

Stunning

The term myocardial stunning was introduced by Braunwald and Kloner[4] in 1982 to describe a temporary post-ischemic myocardial dysfunction in the presence of normal perfusion. Stunning occurs after a short-term, severe reduction or total blockage in coronary blood flow and results in decreased myocardial contraction. This dysfunction will persist for some time following the ischemic event and restoration of blood flow. Depending on the severity and the duration of ischemia, the dysfunction may persist for several hours or even days following the ischemic event. The delayed recovery of contractile function is associated with a normal myocardial perfusion and oxygen consumption, and occurs spontaneously; revascularization is therefore not indicated.

Hibernation

In contrast to stunning, which is a short-term process, myocardial hibernation is a chronic process with impaired myocardial contractile function caused by persistent (relative) reduction in coronary blood flow.

The term hibernation was popularized by Rahimtoola[3] to describe the improvement in contractility in dysfunctional myocardium following revascularization. Hibernating myocardium is caused by a chronically impaired myocardial blood flow, resulting in an imbalance between myocardial oxygen consumption and supply. Hibernation can be considered as a protective mechanism from the heart itself, because the decreased myocardial contractions will lower oxygen demand of the myocardium, which will protect the myocytes from irreversible damage (necrosis). Impaired myocardial contractions in hibernating myocardium can be partially or sometimes completely restored to normal, either by increasing myocardial blood flow or by reducing myocardial oxygen consumption. These findings led to the recognition that in hibernating myocardium, regional and global LV dysfunction is reversible through coronary revascularization.

In the literature, the terms hibernation and viability are sometimes used inconsistently. The term viable implies nothing more than that the myocardium is potentially alive irrespective of contractile function. Hibernation refers to a pathophysiologic mechanism resulting in dysfunction of the myocardium in the presence of viable myocytes.

Identification of hibernating myocardium

The presence of hibernating myocardium should be considered in every patient with CAD and regional or global LV dysfunction. Patients with mildly reduced LV function should also be evaluated as the presence and extent of myocardial hibernation do not always correlate with the severity of LV dysfunction.

Recently, several non-invasive imaging techniques for the identification of hibernating myocardium have been introduced: nuclear imaging techniques, echocardiography, and magnetic resonance imaging (MRI).

Imaging techniques

Thallium-201

Single photon emission computed tomography (SPECT) using thallium-201 was the first technique to be used for the detection of myocardial hibernation.

At first, thallium-201 was considered as a perfusion tracer, because it is dependent on regional flow for uptake in the myocardium. However, it was later found that uptake is also dependent on intact sarcolemmal membranes and adequate membrane ATP stores, and therefore it can also be considered as a marker of viability. Since thallium-201 was initially thought to reflect perfusion, perfusion defects observed immediately after injection were considered to reflect regional infarction, but some of these defects disappeared after several hours. The segments that showed a reversible thallium defect often improved after revascularization and these segments were thus an important sign of the presence of myocardial viability. This protocol is referred to as thallium-201 rest-redistribution imaging.

More recently, reinjection of a second, smaller dose of thallium-201 immediately following the redistribution images was found to improve the detection of viable tissue. This method has been shown to identify viable territories in as many as 50–70% of regions that were previously classified as scar by standard redistribution imaging. The main disadvantage of thallium is the relatively high radiation exposure for patients and hospital staff compared with newly introduced perfusion tracers.

SPECT with technetium-99m labeled tracers

The uptake and retention of technetium-99m labeled tracers is dependent on myocardial perfusion, cell membrane integrity, and mitochondrial function. Most studies for the assessment of viability have used technetium-99m sestamibi, but studies with technetium-99m tetrofosmin showed comparable results for this tracer in the assessment of viability. Most frequently, technetium-99m labeled tracers are injected under resting conditions. In these studies, dysfunctional segments with a tracer uptake of more than 50–60% are considered hibernating.[5] Compared with thallium-201, technetium-99m has a relative lack of redistribution and therefore the use of technetium-99m for the detection of hibernating myocardium requires a second injection. Technetium-labeled tracers show comparable results with thallium-201 in the prediction of hibernation. However, thallium-201 is superior to technetium-99m labeled tracers for the prediction of hibernating myocardium in patients with severely impaired ventricular function (LV ejection fraction less than 25%).

Positron emission tomography with FDG

18F-fluoro-2-deoxy-D-glucose (FDG) positron emission tomography (PET) is traditionally considered as the gold standard for viability assessment. FDG is a glucose analog that is taken up by viable cardiac myocytes in the same way as glucose, but its subsequent metabolism is blocked and it remains within the myocyte.[6] Ischemic myocardial cells utilize proportionally more glucose than non-ischemic cells. Thus, the administration of a glucose analog, FDG, in conjunction with a blood flow agent differentiates normal, hibernating, and

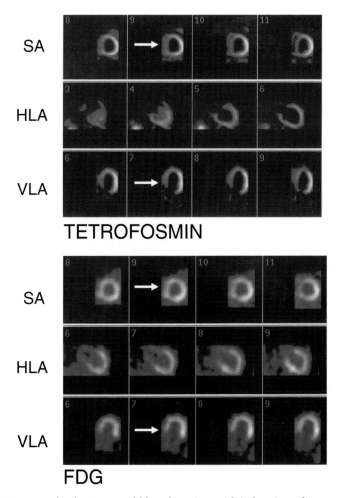

SA

HLA

VLA

TETROFOSMIN

SA

HLA

VLA

FDG

Figure 17.1 Example of a 65-year-old female patient with ischemic cardiomyopathy and hibernating myocardium (left ventricular ejection fraction 11%, end-diastolic volume 538 mL). SPECT perfusion imaging at rest (technetium-99m tetrofosmin) shows large perfusion defects in the territory of the left anterior descending coronary artery. FDG SPECT shows preserved tracer uptake in the septum (white arrows); the perfusion–FDG mismatch indicates an extensive area of hibernation, and revascularization should be considered. HLA, horizontal long axis; SA, short axis; VLA, vertical long axis.

necrotic myocardium with reasonable accuracy. Hibernating myocardium is defined as the presence of viable myocytes (enhanced FDG uptake) in regions of decreased blood flow (referred to as perfusion–FDG mismatch; Fig. 17.1). Scar tissue exhibits a concordant reduction in perfusion and FDG uptake (perfusion–FDG match; Fig. 17.2). Recently, much effort has been invested in the development of SPECT systems equipped with 511 keV collimators, in order to allow for FDG imaging. Direct comparisons between FDG PET and FDG SPECT have demonstrated excellent agreement between the two techniques for the assessment of myocardial viability.[7]

Dobutamine stress echocardiography

Dobutamine stress echocardiography evaluates the so-called contractile reserve of dysfunctional myocardium in response to inotropic agents. Hibernating myocardium will show improved contractions after administration of an inotropic agent, such as dobutamine, as assessed by simultaneous transthoracic echocardiography. Atropine may also be given to enhance the diagnostic value of this technique.

The predictive value for hibernating myocardium is highest with the occurrence of a biphasic response. At low-dose dobutamine (5 mg/kg/min) the contractile reserve is recruited, thus improving contractility, while high-dose dobutamine causes subendocardial ischemia, resulting in a reduction in contractility.[8] The accuracy of dobutamine stress echocardiography is dependent on operator experience and it is sometimes not possible to visualize each myocardial segment.

Dobutamine stress magnetic resonance imaging

Dobutamine stress MRI relies on the same principles for assessing contractile reserve as described earlier with stress echocardiography. Usually only low-dose dobutamine is used for the detection of myocardial hibernation. Hibernating segments are defined as those segments with a certain end-diastolic wall thickness (more than 5.5 mm) and evidence of dobutamine-induced systolic wall thickening (more than 1 mm). The advantages of stress MRI over stress echocardiography are the higher spatial resolution and reproducibility, but MRI is relatively time-consuming and not suitable for patients with severe claustrophobia or for patients with pacemakers.[9]

Contrast-enhanced magnetic resonance imaging

Contrast-enhanced MRI is a relatively new but increasingly popular technique for the detection of myocardial hibernation. Gadolinium-DTPA is injected, and after a period of 10–15 min areas of scarred myocardium will show hyperenhancement, whereas regions that fail to hyperenhance are considered viable. This technique is based on the fact that gadolinium-DTPA is able to exchange rapidly between intravascular space and intracellular matrix (as in scar tissue), but it does not pass through the intact cellular membrane of a viable myocyte.

Myocardial hibernation is present in those areas without hyperenhancement and a reduced contractility on cine MRI. It is considered to be more sensitive for the detection of non-transmural infarctions than other imaging modalities.

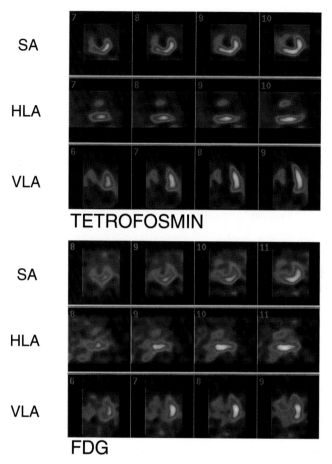

SA

HLA

VLA

TETROFOSMIN

SA

HLA

VLA

FDG

Figure 17.2 Example of a 78-year-old male patient with ischemic cardiomyopathy without hibernating myocardium (left ventricular ejection fraction 15%, end-diastolic volume 236 mL). SPECT perfusion imaging at rest using technetium-99m tetrofosmin shows large perfusion defects in the anterior, apical, and septal regions. Metabolic imaging with FDG shows a complete match with the perfusion images, indicating scar tissue; this patient will not benefit from revascularization. HLA, horizontal long axis; SA, short axis; VLA, vertical long axis.

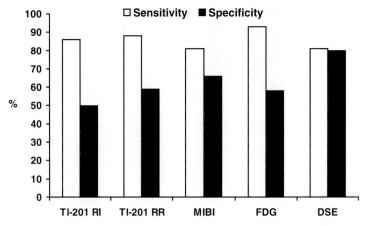

Figure 17.3 Sensitivity and specificity of several viability techniques to predict improvement in regional left ventricular function after revascularization. DSE, dobutamine stress echocardiography; FDG, F18-fluorodeoxyglucose; MIBI, sestamibi; Tl-201 RI, thallium-201 reinjection; Tl-201 RR, thallium-201 rest-redistribution. (Adapted from Bax *et al.*[2])

Contrast-enhanced MRI has the same disadvantages as described above for dobutamine stress MRI.[10]

Prediction of improvement

Each myocardial imaging technique designed for the detection of myocardial hibernation has its own benefits and limitations. FDG PET traditionally shows the highest predictive value for recovery of contractility following revascularization. However, this technique is relatively expensive, and PET scanners are not widely available. Nuclear imaging techniques based on SPECT, using thallium-201 or technetium-99m labeled agents, also show a high sensitivity but a relatively low specificity for the prediction of contractile recovery. Stress echocardiography has a somewhat lower sensitivity, but in the hands of an experienced operator, specificity is relatively high compared with other techniques (Fig. 17.3). The sensitivity and specificity of low-dose dobutamine stress MRI are reported as approximately 88% and 87%, respectively.[10] Currently, there are few data available directly comparing contrast-enhanced MRI with other viability imaging tests for its prediction of improvement following revascularization. Further large studies are needed to evaluate the use of contrast-enhanced MRI for the assessment of myocardial hibernation. However, early trials show promising results, with a sensitivity of 82% for predicting contractile recovery.

Conclusions

LV dysfunction resulting from CAD is becoming a major clinical problem in cardiology. In patients with hibernating myocardium, coronary revascularization is likely to result in improved regional contractility and global LV function. However, dysfunctional LV segments consisting of scarred myocardium will not improve in contractility. Thus, accurate assessment of patients with ischemic cardiomyopathy is required to select those patients who are likely to benefit from coronary revascularization. Accordingly, patients with LV dysfunction and a high likelihood for CAD should be screened for the presence of hibernating myocardium. Several non-invasive imaging modalities for the detection of hibernating myocardium are currently available. Each imaging modality discussed in this chapter offers a good or excellent sensitivity and specificity, and therefore the choice will largely depend on local availability, experience, and patient characteristics.

SPECT imaging with thallium-201, technetium-99m and stress echocardiography are generally considered as first-step imaging modalities. The nuclear imaging techniques based on SPECT show a somewhat higher sensitivity, but stress echocardiography offers a higher specificity.

PET scanning with FDG is traditionally considered as the gold standard for the detection of myocardial viability but, because of its high costs and limited availability, this is normally reserved for those cases in which SPECT and/or stress echocardiography are inconclusive. However, if PET scanning is readily available it is a good alternative.

Stress MRI will normally be reserved for those patients in whom additional information is needed following stress echocardiography. Contrast-enhanced MRI is a relatively new technique showing promising results in recent trials, and is expected to become more popular in the future, especially when MRI becomes more widely available for cardiac patients.

Case Presentation (Continued)

Extensive evaluation of the patient with heart failure was performed. Transthoracic echocardiography showed a severely dilated left ventricle (end-systolic and end-diastolic volumes 372 and 427 mL, respectively) with a severely reduced left ventricular ejection fraction (12%), diffuse severe hypo- to akinesia and severe mitral regurgitation (Figs 17.4 and 17.5; Video clips 17 and 18 👁). Cine MRI images showed also a severely dilated left ventricle with diffuse hypo- to akinesia (Fig. 17.6; Video clips 19–21 👁). Coronary angiography showed an occlusion of the right and left anterior descending coronary arteries. The LIMA-graft and the venous jump-graft were patent, although the run-off of the LIMA-graft was poor (Figs 17.7 and 17.8; Video clips 22 and 23 👁). Next, the presence of viability was evaluated using SPECT imaging with technetium-99m tetrofosmin and FDG (Fig. 17.9). A large perfusion defect is present in the inferior wall extending to the septum and the posterolateral regions. The inferior and posterolateral regions show concordantly reduced FDG uptake, indicating scar tissue. The septum has increased FDG uptake, indicating viable tissue. A second perfusion defect is present in the anterior wall, with partially preserved FDG uptake, indicating some residual viability. Contrast-enhanced MRI confirmed the SPECT findings and showed extensive areas of hyperenhancement (white regions; Fig. 17.10) in the inferior wall, extending to part of the septum and posterolateral wall, indicating scar tissue; the anterior wall also shows partial scar tissue. Part of the septum and the lateral wall do not show hyperenhancement, and these areas thus contain viable tissue.

Based on the findings, revascularization of the septum may result in improvement of function. However, the grafts are patent, a simple percutaneous transluminal coronary angioplasty (PTCA) was technically not feasible, and a second thoracotomy for surgical revascularization could potentially damage the LIMA-graft. Accordingly, the option of revascularization was rejected. Next, echocardiography using tissue Doppler imaging was performed to assess left ventricular dyssynchrony (Fig. 17.11). Tissue Doppler imaging showed a delay in peak systolic velocity between the septum and the lateral wall (referred to as septal-to-lateral delay) of 240 ms, indicating severe left ventricular dyssynchrony (Fig. 17.12). Accordingly, the patient was referred for implantation of a biventricular pacemaker. Tissue Doppler imaging, performed immediately after pacemaker implantation, showed a dramatic reduction in left ventricular dyssynchrony, evidenced by a septal-to-lateral delay of 10 ms. Six months after implantation the patient was in New York Heart Association Class II, and the 6-min walking distance had increased to 360 m, associated with a significant reverse remodeling of the left ventricle (left ventricular end-systolic and end-diastolic volumes 309 and 389 mL, respectively).

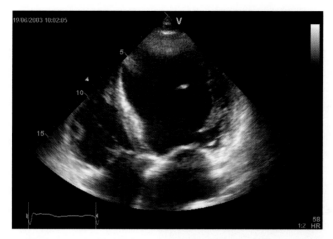

Figure 17.4 Two-dimensional transthoracic echocardiography: four-chamber view showing a severely dilated left ventricle with end-systolic and end-diastolic volumes of 372 and 427 mL, respectively; the left ventricular ejection fraction was 12%. See also Video clip 17 👁.

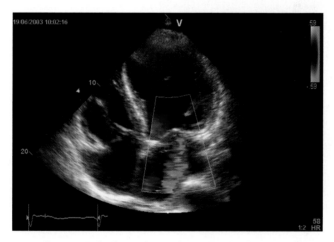

Figure 17.5 Two-dimensional echocardiography with color flow Doppler, showing severe mitral regurgitation. See also Video clip 18 👁.

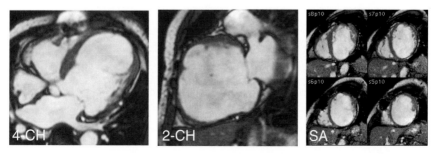

Figure 17.6 Cine MRI images showing a severely dilated left ventricle with diffuse hypo- to akinesia. 4-CH, four-chamber view (Video clip 19); 2-CH, two-chamber-view (Video clip 20); SA, short-axis view (Video clip 21) 👁.

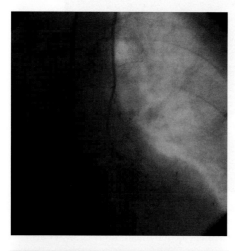

Figure 17.7 Angiography of the LIMA-graft showing patency of the graft, with a poor run-off to the left anterior descending artery. See also Video clip 22 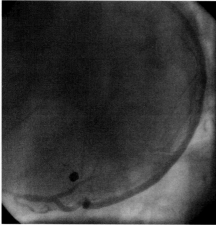.

Figure 17.8 Angiography shows patency of the venous jump-graft, with adequate run-off. See also Video clip 23.

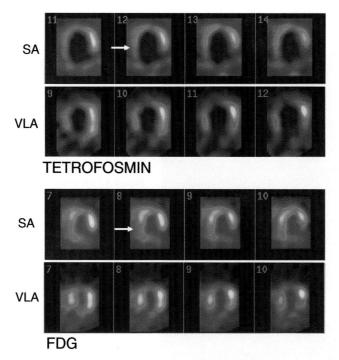

TETROFOSMIN

FDG

Figure 17.9 SPECT imaging with technetium-99m tetrofosmin and FDG SPECT showing large perfusion defects in the septum, inferior and posterolateral regions, with a mismatch pattern in the septum, indicating viability (white arrows). HLA, horizontal long axis; SA, short axis; VLA, vertical long axis.

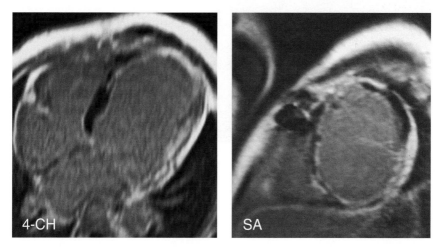

Figure 17.10 Contrast-enhanced MRI showing extensive areas of hyperenhancement (white regions) in the inferior wall, extending to part of the septum and posterolateral wall, indicating scar tissue; the anterior wall also shows partial scar tissue. Part of the septum and the lateral wall do not show hyperenhancement, and these areas thus contain viable tissue. 4-CH, four-chamber view; 2-CH, two-chamber-view; SA, short-axis.

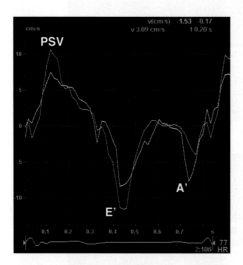

Figure 17.11 Tissue Doppler imaging. Tracing derived from a normal individual with the samples placed in the basal part of the septum (yellow curve) and the lateral wall (green curve), illustrating perfect synchrony. E' and A', diastolic parameters; PSV, peak systolic velocity.

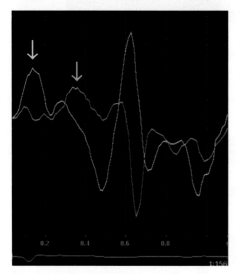

Figure 17.12 Tissue Doppler image of a patient with severe heart failure and dilated cardiomyopathy. The sample volumes are placed in the basal parts of the septum and lateral wall, and tracings are derived (yellow curve, septum; green curve, lateral wall; arrows indicate peak systolic velocity). The septal-to-lateral delay is 240 ms, indicating severe left ventricular dyssynchrony.

References

1 Chatterjee K, Swan HJC, Parmley WW, Sustaita H, Marcus HS, Matloff J. Influence of direct myocardial revascularization on left ventricular asynergy and function in patients with coronary heart disease: with and without previous myocardial infarction. *Circulation* 1973;**47**:276–86.

2 Bax JJ, Wijns W, Cornel JH, Visser FC, Boersma E, Fioretti PM. Accuracy of currently available techniques for prediction of functional recovery after revascularization in patients with left ventricular dysfunction due to chronic coronary artery disease: comparison of pooled data. *J Am Coll Cardiol* 1997;**30**:1451–60.

3 Rahimtoola SH. The hibernating myocardium. *Am Heart J* 1989;**117**:211–21.

4 Braunwald E, Kloner RA. The stunned myocardium: prolonged, postischemic ventricular dysfunction. *Circulation* 1982;**66**:1146–9.

5 Bonow RO, Dilsizian V. Thallium-201 and technetium-99m-sestamibi for assessing viable myocardium. *J Nucl Med* 1992;**33**:815–8.

6 Tillisch J, Brunken R, Marshall R, *et al*. Reversibility of cardiac wall-motion abnormalities predicted by positron emission tomography. *N Engl J Med* 1986;**314**:884–8.

7 Bax JJ, Patton JA, Poldermans D, Elhendy A, Sandler MP. 18-Fluorodeoxyglucose imaging with positron emission tomography and single photon emission computed tomography: cardiac applications. *Semin Nucl Med* 2000;**30**:281–98.

8 Cornel JH, Bax JJ, Elhendy A, *et al*. Biphasic response to dobutamine predicts improvement of global left ventricular function after surgical revascularization in patients with stable coronary artery disease: implication of time course of recovery on diagnostic accuracy. *J Am Coll Cardiol* 1998;**31**:1002.

9 Baer FM, Voth E, Schneider CA, Theissen P, Schicha H, Sechtem U. Comparison of low-dose dobutamine-gradient-echo magnetic resonance imaging and positron emission tomography with [18F] fluorodeoxyglucose in patients with chronic coronary artery disease: a functional and morphological approach to the detection of residual myocardial viability. *Circulation* 1995;**91**:1006–15.

10 Kim RJ, Wu E, Rafael A, *et al*. The use of contrast-enhanced magnetic resonance imaging to identify reversible myocardial dysfunction. *N Engl J Med* 2000;**343**:1445–53.

Section four
Uncommon entities

CHAPTER 18

Cardiac tumors

Joshua Lehrer-Graiwer and Charles B. Higgins

Introduction

Primary tumors are rare. Secondary tumors, either metastatic or direct extension of primary tumors of another organ, are about 40 times more frequent than primary cardiac tumors.

Echocardiography is the most widely used modality for the initial investigation of cardiac and paracardiac masses. It is portable, cost-effective, and provides functional information. Transesophageal echocardiography provides improved imaging of smaller masses, particularly in the atria, atrial appendages, or associated with valvular structures. Contrast-enhanced echocardiography improves visualization of intracardiac masses and contrast perfusion imaging is an emerging technique that may aid in differentiating cardiac masses. All forms of echocardiography, however, are limited in their evaluation of cardiac masses by acoustic windows and poor soft-tissue contrast.

Computed tomography (CT) and magnetic resonance imaging (MRI) can determine the presence and extent of cardiac and paracardiac tumors. These modalities, especially MRI, can also provide characterization of the mass. Although CT may be adequate for the evaluation of cardiac and paracardiac masses, MRI is usually employed for this purpose. Consequently, this chapter focuses upon the findings of MRI.

Because of a wide field of view, which encompasses the cardiovascular structures, mediastinum, and adjacent lung simultaneously, CT and MRI can display the intracardiac and extracardiac extent of tumors. In addition, the capability of imaging in multiple planes makes MRI especially suited for the demarcation of the spatial relationship of a mass to cardiac and mediastinal structures. The multiplanar approach overcomes the volume averaging problem at the diaphragmatic interface encountered with a solely transaxial imaging technique such as CT. These features permit a clear delineation of the possible infiltration of a mass lesion into cardiac and adjacent mediastinal structures. In addition, MRI allows the assessment of functional parameters, such as ventricular wall thickening, ejection fraction, or flow velocity in adjacent vessels. Therefore, the impact of a tumor on cardiovascular function can be evaluated.

In clinical practice, MRI is most often used to verify or exclude a possible mass suggested initially by echocardiography. Echocardiography clearly depicts cardiac morphology and provides an assessment of functional parameters.

However, the effectiveness of transthoracic echocardiography is limited by the acoustic window, which may depend upon obesity or lung disease. Transesophageal echocardiography overcomes this problem but is semi-invasive. The soft-tissue contrast achieved with echocardiography remains limited in comparison with that obtained with MRI. Although definitive differentiation between benign and malignant tumors is not always feasible by MRI, the combination of imaging characteristics of a cardiac mass may render a specific tissue diagnosis highly probably in some cases.

Techniques

Computed tomography

Multislice or spiral single-slice CT scans in the axial plane after contrast enhancement is used to identify and determine the extent of masses. For this evaluation, electron beam CT or retrospectively electrocardiography (ECG) gated multislice CT acquisition are optimal but not essential. Collimation is usually 5 mm. Retrospective reconstruction of volumetric data in the sagittal or coronal plane may be useful.

Magnetic resonance imaging

ECG-gated transaxial T1-weighted spin-echo images of the entire thorax are initially acquired for the evaluation of suspected cardiac or paracardiac masses. In addition, such images are frequently acquired in the sagittal or coronal plane to delineate the regions that are displayed suboptimally in the transaxial plane, such as the diaphragmatic surface of the heart. Contrast between intramural tumor and normal myocardium may be low on non-enhanced T1-weighted images. Transaxial T2-weighted spin-echo images are acquired to enhance the contrast between myocardium and tumor tissue, which usually has a longer T2 relaxation time, and to delineate possible cystic or necrotic components of a mass. The comparison of signal intensities of a mass lesion on T1-weighted and T2-weighted images may allow tissue characterization. The administration of Gd-DTPA (gadolinium diethylenetriamine penta-acetic acid) usually improves the contrast between tumor tissue and myocardium on T1-weighted images and may facilitate tissue characterization. Hyperenhancement of tumor tissue with MR contrast agents indicates either a high degree of vascularity of the mass or an enlarged extracellular space of tumor tissue in comparison with normal myocardium.

In patients with cardiac tumors, cine MRI provides valuable information regarding the movement of the cardiac mass relative to cardiovascular structures. Because cine MR images are acquired with steady state free precession or gradient-echo sequences, a different contrast is obtained than with the spin-echo technique.

Benign primary cardiac tumors

Approximately 80% of all primary cardiac tumors are benign. Although these tumors do not metastasize or invade locally, they may lead to significant morbidity and mortality by causing arrhythmias, valvular obstruction, or embolism. An intramyocardial location can interfere with normal conduction pathways and produce arrhythmias, obstruct coronary blood flow, or diminish compliance or contractility through replacement of myocardium.

Myxoma

Myxoma, the most common benign cardiac tumor, accounts for 25% of primary cardiac masses. It is located in the left atrium (LA) in 75% and in the right atrium (RA) in 20% of cases. This tumor is usually spherical in shape, but the shape may vary during the cardiac cycle because of its gelatinous consistency (Fig. 18.1). LA myxomas are typically attached by a narrow pedicle to the area of the fossa ovalis. Infrequently, myxomas have a wide base of attachment to the atrial septum. However, a wide mural attachment is more frequently encountered with malignant tumors. The extent of attachment may be difficult to assess for large tumors, which nearly fill the entire cavity so that they are compressed against the septum. As a result, the tumor appears to have broad contact with the atrial septum on static MRI. T1 and T2 spin-echo images may show a wider attachment than cine images because of slow-flow signal around the tumor, interfering with contour delineation. Cine MRI permits an evaluation of tumor motion and may help to identify the site and length of attachment of the tumor to the wall(s) of cardiac chamber(s).

Usually, myxomas display intermediate signal intensity (isointense to the myocardium) on T1-weighted spin-echo images. On T2-weighted spin-echo images, myxomas usually have higher signal intensity than myocardium. However, myxomas with very low signal intensity have also been observed. Fibrous

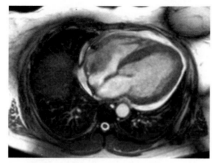 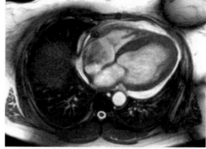

Figure 18.1 Myxoma. Cine magnetic resonance images (MRI) (balanced steady state free precession) in axial plane displays a right atrial myxoma in diastole (left) and systole (right). The motion of the tumor is evident with movement into the tricuspid valve during diastole. There is a moderate pericardial effusion.

stroma, calcification, and the deposition of paramagnetic iron following interstitial hemorrhage can reduce the signal intensity of the tumor on T2-weighted spin-echo images. Rarely, myxomas have been reported to be invisible on spin-echo images because of a lack of contrast with the dark blood pool. Such tumors can be delineated with cine MRI, on which they appear with high contrast against the surrounding bright blood. Most myxomas show increased signal intensity after the administration of Gd-DTPA on T1-weighted images.

Lipoma and lipomatous hypertrophy of the atrial septum

Lipomas are reported to be the second most common benign cardiac tumor in adults but may actually be the most common. They may occur at any age but are encountered most frequently in middle-aged and elderly adults. Lipomas consist of encapsulated mature adipose cells and fetal fat cells. The tumor consistency is soft, and lipomas may grow to a large size without causing symptoms. Lipomas are typically located in the RA or atrial septum. They arise from the endocardial surface and have a broad base of attachment. Lipomas have the same signal intensity as subcutaneous and epicardial fat on all MRI sequences. Because fat has a short T1 relaxation time, lipomas have high signal intensity on T1-weighted images, which can be suppressed with fat saturating pulse sequences (Fig. 18.2). Usually, they appear with homogeneous signal intensity but may have a few thin septations. They do not enhance after the administration of contrast material. On T2-weighted images, lipomas have intermediate signal intensity.

Lipomatous hypertrophy of the atrial septum is considered to be an entity distinct from intracavitary lipoma. Lipomatous hypertrophy is distinct from

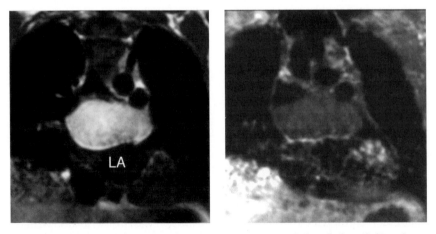

Figure 18.2 Lipoma. ECG-gated spin-echo images in coronal plane before (left) and after fat saturation (right) of a mass situated above the left atrium (LA). Signal of the mass is suppressed with fat saturation.

true lipoma as the fatty tissue is not encapsulated and infiltrates through the tissue of the atrial septum. Signal intensity on MRI is similar to that of lipomas.

Papillary fibroelastoma

Papillary fibroelastoma is a rare, benign, primary cardiac tumor consisting of small avascular fronds of connective tissue lined by endothelium and attached to the cardiac valves. Symptoms are usually related to distal embolization of thrombi. Because of their high content of fibrous tissue, they have low signal intensity on T2-weighted images. Although the diagnosis of these valvular tumors is challenging, recent advances in fast cine MRI have improved diagnostic accuracy. Cine MRI can be used to assess the effect of valvular tumors on valve function. Papillary fibroelastoma may be distinguished from myxoma on gradient echo MRI imaging by a signal intensity slightly lower than myocardium, compared with an isointense signal for myxoma.

Rhabdomyoma

Rhabdomyomas are the most common cardiac tumors in children, comprising 40% of all cardiac tumors in this age group, and the most common cardiac tumor associated with tuberous sclerosis. Rhabdomyomas vary in size and are frequently multiple. They are characterized by an intramural location and involve equally the left ventricle (LV) and right ventricle (RV). Small, entirely intramural tumors may be difficult to identify. Rhabdomyomas may demonstrate signal intensity similar to that of normal myocardium on spin-echo images as well as hyperenhancement after the administration of gadolinium contrast media. In a case series of six rhabdomyomas, gadolinium contrast media was required in all cases to depict tumor contour clearly. As a result of well-established echocardiographic criteria for rhabdomyoma diagnosis, MRI is currently restricted to a minority of cases where echocardiography fails to adequately depict the tumor.[1]

Fibroma

Fibroma is the second most common benign cardiac tumor in children. It is a connective tissue tumor composed of fibroblasts interspersed among collagen fibers. It arises within the myocardial walls. Unlike most other primary cardiac tumors, fibromas usually do not display cystic changes, hemorrhage, or focal necrosis, but dystrophic calcification is common. Fibromas may cause arrhythmias and have been reported to be associated with sudden death. Approximately 30% of these tumors remain asymptomatic and may be discovered incidentally. Fibromas occur most often within the septum or anterior wall of the RV and can reach a large diameter (Fig. 18.3). On T2-weighted MRI, they are characteristically hypointense to the surrounding myocardium. On T1-weighted images, fibromas may appear isointense to the myocardium. Fibromas show delayed hyperenhancement of the periphery of the tumor early after the administration of Gd-DTPA. Administration of Gd-DTPA has been effective

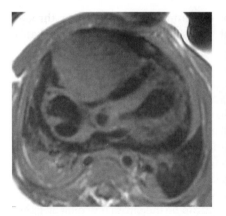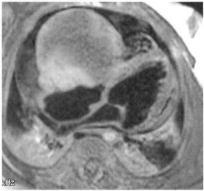

Figure 18.3 Fibroma. ECG-gated T1-weighted spin-echo transaxial images before (left) and after (right) gadolinium chelate in an infant. The periphery of the huge mass shows hyperenhancement. The mass bulges off the free wall of the right ventricle.

for demarcating these intramural tumors more clearly from normal myocardium (Fig. 18.3). Hyperenhancement of compressed myocardium at the margin of the tumor facilitates delineation of the borders of the non-enhancing tumor. Delayed hyperenhancement (15–20 min after administration) of the entire mass has also been observed.

The differential diagnosis for intramural masses in children is rhabdomyoma versus fibroma. If the tumor is solitary, has low signal intensity on T2-weighted images, and delayed hyperenhancement, fibroma is more likely. If multiple tumors are present with high intensity on T2-weighted images, rhabdomyomas are the likely diagnosis. The presence of dystrophic calcifications argues strongly for fibroma over rhabdomyoma.

Pheochromocytoma

Pheochromocytomas arise from neuroendocrine cells clustered in the visceral paraganglia in the posterior wall of the LA, roof of the RA, atrial septum, behind the ascending aorta, and along the coronary arteries, but are predominantly encountered in and around the LA (Fig. 18.4). Most are located outside of the cardiac chamber. The average age at diagnosis is 30–50 years. Cardiac pheochromocytomas are usually benign. Pheochromocytomas are generally highly vascular. The average size at diagnosis is 3–8 cm. Pheochromocytomas are hyperintense to the myocardium on T2-weighted and isointense or hyperintense on T1-weighted images (Fig. 18.4). After the administration of Gd-DTPA, they show strong signal enhancement because of their high vascularity. Enhancement may be heterogeneous, with central non-enhancing areas, related to tumor necrosis.

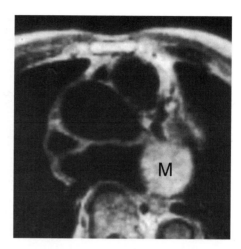

Figure 18.4 Pheochromocytoma. ECG-gated T1-weighted spin-echo images show a high signal intensity mass (M) adjacent to the left atrium.

Hemangioma

Cardiac hemangiomas are composed of endothelial cells that line interconnecting vascular channels. These vascular cavities are separated by connective tissue. According to the size of the vascular channels, hemangiomas are divided into capillary, cavernous, or venous types. Calcification, which can easily be identified on CT, is often present in these tumors. Hemangiomas may involve the endocardium, myocardium, or epicardium. They have been found in all chambers and also the pericardium. Hemangiomas typically demonstrate high signal on T2-weighted images and intermediate to high signal on T1-weighted images (Fig. 18.5). Because of interspersed calcifications and possible flow voids at areas of blood flow in the channels of hemangiomas, they may have inhomogeneous signal intensity. They usually show intense enhancement after the administration of a gadolinium contrast medium because of their rich vascularity.

Malignant primary cardiac tumors

One-quarter of primary cardiac tumors are malignant; sarcomas comprise the largest number, followed by primary cardiac lymphomas. The features of malignant cardiac tumors are involvement of more than one cardiac chamber; extension into pulmonary veins, pulmonary arteries, or vena cavae, wide point of attachment to the wall of a chamber(s); necrosis within the tumor; extension outside the heart; and hemorrhagic pericardial effusion. A combined intramural and intracavitary location is another suggestive feature of malignant tumors (Fig. 18.6). Univariate and multivariate analysis of a large series of tumors identified morphologic features on MRI such as right-sided cardiac location, inhomogeneity of the tumor, and presence of pericardial effusion as strong predictors of malignancy.[2]

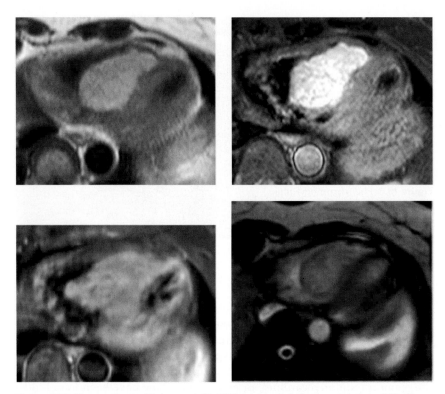

Figure 18.5 Hemangioma. T1 (upper left), T2 fat saturation (upper right), and T1 after gadolinium chelate (lower left) spin-echo images and a gradient-echo cine MRI (lower right) demonstrate a large mass originating in the septum and bulging into the right ventricular cavity. The mass has high signal on all sequences.

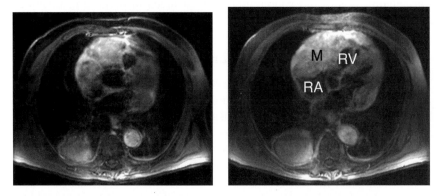

Figure 18.6 Lymphoma. T1-weighted spin-echo image with fat saturation after gadolinium chelate at level of right atrium (left), and right ventricle (right) mass (M) invades the right atrial cavity and right ventricular wall. RA, right atrium; RV, right ventricle.

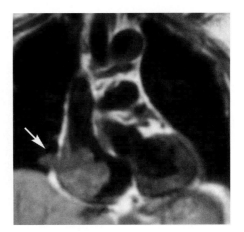

Figure 18.7 Angiosarcoma. ECG-gated spin-echo image in coronal plane shows a large tumor in the right atrium extending through the atrial wall (arrow). The wide field of view of the coronal plane demonstrates the extent of this angiosarcoma.

Angiosarcoma

Angiosarcomas are the most common malignant cardiac tumors in adults and constitute one-third of malignant cardiac tumors (Fig. 18.7). They occur predominantly in men aged 20–50 years. This entity has been divided into two clinicopathologic forms. Most frequently, angiosarcomas are found in the RA (Fig. 18.7). In this form, no evidence of Kaposi sarcoma is found. Another form is characterized by involvement of the epicardium or pericardium in the presence of Kaposi sarcoma. These lesions are usually small, localized, and asymptomatic. This form is associated with the acquired immunodeficiency syndrome. Angiosarcomas consist of ill-defined anastomotic vascular spaces that are lined by endothelial cells and avascular clusters of moderately pleomorphic spindle cells surrounded by collagen stroma. T1-weighted spin-echo imaging usually demonstrates heterogeneous signal intensity of the tumor with focal areas of high signal intensity, which presumably represent hemorrhage. T2-weighted spin-echo imaging usually demonstrates high signal intensity. However, angiosarcomas can also have homogeneous signal intensity. The hypointense layer on GRE images with significant phase shift represents susceptibility effect caused by intratumor hemorrhage. After the administration of contrast medium, angiosarcomas show hyperenhancement. Some of the tumors show regions of low signal intensity on both T1- and T2-weighted images. These central regions have high signal intensity on cine gradient-echo images and represent vascular channels. This finding is often described as a "cauliflower" appearance. Cases with diffuse pericardial infiltration have been found to show linear hyperenhancement along vascular spaces, described by some authorities as a "sunray" appearance.

Rhabdomyosarcoma and other sarcomas

Rhabdomyosarcomas are the most common malignant cardiac tumors in children. They can arise anywhere in the myocardium. Rhabdomyosarcomas are

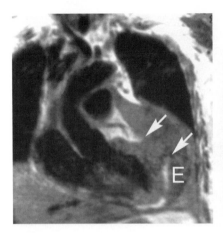
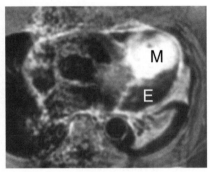

Figure 18.8 Rhabdomyosarcoma. Coronal (left) and transaxial after gadolinium chelate (right) spin-echo images. Coronal images show a loculated pericardial effusion (E) with high intensity on T1-weighted image (hemorrhagic effusion). The epicardial fat line (arrows) is disrupted by the tumor extending into the pericardial space. Transaxial image after contrast media shows the tumor (M) demonstrated by the marked enhancement, while the pericardial effusion (E) is not enhanced.

often multiple. Their signal intensity on MRI is variable. Rhabdomyosarcomas may be isointense to the myocardium on T1- and T2-weighted images, but areas of necrosis can exhibit heterogeneous signal intensity and patchy hyperenhancement after the administration of Gd-DTPA (Fig. 18.8). Extracardiac extension into the pulmonary arteries and descending aorta has been clearly delineated with MRI.

Other possible primary sarcomas are fibrosarcomas, osteosarcomas, leiomyosarcomas, and liposarcomas. These are all rare tumors, comprising approximately 4% of primary cardiac masses. The signal intensity characteristics of these entities are non-specific. Most of these tumors show signal intensity isointense to normal myocardium on T1-weighted images and hyperintense on T2-weighted images. Typically, there is increased signal intensity on T1-weighted images after the administration of Gd-DTPA.

Lymphoma
Primary cardiac lymphoma is less common than secondary lymphoma involving the heart, which usually represents the spread of non-Hodgkin lymphoma. Primary lymphoma of the heart most often occurs in immunocompromised patients and is highly aggressive. Almost all primary cardiac lymphomas are B-cell lymphomas. Although primary cardiac lymphoma is rare, it is mandatory to consider this entity in the diagnosis of malignant cardiac tumors because early chemotherapy is usually effective. These tumors arise most often on the right side of the heart, especially in the RA, but have also been found in the other chambers (Fig. 18.6). A large pericardial effusion is frequently present, often

with accompanying pericardial thickening. Variable morphology of the masses has been described. Lymphomas may appear hypointense to the myocardium on T1-weighted and hyperintense on T2-weighted images. After the administration of Gd-DTPA, homogeneous or heterogeneous enhancement of the tumor, depending on the presence of necrosis, may be seen.

Secondary cardiac tumors

Secondary tumors of the heart and pericardium are approximately 40-fold more frequent than primary tumors. Three routes of spread to the heart can be discerned:

1 Direct extension from intrathoracic tumors (mediastinum and lungs)
2 Extension of abdominal malignancies through the inferior vena cava into the RA (renal, adrenal, and hepatic carcinomas)
3 Metastasis

Direct extension from adjacent tumors
Tumors of the lung and mediastinum can infiltrate the pericardium and heart directly. It is important to recognize invasion of the heart because such a tumor is usually non-resectable. In mediastinal lymphoma, possible invasion of the pericardium can change the staging of the tumor. MRI is especially suited for delineating paracardiac tumors and possible extension into the heart because of its wide field of view. MRI clearly shows extension of these tumors to the cardiac structures and may show evidence of hemorrhagic or non-hemorrhagic pericardial effusion. MRI is more effective in demonstrating invasion of the pericardium and myocardium in advanced lung cancer.

Transvenous extension into the heart
Another site for the entry of secondary tumors into the heart is tumor extension through large veins connecting with cardiac chambers. Tumor thrombus arising from carcinoma of the kidney, liver, or adrenal gland can extend through the inferior vena cava into the RA, and primary carcinoma of the thymus can extend through the superior vena cava. The evaluation of the possible attachment of such tumors to the atrial wall is mandatory for surgical planning. If the atrial walls are not infiltrated, complete resection of the tumor may still be possible.

Metastasis
Melanomas, leukemias, and lymphomas are the tumors that most frequently metastasize to the heart, but cardiac metastases can arise from almost any malignant tumor in the body. Melanomas have the highest frequency of seeding into the heart and are frequently found in the heart at autopsy. The mechanism of metastatic spread of tumors to the heart is either direct seeding to the endocardium, passage of tumor emboli through the coronary arteries, or retrograde lymphatic spread through bronchomediastinal lymphatic channels. MRI is

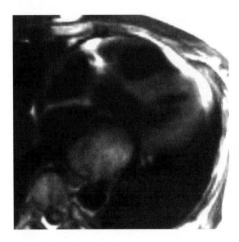

Figure 18.9 Metastasis to the left atrium. ECG-gated T1-weighted spin-echo transaxial images.

highly effective for delineating the location and extent of metastatic tumors in cardiac chambers and assessing the potential for surgical resection (Fig. 18.9).

Intracardiac thrombus

Thrombus is the most common intracardiac mass, involving most frequently the LV or LA, and may be difficult to distinguish from an intracardiac tumor.

On spin-echo images, the signal intensity of thrombus can vary from low to high depending on age-related changes in the composition of the thrombus. The signal intensity of thrombus can with time be influenced by paramagnetic hemoglobin breakdown products, such as intracellular methemoglobin and hemosiderin, or superparamagnetic substances, such as ferritin. Fresh thrombus usually shows high signal intensity on T1- and T2-weighted spin-echo images, whereas older thrombus has low signal intensity on T1- and T2-weighted images. Intracavitary high signal on spin-echo images caused by slowly flowing blood may be difficult to distinguish from thrombus. However, this problem can be overcome either by using the spin-echo sequences after inversion recovery pulses to null intracavitary signal or by using cine MRI.

Differentiation between tumor and blood clot

The distinction between clot and tumor is more reliably attained with gradient-echo sequences. The gradient-echo technique is more sensitive to susceptibility and T2* effects than is the spin-echo technique. As the various blood degeneration products pass through the different stages of magnetic susceptibility, they continue to cause shortening of T2* relaxivity; the result is low signal intensity of the thrombus on gradient-echo images (Fig. 18.10). An exception to this generalization is fresh thrombus, which can have high signal intensity.

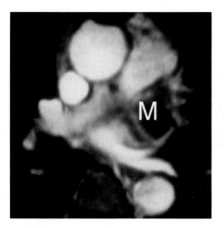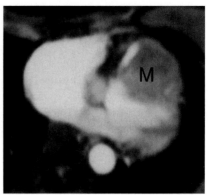

Figure 18.10 LA appendage thrombus (left) and metastatic tumor of the right ventricle (right). Transaxial gradient-echo (cine MRI) shows a mass (M) filling the left atrial appendage with low intensity. The mass (M) in the right ventricle has intermediate signal intensity.

Tumor tissue usually is hyperintense in comparison with myocardium and skeletal muscle on T2-weighted spin-echo images and cine MRI. However, some myxomas containing substantial iron produce low signal and so mimic thrombus.

Another method for differentiating between tumor and clot is to use Gd-DTPA-enhanced T1-weighted images. Thrombus does not enhance after the administration of Gd-DTPA, whereas tumors show enhancement (Fig. 18.8). Tumor can usually be differentiated from thrombus by using gradient-echo and T1-weighted spin-echo images after the administration of Gd-DTPA.

References

1 Kaminaga T, Takeshita T, Kimura, I. Role of magnetic resonance imaging for evaluation of tumors in the cardiac region. *Eur Radiol* 2003;**13**(Suppl 4):L1.
2 Hoffman U, Globits S, Schima W, *et al.* Usefulness of magnetic resonance imaging of cardiac and paracardiac masses. *Am J Cardiol* 2003;**92**:890.

Further reading

Araoz PA, Mulvagh SL, Tazlaar HD, *et al.* CT and MR imaging of benign primary cardiac neoplasms with echocardiographic correlation. *Radiographics* 2000:**20**:1303.
Araoz PA, Eklund HE, Welch TJ, *et al.* CT and MR imaging of primary cardiac malignancies. *Radiographics* 1999;**19**:1421.
Barakos JA, Brown JJ, Higgins CB. MR imaging of secondary cardiac and pericardiac lesions. *Am J Roentgenology* 1989;**153**:47–50.
Fujita N, Caputo GR, Higgins CB. Diagnosis and characterization of intracardiac masses by magnetic resonance imaging. *Am J Card Imaging* 1994;**8**:69.

Mader MT, Poulton TB, White RD. Malignant tumors of the heart and great vessels: MR imaging appearance. *Radiographics* 1997;**17**:145.

Meng Q, Lai H, Lima J, *et al.* Echocardiographic and pathologic characteristics of primary cardiac tumors: a study of 149 cases. *Int J Cardiol* 2002;**84**:69.

Schvartzman PR, White RD. Imaging of cardiac and paracardiac masses. *J Thorac Imaging* 2000;**15**:265.

Siripornpitak S, Higgins CB. MRI of primary malignant cardiovascular tumors. *J Comput Assist Tomogr* 1997;**21**:462.

CHAPTER 19

Evaluation of the transplanted heart

Oberdan Parodi, Maria Frigerio, and Benedetta De Chiara

Introduction

Cardiac transplantation is an established treatment for advanced heart failure. Clinical experience and progress in immunosuppression have increased recipient survival to more than 80% at 1 year; 10-year survival is more than 50% at many centers.[1] Common complications after heart transplantation (HTx) include acute rejection, infections, cardiac allograft vasculopathy (CAV), and lymphoproliferative disorders and other malignancies, as well as other conditions mainly related to side-effects of immunosuppressive drugs (Fig. 19.1). This chapter summarizes briefly the role of cardiac imaging techniques for the diagnosis of acute rejection, and will provide a more in-depth review of current techniques for invasive and non-invasive evaluation of CAV.

Case Presentation

A 55-year-old man with idiopathic dilated cardiomyopathy underwent heart transplantation in 1999, from a donor of the same age and gender. The patient had cytomegalovirus infection and one treated acute rejection episode in the early postoperative months. One year after heart transplantation, the resting ECG showed an incomplete right bundle branch block, and further evaluation was sought for surveillance for rejection and allograft vasculopathy.

Diagnosis of acute cardiac allograft rejection

Acute rejection is an important cause of death in HTx recipients, accounting for 20% of the deaths occurring in the first post-transplant year, and up to 15% thereafter.[1] Nevertheless, the majority of acute rejections can be safely managed, providing diagnosis precedes the occurrence of graft dysfunction. Minor clinical signs of acute cardiac allograft rejection may be absent and are non-specific (Table 19.1). Thus, surveillance for preclinical diagnosis is of utmost importance.

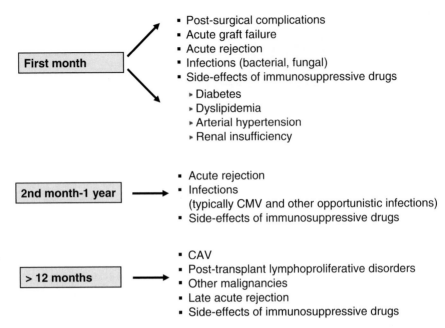

First month →
- Post-surgical complications
- Acute graft failure
- Acute rejection
- Infections (bacterial, fungal)
- Side-effects of immunosuppressive drugs
  - ▸ Diabetes
  - ▸ Dyslipidemia
  - ▸ Arterial hypertension
  - ▸ Renal insufficiency

2nd month-1 year →
- Acute rejection
- Infections
  (typically CMV and other opportunistic infections)
- Side-effects of immunosuppressive drugs

> 12 months →
- CAV
- Post-transplant lymphoproliferative disorders
- Other malignancies
- Late acute rejection
- Side-effects of immunosuppressive drugs

Figure 19.1 Common complications after cardiac transplantation. Side-effects of immunosuppressive drugs occur early after heart transplantation and contribute to endothelial dysfunction and progression of cardiac transplant vasculopathy. CAV, coronary allograft vasculopathy; CMV, cytomegalovirus.

Table 19.1 Clinical symptoms and signs of acute cardiac allograft rejection.

None
Malaise, fatigue
Fever
Tachycardia
Supraventricular arrhythmias, conduction disturbances
Reduced QRS amplitude (peripheral leads)
Reduced systolic blood pressure
Reduced pulse pressure
Dyspnea
Congestive heart failure
Sudden death

Endomyocardial biopsy (EMB) is the most widely used and reliable tool for the diagnosis of acute rejection. Acute cardiac allograft rejection may show a wide spectrum of lesions with standard staining (hematoxylin and eosin), ranging from sparse perivascular or interstitial infiltrates of small lymphocytes, to more widespread and aggressive infiltration of large, activated lymphocytes, associated or not with granulocytes, with various degrees of myocyte disruption and necrosis, up to severe, extensive necrosis, associated with edema, polymorphonuclear infiltrates and hemorrhages. A less common but ominous condition is the so-called "humoral" or "vascular" rejection, which can be briefly defined as an immunomediated, acute graft dysfunction despite a normal ("negative") EMB. The main limitations of EMB are patient discomfort, risk of complications (less than 1% when performed by skilled personnel: right ventricle perforation, tricuspid leaflet disruption, bleeding, pneumothorax), costs, and sampling error. Despite the debates about rejection classification, the disagreement observed between pathologists in EMB interpretation, and the uncertainties regarding therapeutic implications of the EMB results (except in case of very low- or high-grade rejections), EMB remains the cornerstone for rejection surveillance at most HTx centers. Nevertheless, various non-invasive alternative techniques have been evaluated, with the aim of reducing the need for repeated EMBs, to optimize their timing, and to add information relevant for clinical management.

Echocardiography is the most extensively used diagnostic technique for noninvasive monitoring of HTx recipients. During the first postoperative weeks, the echocardiogram reflects the mutual adaptation of the donor's heart and of the recipient's hemodynamic profile to the new condition, and postoperative sequelae: right ventricular dilatation, tricuspid regurgitation, paradoxic septal motion, and pericardial effusion are common. After 1 month, the echocardiographic pattern remains quite stable in the absence of significant rejection in most patients, generally up to 1 year. In the long term, the effects of hypertension and CAV may interfere with echocardiographic findings. The main features of acute rejection are alterations of indexes of left ventricular (LV) diastolic function, commonly detected by pulsed wave Doppler (reduction of pressure half-time and of isovolumic relaxation time), increased wall thickness, increased myocardial echogenicity, dilated right ventricle, and increased pericardial effusion. LV systolic dysfunction is less frequent, is prognostically unfavorable, and is more often associated with high-grade rejection or with biopsy-negative (humoral/vascular) rejection. The accuracy of echocardiographic findings may vary according to the operators' experience and patient body structure; obesity, not uncommon after HTx, may reduce the quality of echocardiography. Recently, tissue Doppler imaging (TDI) has been proposed for early detection of rejection-related diastolic dysfunction in HTx recipients; high sensitivity (93%) and high negative predictive value (96%) have been reported, with a favorable impact on the number of EMBs as well as prognostic implications.[2]

Magnetic resonance imaging (MRI) has been more recently explored, both in experimental and human research. Labeling of macrophages with dextran-coated, ultrasmall, superparamagnetic iron oxide (USPIO) particles can be used to detect the accumulation of macrophages in rejecting tissue.[3] Furthermore, USPIO can be used alone (i.e. not in macrophages) because blood pool contrast agents leak into the interstitial space in areas of inflammation associated with rejection, where the vessels display increased permeability. Moreover, the myocardial T2 relaxation time, determined using a black-blood MRI sequence, has been demonstrated to predict acute heart transplant rejection in humans.

An intriguing radioisotope technique is represented by myocardial scintigraphy with radiolabeled (indium-111 pentetreotide) somatostatin receptor analogue.[4] The pathophysiologic hypothesis is that somatostatin receptors are expressed on activated lymphocytes and up-regulated during cardiac allograft rejection. It is noteworthy that somatostatin receptor imaging seems to predict impending rejection at least 1 week before the EMB becomes positive, because of the interval between lymphocyte activation and relevant myocardial infiltration or damage. The possibility of anticipating the occurrence of EMB-proven rejection by means of analysis of gene expression in the peripheral blood is currently under evaluation.

Another interesting approach, which implies the possibility of telemonitoring of HTx recipients, is represented by continuous recording of high-resolution, intramyocardial electrocardiogram (ECG) by means of special electrodes implanted at the time of transplantation.

However, these innovative approaches have not yet gained widespread clinical use. At present, echocardiography is used at most HTx centers as an adjunct to clinical, laboratory, ECG, and EMB data: it is helpful in deciding if and how to change the immunosuppressive regimen and for planning patient follow-up, but it is not a substitute for EMB except in small pediatric patients.

Case Presentation (Continued)

Echocardiographic evaluation demonstrated normal regional and global left ventricular function (ejection fraction 0.59) and diastolic parameters. A routine biopsy was normal. However, further evaluation was sought for allograft vasculopathy.

Coronary allograft vasculopathy

CAV is the main factor limiting long-term survival after transplantation, and accounts for more than 20% of later mortality.[1] Pretransplant conditions, donor characteristics, and events occurring during the first post-transplant year and thereafter are implicated in the pathogenesis of CAV (Table 19.2).[5] The initial endothelial dysfunction and injury are followed by intimal hyperplasia and vascular smooth muscle cell proliferation. The process has been angiographically documented in 40–50% of patients surviving 5 years after transplantation.[1] The histologic hallmark of CAV (intimal proliferation in graft coronary arteries) can be observed in all surviving recipients as soon as 1 year after HTx; its *in vivo* equivalent can be appreciated by means of intracoronary ultrasound (ICUS). Unfortunately, warning anginal symptoms are often absent, as a result of car-

Table 19.2 Factors involved in the pathogenesis of coronary allograft vasculopathy.

Immune mechanisms		Non-immune mechanisms
Recurrent/persistent acute rejection		Older donor age
Vascular/humoral rejection		Hyperlipidemia
HLA mismatch		Hypertension
		Diabetes
	Ischemia reperfusion injury*	
	CMV infection*	

* These factors are in an intermediate position, because they may be considered partially "immune" inasmuch as they imply exposure of endothelial antigens and/or activation of immune reaction.
CMV, cytomegalovirus.

diac denervation; clinical manifestations of CAV are frequently severe, and include congestive heart failure, myocardial infarction, life-threatening ventricular arrhythmias, and sudden death.

Treatment of CAV remains a difficult challenge. The solution for severe, diffuse disease is retransplantation, although this option is limited by donor availability. Focal stenoses can be approached by percutaneous angioplasty and stenting, with satisfactory angiographic short-term results, but little is known regarding long-term success and the prognostic relevance of these procedures. Recently, the use of proliferation inhibitors (sirolimus and everolimus) appears promising for preventing, stopping, and perhaps reversing intimal proliferation. This section describes the advantages and limitations of non-invasive approaches, the place of invasive techniques in the detection of CAV and in prognostic stratification of HTx recipients, and the potential of new imaging modalities.

Non-invasive testing

The availability of accurate non-invasive tests for diagnosis of the presence (and of the functional and prognostic relevance) of CAV is highly desirable for clinical, organizational, and economic reasons. Moreover, non-invasive tests may provide information regarding microvascular circulation, which can be impaired after HTx. Unfortunately, the sensitivity and specificity of non-invasive tests for diagnosis of CAV is difficult to establish in relation to angiography, because anatomic narrowing does not always induce ischemia and, conversely, ischemia may occur in patients with small vessel coronary artery vasculopathy undetected by angiography. The diffuse nature of CAV may result in balanced ischemia that is difficult to recognize by imaging modalities, such as perfusion scintigraphy, which are based on intrapatient comparison of different myocardial areas. Moreover, new events (e.g. late acute rejection) may occur at any time after HTx, and may accelerate the progression of CAV, thus limiting the predictive value of any test, irrespective of its accuracy. However, for the individual patient, a positive non-invasive test indicating inducible myocardial ischemia may have powerful prognostic value.

Stress electrocardiography

Most transplant patients have resting ECG abnormalities (mostly incomplete right bundle branch block and T-wave inversion) that make the interpretation of stress ECG less sensitive and specific than in general population. Furthermore, sensitivity is reduced because angina is rarely present, and the target heart rate during exercise usually is not achieved because of heart denervation and, in some patients, inadequate physical conditioning. Reported sensitivity and specificity of exercise ECG for the detection of CAV are in the ranges 0–38% and 77–100%, respectively. Ambulatory ECG monitoring is similarly insensitive. Arterial hypotension during exercise is quite specific for significant CAV. Additional information may be provided by ECG data when combined with imaging techniques. In our experience, the appearance of complete right bundle branch block increases the specificity of myocardial perfusion defects for predicting CAV; a blunted heart rate response during dipyridamole-induced vasodilatation predicts stress perfusion defects, and higher probability of cardiac events during follow-up.

Echocardiography

Baseline ejection fraction (EF) and regional wall motion are generally normal in HTx recipients, even in the presence of CAV. Thus, regional wall motion abnormalities and/or a reduced ejection fraction have a low sensitivity for diagnosis of CAV (50–60%), although their prevalence is higher in HTx patients with CAV. Spes et al.[6] reported that resting wall motion abnormalities in any left ventricular territory had a 90% positive predictive value and an 88% specificity, but only a 57% sensitivity in detecting CAV. Furthermore, normal resting echocardiography had a 90% negative predictive value for cardiac events. In a previous study,[7] we showed that normal resting wall motion at echocardiography coupled to normal stress myocardial perfusion scintigraphy ruled out the presence of significant CAV. Conversely, resting wall motion abnormalities and perfusion defects strongly predicted cardiac events. Resting echocardiography alone detected significant CAV only in 50% of cases, but it was an independent prognostic determinant of cardiac events. The addition of a pharmacologic stress (e.g. dipyridamole or dobutamine) may improve the limited sensitivity of resting echocardiography for detection of CAV (Table 19.3). Ciliberto et al.[8] first reported that high-dose dipyridamole stress echocardiography is useful for identifying patients with significant CAV, and more recently found that dipyridamole-induced wall motion abnormalities were associated with adverse prognosis.[9] Dobutamine stress echocardiography (DSE) provides accurate diagnosis as well as useful prognostic information in cardiac transplant recipients.[6] Dobutamine increases contractility, heart rate, and wall stress in a dose-dependent fashion, an attractive approach to evaluate both microvasculature and epicardial coro-

Table 19.3 Accuracy of stress echocardiography in the detection of coronary allograft vasculopathy.

Study	Journal	Year	Patients (n)	Stress	Sensitivity (%)	Specificity (%)
Derumeaux et al.	J Am Coll Cardiol	1995	37	Dobutamine	86	91
Herregods et al.	J Heart Lung Transplant	1994	28	Dobutamine	0	100
Akosah et al.	J Heart Lung Transplant	1994	41	Dobutamine	95	55
Ciliberto et al.	Eur Heart J	1993	80	Dipyridamole	32	100
Spes et al.	Am J Cardiol	1996	46	Dobutamine	79	83
Collings et al.	J Heart Lung Transplant	1994	51	Exercise	25	86
Cohn et al.	Am J Cardiol	1996	51	Exercise	15	85
Spes et al.	Circulation	1999	109	Dobutamine	94	57

nary vessels in HTx patients. DSE is more sensitive than exercise echocardiography because the transplanted heart is more responsive to catecholamine stimulation than a normal heart, while the exercise-induced increase in heart rate is limited. Spes et al.[6] suggested that serial routine coronary angiography could be deferred in HTx recipients with normal DSE, because the prognostic value of this test is comparable to that of ICUS. Therefore, resting echocardiography plus DSE appear a reliable method for routine surveillance of patients after HTx. As usual, echocardiography may be limited by poor image quality in obese patients, and its accuracy relies upon the operator's experience.

Myocardial perfusion scintigraphy

Stress myocardial scintigraphy with thallium-201 or technetium-99m labeled perfusion tracers and single photon emission computed tomography (SPECT) has a well-established role in detection of atherosclerotic coronary lesions in patients with known or suspected ischemic heart disease. In HTx recipients, stress myocardial scintigraphy provides a low-to-moderate sensitivity and a good specificity for the detection of CAV, with exercise testing performing better than a dipyridamole test (Table 19.4). However, the limitations of exercise testing in HTx patients have been already described. Moreover, most published studies utilized a qualitative (visual) assessment of perfusion defects, or a semi-quantitative evaluation of myocardial tracer distribution, without any reference to maps of normal regional perfusion pattern. The limited sensitivity of the technique reported by these studies might be related to the lack of quantitative as-

Table 19.4 Accuracy of stress myocardial scintigraphy in the detection of coronary allograft vasculopathy.

Study	Journal	Year	Patients (n)	Stress	Sensitivity (%)	Specificity (%)
Smart et al.	Am J Cardiol	1991	57	Dipyridamole	21	88
Redonnet et al.	Transplant Proc	1995	43	Dipyridamole	58	64
Ciliberto et al.	Eur Heart J	1993	50	Exercise	67	100
Rodney et al.	J Heart Lung Transplant	1994	25	Exercise	77	100
Smart et al.	Transplant Proc	1991	35	Exercise	21	81
Valantine et al.	Circulation	1988	20	Exercise	36	78
McKillop et al.	Clin Radiol	1981	7	Exercise	100	0
Mairesse et al.	J Heart Lung Transplant	1995	37	Exercise	NA	84–92
Ambrosi et al.	Eur Heart J	1994	34	Exercise	NA	97
Carlsen et al.	J Heart Lung Transplant	2000	67	Dip /Exercise	80	92
Ciliberto et al.	Eur Heart J	2001	78	Dipyridamole	92	86

NA, not assessed.

sessment of the regional tracer uptake. More recently, we evaluated the accuracy of high-dose dipyridamole sestamibi SPECT in the detection of CAV and in prognostic stratification utilizing a semi-quantitative technique corrected for bull's eye maps of perfusion normalcy rates in 78 HTx recipients.[7] Our findings indicate that this approach is sensitive in the detection of significant CAV (sensitivity 92%), and that its combination with resting echocardiography can be a safe and reasonable non-invasive approach for prediction of long-term prognosis after HTx. In this study, concordant negative tests occurred in over two-thirds of cases, in whom non-invasive testing had an optimal accuracy in ruling out significant CAV (specificity 82%, negative predicting value 100%). These patients also had a high event-free survival. Conversely, a significant CAV was present in 100% of the five patients with abnormalities in both non-invasive tests. Patients with abnormal resting echocardiography had a 10-fold relative risk of cardiac events at follow-up, while a positive dipyridamole SPECT conferred a 4 : 1 relative risk of cardiac events. Thus, the association of these tests may be useful to rule out the need for coronary angiography when both are negative, and to recommend it when at least one is positive. In our hands, the sensitivity of this imaging approach for significant CAV favorably compares with previous studies that used either dipyridamole or exercise thallium-201 scans[10] or visual interpretation of exercise myocardial perfusion imaging by technetium-99m labeled compounds.[11] High-dose dipyridamole may augment the differences in regional tracer distribution among areas with different coronary vasodilating capability, improving the detection of minor coronary lesions. It is not yet clearly established which stressor is preferable in the evaluation of blunted coronary flow reserve in heart transplant recipients. In our experience, the dipyridamole test is safe, reproducible, and feasible (in up to 95% of transplanted patients), and it provides good sensitivity in CAV detection and relevant prognostic information when associated to quantitative evaluation of myocardial tracer uptake.

To refine the capability of detecting perfusion defects by quantitative bull's eye imaging in this specific patient population, an ongoing study is being carried out at our institution, where correction for normal perfusion has been performed utilizing a map obtained from a database of transplanted patients with normal cardiac function, no rejection, and normal coronary angiography, who underwent dipyridamole SPECT imaging 1 year after HTx. This approach may optimize the rest and stress regional cut-off values used for definition of normalcy versus perfusion defects.

Regional perfusion and coronary flow reserve may be accurately measured in HTx recipients by positron emission tomography in conjunction with flow tracers (^{13}N-ammonia, ^{15}O-water). The diffuse nature of CAV is a challenge for all cardiac imaging techniques. Absolute measurements of myocardial blood flow and coronary flow reserve may circumvent the limitations of other imaging techniques, which explore regional myocardial differences by means of relative tracer distribution. However, the accuracy of positron emission tomography in the detection of CAV has not yet been tested, probably also because this technique is expensive and is not always clinically feasible, and not widely available.

Invasive techniques
Coronary angiography

After recognition of the occurrence and clinical relevance of CAV, annual coronary angiography has been utilized to monitor its development and progression. The classification of angiographic abnormalities of the transplanted heart was proposed by Gao *et al.* in 1988.[12] Three types of coronary lesions were defined:

1 Type A, with discrete, tubular or multiple stenoses, which resembles coronary artery disease of the native heart

2 Type B, characteristic of HTx recipients, which is subclassified as B_1 (sharp onset of distal diffuse concentric narrowing and obliteration, with apparently normal or nearly normal proximal segments) or B_2 (progressive, concentric tapering from proximal to distal segments, with some residual flow in the periphery)

3 Type C, with relative proximal dilatation and irregular narrowing of distal branches, which may show non-tapered, abrupt interruption.

Several studies have demonstrated the prognostic relevance of CAV as detected by coronary angiography in large patient cohorts. After 3–4 years, the relative risk of any cardiac event is more than tripled in patients with angiographic evidence of obstructive disease compared with those without evidence of disease. However, coronary angiography has several major limitations: it is invasive, requires hospitalization, and the nephrotoxicity of contrast agents may be harmful in HTx recipients, who may suffer from drug-induced renal insufficiency. Moreover, the organizational and economic burden of annual coronary angiography of an increasing population of long-term HTx recipients is not negligible. The main limitation of coronary angiography is represented by its "lumenographic" approach, which is insensitive in detecting a diffuse, concentric disease. Thus, angiography may underestimate the severity of CAV.

Intracoronary ultrasound

The ICUS technique provides images of both the lumen and the vessel wall, and is at the present time the best tool for early diagnosis and quantification of CAV. According to the experience of the Stanford HTx program, an intimal thickening of more than 0.3 mm is associated with a significantly reduced probability of survival and an increased risk for cardiac events during follow-up, regardless of angiographic findings.[13] Furthermore, functional impairment, such as decreased coronary blood flow reserve, can be evaluated by ICUS and is more frequently associated to intimal thickening. Increased intimal thickening is currently proposed as the best surrogate end-point for therapies aimed at limiting or reversing the evolution of CAV.[14]

Unfortunately, ICUS also has some limitations: it implies more risks with respect to standard angiography (vessel spasm, dissection, and complications related to guidewire manipulation); and it is expensive and time-consuming. Standardization of the procedure facilitates comparison of serial examinations, and interobserver agreement is good among trained personnel. The characteristics of the probe do not allow the examination of peripheral segments. However, it is likely that given the diffuse nature of CAV, measurements of wall thickness from one artery should reflect the overall extent of the disease, or at least its prognostic relevance.

ICUS represents the contemporary gold standard for the diagnosis and serial evaluation of CAV, particularly when therapies targeted at CAV (e.g. proliferation inhibitors such as sirolimus or everolimus, extensive use of statins irrespective of cholesterol values) become available or are under evaluation. Unfortunately, its invasive nature and costs continue to limit its use.

Case Presentation (Continued)

The patient also underwent dipyridamole technetium-99m sestamibi SPECT. At the time of the examination he was treated with a triple-drug immunosuppression protocol (cyclosporine, prednisone, and azathioprine). Dipyridamole myocardial perfusion scintigraphy showed a fixed perfusion defect in inferior wall and a slight reversible antero-apical defect; quantitative analysis better clarified the reduction of tracer uptake (under the physiologic threshold) in the antero-apical segments (Fig. 19.2). Coronary angiography did not show any coronary artery lesion; ICUS was employed to assess vascular composition of the left descending coronary artery. An obvious intimal proliferation of this vessel was found, confirming the scintigraphic findings (Fig. 19.3); conversely, no abnormalities were detected in the right coronary artery, suggesting that the fixed perfusion defect in the inferior wall was likely a result of previous acute rejections. The patient underwent aggressive pharmacologic treatment with statins, alpha- and beta-blockers. At 4-year follow-up, myocardial stress scintigraphy did not show any progression of CAV, and no cardiac event occurred.

This case illustrates how careful observation of transplanted patients by imaging techniques in the first 1–2 years after transplantation may help select patients for treatments that appear to slow the progression of established CAV.

New imaging modalities
Magnetic resonance imaging

Magnetic resonance perfusion imaging (MRPI) using gadolinium-based contrast agents has recently been validated as a clinical tool to quantify myocardial perfusion. Using MRPI, it is possible to quantify myocardial perfusion reserve, a parameter that mirrors coronary flow reserve as a measure of the functional significance of epicardial lesions in the pertinent perfusion territories. Because resting endomyocardial : epimyocardial perfusion ratio decreases with impaired coronary circulation, calculation of this index by MRPI may represent a simple measurement of myocardial perfusion at rest that could be sufficient to detect early CAV. Perfusion imaging during rest and adenosine- or dipyridamole-induced hyperemia can be performed in the same session. Adenosine or dipyridamole are intravenously infused according to protocols commonly used in echocardiography and nuclear medicine laboratories. Perfusion is usually determined in three LV short-axis slices. The first slice is located close to the base of the heart just below the aortic outflow tract, the second in the middle of the LV, and the third close to the apex just below the base of the papillary muscles. A single-shot gradient-echo sequence with saturation recovery magnetization preparation for T1 weighting and linear k-spacing is used for imaging. Temporal resolution allows acquisition of one image in each of the three selected slices within one heart beat up to a heart rate of 110 b/min. Sixty images per

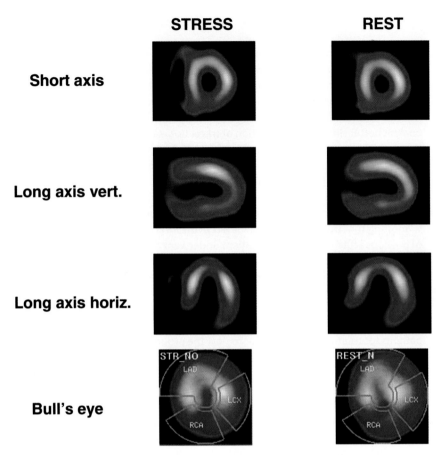

Figure 19.2 Myocardial single photon emission computed tomography (SPECT) imaging in the short- and long-axis views and bull's eye analysis of the case report. A fixed perfusion defect in the inferior wall and a slight reversible antero-apical defect is detectable at visual inspection; quantitative analysis better clarifies the reversible reduction of tracer uptake (under the physiologic threshold) in the antero-apical segments.

slice location are usually acquired with a spatial resolution of 2–3 mm. Patients are asked to hold their breath at end expiration for the first 15–20 s of each perfusion scan, such that the tracking of the first pass of the bolus at the three chosen slice locations is not affected by respiratory motion. Immediately after initiation of the sequence, a compact bolus of 0.03 mmol/kg bodyweight gadolinium-DTPA is injected over an antecubital vein at a rate of 7 mL/s using a power injector. Analysis of MRPI curves for calculation of myocardial perfusion reserve has been described previously in details, and its application for the detection of CAV provided interesting findings.[15] A significant correlation was found between invasive measurement of coronary flow reserve and the non-

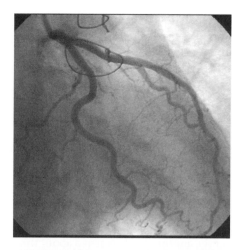

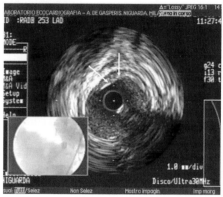

Figure 19.3 Angiograms of the left coronary artery (upper panel) and intracoronary ultrasound (lower panel) in the same patient. Note that the angiogram does not reveal any significant abnormalities, whereas intracoronary ultrasound demonstrates significant intimal thickening (arrows). No abnormalities were detected in the right coronary artery by both coronary angiography and intracoronary ultrasound, despite obvious stable perfusion defects in the inferior wall at myocardial scintigraphy.

invasive evaluation of resting endomyocardial : epimyocardial perfusion ratio. HTx patients with CAV showed a reduced myocardial perfusion reserve and resting endomyocardial : epimyocardial perfusion ratio. When patients with left ventricular hypertrophy and/or prior rejection were excluded, a normal resting endomyocardial : epimyocardial perfusion ratio was able to exclude CAV (negative predictive value 100% with a cut-off value of 1.3), suggesting that further stress tests or invasive examinations are not required. A myocardial perfusion reserve of more than 2.3 as assessed with adenosine infusion excluded CAV (negative predictive value 100%) in the overall population, suggesting that this test is useful in HTx recipients with left ventricular hypertrophy and/or history of acute rejection(s).

These data were obtained in a small sample of HTx patients; if confirmed in larger cohorts, MRPI might be a good method for routine non-invasive surveillance for CAV after HTx. The potential of dobutamine stress MRI has not yet been evaluated in HTx recipients.

Electron beam computed tomography

Recently, electron beam computed tomography (EBCT) has been proposed in the setting of HTx recipients. Contrary to the notion that coronary artery calcification is an atypical or late feature of CAV, quantification of coronary calcification by EBCT has recently been reported to correlate closely with the occurrence of coronary artery lesions in HTx recipients. Calcium scores revealed close correlation with the ICUS degree of intimal proliferation and showed high sensitivity (94%) and rather good specificity (79%) for detecting CAV;[16] in addition, EBCT appeared to be associated with coronary events after HTx. Because of its relatively low cost, EBCT could be useful to detect the presence of CAV non-invasively, and to select high-risk patients for invasive procedures; moreover, it could serve for follow-up purposes. However, types B_2 and C distal coronary artery lesions might be underestimated by this approach, and the functional significance of these calcifications cannot be ascertained. Very recently, another study warned about the lack of usefulness of EBCT in detecting documented CAV,[17] confirming the concerns reported above. Finally, the radiation exposure of CT should be considered before recommending a widespread indication for this technique.

Practical implication of cardiovascular imaging in heart transplantation

Follow-up of HTx recipients is a complex task for both physicians and the patient, and non-invasive tests that could diagnose or anticipate significant cardiac events, such as acute rejection or clinically relevant CAV, are certainly warranted. At present, the diagnosis of acute rejection still relies upon routine or extemporary EMBs. Echocardiography at rest is useful for increasing the clinical suspicion of rejection, for monitoring its impact on cardiac function, and for optimizing the timing of follow-up biopsies. In the long-term, resting and stress (with dobutamine) echocardiography may raise the suspicion for CAV, and provides prognostic information. It is of utmost importance to compare each echocardiogram with previous examinations, and the specific experience of the reviewer in follow-up of HTx patients is relevant to the reliability of echocardiographic findings. DSE is important in prognostication after HTx,[6] and provides a good accuracy for detecting significant CAV.[10] However, early vasculopathy not associated with obvious impairment of coronary flow reserve may be missed. ICUS appears the best tool for early recognition of these problems. Nevertheless, non-invasive assessment of (initially) blunted coronary flow reserve by myocardial perfusion scintigraphy at maximal coronary artery vasodilatation is feasible and validated in ischemic heart disease. Myocardial perfusion scintigraphy with high-dose dipyridamole has a role in detecting CAV, with the advantage of being less patient- and operator-dependent than echocardiography. The use of a reference map for normalcy derived from "healthy" HTx recipients (i.e. without either CAV or history of acute rejections) instead of from healthy non-transplant individuals could increase its accuracy.

However, the diffuse nature of CAV may result in balanced ischemia that is difficult to recognize even by quantitative perfusion imaging. Among recently introduced imaging techniques, MRI appears promising for diagnosis of both acute rejection and CAV, but more experience and data are needed.

In general, the evaluation of any non-invasive technique for the diagnosis of CAV meets some problems. First of all, a reference "gold standard" must be defined: at present, ICUS is the best technique for characterizing the specific morphology of CAV, but in practice it is not widely employed. The use of coronary angiography could result in an inappropriate classification of some cases as false-positive by other imaging modalities, because of the low sensitivity of angiography in detecting diffuse disease. In theory, this problem could be circumvented by testing the imaging technique with respect to the occurrence of relevant clinical events (e.g. death, heart failure, myocardial infarction, reduction in EF) during follow-up. This approach is attractive, but it must be kept in mind that the same events can occur as a consequence of other causes (e.g. acute rejection, complication of long-standing hypertension and/or renal failure). Acute rejection, especially if occurring late after HTx, may promote acceleration of the immune process of CAV, thus frustrating the ability of non-invasive tests to predict patient course beyond characterizing his or her status at the time of the test.

In practice, it must be kept in mind that sensitivity should be selected, rather than specificity, when choosing a technique for non-invasive screening of HTx recipients during long-term follow-up. In fact, despite the limitations of therapeutic options, the diagnosis of CAV is relevant for the following reasons:

1 HTx recipients form a small, heterogeneous, and very challenging and costly patient cohort. The more we learn about the mechanisms of disease, the greater the probability of finding a strategy for prevention and treatment, in terms of general and individualized protocols.

2 Patients desire prognostic information, even if there are no direct therapeutic consequences.

3 Perhaps most important, new immunosuppressive therapies are emerging (proliferation inhibitors: sirolimus and everolimus) that could improve our capability to prevent and treat CAV, when utilized either in *de novo* patients or as "rescue" after CAV has been diagnosed. The use of reliable non-invasive tests for monitoring of CAV and prediction of its consequences on patient outcome will facilitate the evaluation of their efficacy in clinical practice.

References

1 Taylor DO, Edwards LB, Boucek MM, *et al.* The registry of the International Society for Heart and Lung Transplantation: twenty-first official adult heart transplant report, 2004. *J Heart Lung Transplant* 2004;**23**:796–803.
2 Dandel M, Hummel M, Muller J, *et al.* Reliability of tissue Doppler wall motion monitoring after heart transplantation for replacement of invasive routine screenings by optimally timed cardiac biopsies and catheterizations. *Circulation* 2001;**104**:1184–91.

3 Kanno S, Wu YJ, Lee PC, *et al.* Macrophage accumulation associated with rat cardiac allograft rejection detected by magnetic resonance imaging with ultrasmall superparamagnetic iron oxide particles. *Circulation* 2001;**104**:934–8.

4 Aparici CM, Narula J, Puig M, *et al.* Somatostatin receptor scintigraphy predicts impending cardiac allograft rejection before endomyocardial biopsy. *Eur J Nucl Med* 2000;**27**:1754–9.

5 Vassalli G, Gallino A, Weis M, *et al.* Alloimmunity and non-immunologic risk factors in cardiac allograft vasculopathy. *Eur Heart J* 2003;**24**:1180–8.

6 Spes HC, Klauss V, Mudra H, *et al.* Diagnostic and prognostic value of serial dobutamine stress echocardiography for non-invasive assessment of cardiac allograft vasculopathy: comparison with coronary angiography and intravascular ultrasound. *Circulation* 1999;**100**:509–15.

7 Ciliberto GR, Ruffini L, Mangiavacchi M, *et al.* Resting echocardiography and quantitative dipyridamole technetium-99m sestamibi tomography in the identification of cardiac allograft vasculopathy and the prediction of long-term prognosis after heart transplantation. *Eur Heart J* 2001;**22**:964–71.

8 Ciliberto GR, Massa D, Mangiavacchi M, *et al.* High-dose dipyridamole echocardiography test in coronary artery disease after heart transplantation. *Eur Heart J* 1993; **14**:48–52.

9 Ciliberto GR, Parodi O, Cataldo G, *et al.* Prognostic value of contractile response during high-dose dipyridamole echocardiography test in heart transplant recipients. *J Heart Lung Transplant* 2003;**22**:526–32.

10 Fang JC, Rocco T, Jarcho J, *et al.* Non-invasive assessment of transplant-associated arteriosclerosis. *Am Heart J* 1998;**134**:980–7.

11 Mairesse GH, Marwick TH, Melin JA, *et al.* Use of exercise electrocardiography, technetium-99m-MIBI perfusion tomography, and two-dimensional echocardiography for coronary disease surveillance in a low-prevalence population of heart transplant recipients. *J Heart Transplant* 1995;**14**:222–9.

12 Gao SZ, Alderman EL, Schroeder JS, *et al.* Accelerated coronary vascular disease in heart transplant patients: coronary arteriographic findings. *J Am Coll Cardiol* 1988;**12**:334–40.

13 Rickenbacher PR, Pinto FJ, Lewis NP, *et al.* Prognostic importance of intimal thickness as measured by intracoronary ultrasound after cardiac transplantation. *Circulation* 1995;**92**:3445–52.

14 Kobashigawa JA, Katznelson S, Laks H, *et al.* Effect of pravastatin on outcomes after cardiac transplantation. *N Engl J Med* 1995;**333**:621–7.

15 Muehling OM, Wilke NM, Panse P, *et al.* Reduced myocardial perfusion reserve and transmural perfusion gradient in heart transplant arteriopathy assessed by magnetic resonance imaging. *J Am Coll Cardiol* 2003;**42**:1054–60.

16 Knollmann FD, Bocksch W, Spiegelsberger S, *et al.* Electron-beam computed tomography in the assessment of coronary artery disease after heart transplantation. *Circulation* 2000;**101**:2078–82.

17 Ratliff NB III, Jorgensen CR, Gobel FL, *et al.* Lack of usefulness of electron beam computed tomography for detecting coronary allograft vasculopathy. *Am J Cardiol* 2004; **93**:202–6.

CHAPTER 20

Unusual cardiomyopathies — role of cardiac magnetic resonance imaging

Sanjay K. Prasad, Ravi G. Assomull, and Dudley J. Pennell

Introduction

In the WHO/ISFC classification, cardiomyopathies are classified on the basis of their predominant pathophysiologic features. The best characterized and clinically most prevalent cardiomyopathies are hypertrophic cardiomyopathy (HCM) and dilated cardiomyopathy (DCM). However, there are other less common but clinically important diseases that affect the myocardium. These are either associated with a particular cardiac disorder or are part of a generalized systemic disorder. The latter are termed specific cardiomyopathies. Within the framework of this classification, there are a range of uncommon cardiomyopathies that may present in diverse ways and where diagnosis can be both challenging and frustrating. Examples include predominant restrictive cardiomyopathies such as amyloidosis and Fabry disease; specific cardiomyopathies resulting from sarcoidosis; toxic reactions caused by iron overload; arrhythmogenic right ventricular dysplasia (ARVD); and unclassified conditions including myocardial non-compaction. Accurate diagnosis is important in directing correct treatment strategies. Traditionally, invasive procedures including endomyocardial biopsy have played a key part in diagnosis but carry the problems of associated morbidity and mortality and, importantly, are very prone to sampling errors. More recently, cardiac magnetic resonance imaging (CMR) has had an important role in defining the severity of systolic and diastolic function and in tissue characterization. In many cases, a near definitive diagnosis can be obtained non-invasively with the benefit of serial monitoring and the opportunity to assess therapeutic responsiveness. The non-invasive nature of CMR coupled with the lack of ionizing radiation make it an ideal modality for initial assessment and serial monitoring of many of these conditions.

Amyloidosis

Amyloidosis is a multisystem disease characterized by the deposition of amyloid fibrils in the extracellular compartments of various organs, including the heart, liver, kidneys, and neurologic system. These deposits result in widespread organ dysfunction and death. Classification of amyloidosis is based on the immuno-chemical analysis of the protein fibrils involved. Primary amyloidosis is charac-terized by monoclonal immunoglobulin light-chain amyloid protein deposition and is associated with multiple myeloma. Secondary amyloidosis (AA amyloid) is associated with disorders of chronic inflammation (e.g. rheumatoid arthritis and tuberculosis) and involves the deposition of protein A. The rarest form, fa-milial amyloidosis, is characterized by a mutation in the plasma protein pre-albumin (transthyretin). Up to 50% of patients with amyloidosis have signifi-cant deposition of amyloid in the heart. Although the syndrome of congestive heart failure (CHF) is only seen in approximately 25% of amyloidosis patients, its development is associated with a survival of less than 6 months. In addition, more than half of all amyloidosis-related deaths are attributed to cardiac infiltration.

The hallmark of this disorder is a restrictive cardiomyopathy with the "stiff heart syndrome," characterized by early impairment of diastolic function and relatively preserved systolic function until late in the disease (Fig. 20.1). Typi-cally, there is concentric hypertrophy of the ventricle and interatrial septal thickening. Histologically, there is accumulation of amyloid fibrils mainly in the myocardial interstitium, resulting in interstitial expansion with amyloid pro-

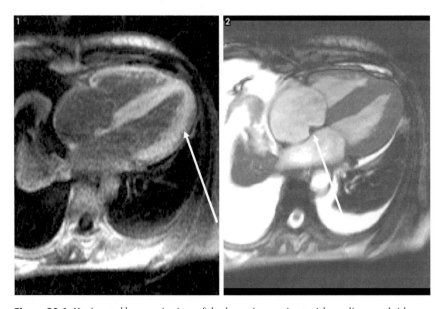

Figure 20.1 Horizontal long-axis view of the heart in a patient with cardiac amyloid. Panel 1 (left) shows images following gadolinium enhancement. There is widespread late enhancement in the left and right ventricles. The degree of late enhancement is al-most transmural with some sparing of the lateral epicardial wall (see pointer). Panel 2 (right) shows gradient echo cine image demonstrating concentric left ventricular hyper-trophy, biatrial dilatation with hypertophy of the intra-atrial septum (see pointer).

tein and associated endomyocardial fibrosis. The restrictive physiology results not only from the physical presence of amyloid infiltrates in the myocardium, but also from direct depression of diastolic function by circulating immunoglobulin light chains. Unlike HCM, left ventricular (LV) systolic and diastolic function is impaired, with a reduced ejection fraction.[1] In contrast to the accelerated early LV diastolic filling found in constrictive pericarditis, cardiac amyloidosis is characterized by an impaired rate of early diastolic filling, which can be detected by flow mapping. Following administration of Gd-DTPA, CMR shows a characteristic pattern of global subendocardial late enhancement coupled with abnormal myocardial and blood-pool gadolinium kinetics.[2] The findings accord with the transmural histologic distribution of amyloid protein and the cardiac amyloid load, and may potentially enable earlier diagnosis and follow-up. The mitral and tricuspid valve leaflets may also be thickened. See Video clips 24–26 ◉.

Fabry disease

This condition, also known as angiokeratoma corporis diffusum universale, is an X-linked recessive disorder of glycosphingolipid metabolism resulting from a deficiency of the lysosomal enzyme alpha-galactosidase A. The disease is characterized by an intracellular accumulation of glycosphingolipids with prominent involvement of the skin and kidneys as well as the myocardium in the classic form. Histologic examination often reveals widespread involvement of the myocardium, vascular endothelium, conducting tissues, and valves, particularly the mitral valve. The major clinical manifestations result from the accumulation of the glycolipid substrate in endothelial cells, with eventual occlusion of small arterioles. The CMR usually reveals increased LV wall thickness producing diastolic dysfunction which is usually mild. Generally, LV systolic function is preserved, and there is mild mitral regurgitation. Delayed enhancement is useful in differentiating Fabry from other hypertrophic processes, as there is a characteristic pattern of mid-wall late enhancement of the basal lateral wall.[3] See Video clips 27–29 ◉.

Sarcoidosis

Sarcoidosis is a multisystem, granulomatous disease of unknown etiology. It may affect almost any organ and is characterized typically by the presence of non-caseating granulomas (Table 20.1). These are composed mainly of an aggregate of epithelioid cells and Langhans or foreign body-type giant cells in the center, surrounded by lymphocytes, plasma cells, and mast cells. It is thought that granuloma formation results from an exaggerated cellular immune response to a variety of antigens or self-antigens which cause CD4 (helper-inducer) T-cell accumulation, activation, and release of inflammatory cytokines. Underlying infectious, environmental, and genetic factors have been implicated, but no clear relationship has been established.

Table 20.1 Guidelines for diagnosing cardiac sarcoidosis, the Japanese Ministry of Health and Welfare, 1993.

• Histological diagnosis
Cardiac sarcoidosis is confirmed when histological analysis of operative or endomyocardial biopsy demonstrates non-caseating granuloma
Or
• Clinical diagnosis
In patients with a histological diagnosis of extracardiac sarcoidosis, cardiac sarcoidosis is suspected when item 1 and one or more of items 2–5 are present
1. Complete RBBB, left-axis deviation, atrioventricular block, VT, premature ventricular contractions (>grade 2 of Lown's classification of PVC), or abnormal Q or ST-T wave abnormalities on the ECG
2. Abnormal wall motion, regional wall thinning, or dilatation of the left ventricle in echocardiographic studies
3. Perfusion defects by 201 Tl-myocardial scintigraphy or abnormal accumulation by 67 Ga-citrate or 99 m TC-myocardial scintigraphy
4. Abnormal intra-cardiac pressure, low cardiac output, or abnormal wall motion or depressed LV ejection fraction in cardiac catheterization
5. Non-specific interstitial fibrosis or cellular infiltration in myocardial biopsy

---

The occurrence of cardiac involvement depends on the population and occurs in 10–27% of sarcoid patients in Europe and the USA but may be as high as 40% in Japan. In the University of Southern California postmortem series, granulomatous lesions in the heart were found in 24 of 123 patients (19.5%) with sarcoidosis who had autopsies performed.

From a cardiac perspective, most sarcoid patients are asymptomatic; clinical evidence of cardiac involvement is present in less than 5% of patients and generally occurs in patients with multisystem disease. Isolated cardiac involvement has been described in a few case reports but is extremely rare and usually precedes future systemic sarcoidosis. The most common presentation is with conduction abnormalities. However, patients may also demonstrate ventricular arrhythmias, mitral regurgitation, CHF, ventricular aneurysms, pericardial effusion, and pericarditis. The two most common causes of mortality are ventricular arrhythmias and heart failure.

Accurate diagnosis by CMR relies on an awareness of which regions of the heart are affected and identifying the extent of the myocardium involved. In 1977, Roberts et al. reported the result of 113 necropsy patients with cardiac sarcoidosis.[4] They found that the LV free wall is the most common location for granulomas and scars, followed by the intraventricular septum, right ventricular (RV) free wall, and then right and left atria. Skold et al. reported the presence of both systolic and diastolic dysfunction in patients with cardiac sarcoidosis documented by CMR.[5] Patients with CHF syndrome may show clinical features of restrictive and/or DCM. Where there is extensive pulmonary parenchymal

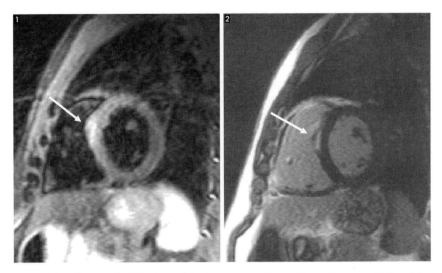

Figure 20.2 Short-axis (SA) view of the heart in a patient with cardiac sarcoid. Panel 1 (left) shows a T2-weighted STIR (short tau inversion recovery) sequence. There is increased signal in the intraventricular septum indicating an area of myocardial edema (see pointer). Panel 2 (right) shows a gadolinium-enhanced sequence of the same SA slice. There is delayed enhancement seen in the same area of the intraventricular septum (see pointer). This area represents fibrosis with an element of myocardial inflammation.

fibrotic involvement, secondary pulmonary hypertension may develop leading to RV hypertrophy and eventually to RV failure.

In active disease, granulomatous infiltrates may show patchy regions of increased signal on T2-weighted images, reflecting myocardial edema or inflammation (Fig. 20.2). Following administration of gadolinium, regional patterns of delayed enhancement can be seen that reflect postinflammatory scarring.[6] The most common pattern is mid-wall enhancement but papillary muscle and subendocardial involvement can also be seen. A late feature of cardiac sarcoid involvement is ventricular dilatation associated with wall thinning and impaired function. CMR can be useful to distinguish the etiology from an idiopathic DCM. Valvular dysfunction resulting from papillary muscle involvement is more common than direct destruction of the valvular leaflets by sarcoidosis and has been observed in up to 68% of patients with cardiac sarcoidosis. Patients may present either with the acute onset of mitral regurgitation and hemodynamic decompensation caused by acute papillary muscle dysfunction or rupture, or with more insidious and chronic state characterized by LV enlargement and compensatory eccentric hypertrophy. CMR can be used to assess accurately the severity of the mitral regurgitation through a combination of flow-mapping and measurement of right and left ventricular stroke volumes. Use of delayed enhancement can also identify papillary muscle involvement.

On a wider front, extracardiac involvement can be imaged. Much less commonly, rare cases of cardiac sarcoidosis mimicking RV dysplasia or hypertrophic cardiomyopathy have been described.

In the serial use of CMR as a method of evaluating and monitoring cardiac sarcoidosis, Vignaux et al.[7] studied 12 patients. CMR abnormalities, consisting of cardiac signal intensity and thickness, were grouped in the following three patterns: nodular; focal increase in signal on Gd-DTPA T1-weighted images; and focal increased signal on T2-weighted images without Gd-DTPA uptake. CMR scans were obtained initially and after a 12-month follow-up interval. In six patients who had received corticosteroid therapy, the CMR improved either partially or completely, whereas the images from the patients who had received no corticosteroid therapy either worsened or remained unchanged. While these findings are encouraging, larger multicentre trials are required that incorporate correlation of myocardial histology with CMR features to ascertain the true sensitivity and specificity of CMR in detection and monitoring of cardiac sarcoid involvement. Currently, there is much interest in the use of CMR to direct biopsies, guide initiation of steroids, and monitor therapeutic response. See Video clips 30 and 31 .

Arrhythmogenic right ventricular cardiomyopathy

Arrhythmogenic right ventricular cardiomyopathy (ARVC) is a genetically determined heart muscle disease that is a recognized cause of sudden death in young people. Replacement of the RV myocardium by adipose and fibrous tissue is characteristic. The natural history of the disease includes four main phases. In the early, "concealed" phase, minor ventricular arrhythmia may occur while morphologic changes remain subtle. Subsequently, overt electrical disorders and RV fibrofatty changes are more apparent. Fibrofatty replacement commences at the epicardium and gradually extends through the myocardium towards the subendocardium. The right ventricular outflow tract (RVOT), apex, and subtricuspid region are most frequently affected. Later, progression of myocardial disease may lead to isolated RV failure. Advanced cases may demonstrate LV involvement with biventricular pump dysfunction.

Possible underlying mechanisms at a cellular level include mutations in desmoplakin and plakoglobin. Both are cell adhesion proteins involved in maintaining the structural integrity of tissues. The RV may be more susceptible to mechanical stress than the LV because of its relatively thin walls. An international task force has proposed guidelines to facilitate the clinical diagnosis of ARVC. Structural, histologic, electrocardiographic, arrhythmic, and genetic features of the disease are incorporated into major and minor criteria. The presence of two major, one major plus two minor, or four minor criteria is considered confirmatory. Morphologic and functional abnormalities that qualify as major criteria include severe dilatation and reduction of RV ejection fraction with minimal or no LV impairment, localized RV aneurysms (dyskinetic areas with diastolic bulging), and severe segmental dilatation of the RV. Minor criteria include mild global RV dilatation and/or reduced ejection fraction with normal LV, mild segmental dilatation of the RV and regional RV hypokinesia.

CMR is well placed to detect the structural and functional abnormalities associated with ARVC, as it enables clear visualization of both the RV and its outflow tract, unlike 2D echocardiography.[8,9] Cine MRI in the short axis and transverse planes offers good depiction of RV dilatation, regional wall motion abnormality, aneurysms, trabecular disarray, and wall thinning. RV volumes can be measured accurately, which is a very useful quantitative indication of early disease. T1-weighted spin-echo images can show fatty replacement. This may be patchy, and care is needed to prevent over-reading because of the normal presence of epicardial fat. Furthermore, intramyocardial fat may be a normal finding in elderly subjects, particularly at the apex of the RV. Overall, CMR is an accurate and reliable means of defining anatomic abnormalities in experienced hands. In the concealed phase of the disease, where structural changes are more subtle, correlation with other clinical information is mandatory. Early data suggest that an abnormal CMR study is of prognostic importance in ARVC. See Video clips 32–34 👁.

Iron overload cardiomyopathy

Iron overload cardiomyopathy is an important global cause of mortality. Beta-thalassemia major is the main predisposing condition, and 60,000 homozygote children are born with this annually. More than 70% of these patients die of heart failure resulting from the tissue iron overload caused by the requirement for repeat blood transfusions. Myocardial iron cannot be predicted from other surrogate measures such as serum ferritin or liver iron, and direct assessment of myocardial iron by biopsy is complicated because of safety issues, and patchy myocardial iron distribution. Recently, iron measurement using myocardial T2* CMR has been shown to be useful[10] (Fig. 20.3). T2* is a measure of magnetic relaxation, and this falls as iron levels rise. The lower limit of normal of myocardial T2* is 20 ms. Classic ventricular remodeling of heart failure occurs in patients with low T2*, with increased volumes and mass but reduced ejection fraction. The important advantage of myocardial T2* as an indicator of myocardial iron overload is that it can be easily recognized early because of the well-defined limit of normality, whereas ventricular function parameters have a much wider variation and early recognition of abnormality can be problematic. T2* CMR has been used to evaluate the myocardial effects of different chelation therapies, and can be completed rapidly in a single breath-hold with excellent reproducibility.[11] Iron overload can also be assessed in primary hemochromatosis.

Left ventricular non-compaction

Isolated non-compaction of the ventricular myocardium is a rare, unclassified cardiomyopathy characterized by an excessively prominent trabecular

2ms 4ms 6ms 8ms

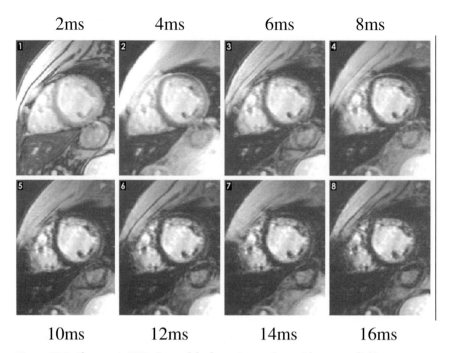

10ms 12ms 14ms 16ms

Figure 20.3 Short-axis (SA) views of the heart in a patient with myocardial iron overload. The eight panels show the same SA slice with images taken at increased echo times using a T2* sequence. The images are all acquired in a single breath-hold and demonstrate significant iron loading at an echo time below 20 ms. This corresponds to clinically severe myocardial iron loading.

meshwork and deep intertrabecular recesses.[12] There is altered structure of the myocardial wall as a result of intrauterine arrest of compaction of the endocardium and myocardium in the absence of any coexisting congenital lesion. There is continuity between the LV cavity and the intratrabecular recesses without evidence of communication to the epicardial coronary artery system. It may have an autosomal dominant pattern of inheritance. Clinical presentation is usually because of heart failure, ventricular dysrhythmias, or embolic events. CMR demonstrates these patterns of abnormal LV trabeculation well and in particular because of differences in signal intensity, readily distinguishes the compacted from the non-compacted layer (Fig. 20.4). The most common sites affected are the LV apical and inferior walls followed by the mid-ventricular lateral wall. LV function is typically impaired with both systolic and diastolic dysfunction. A restrictive filling pattern may be seen. A quantitative approach to diagnosis has been widely used by determining the ratio of maximal thickness of the non-compacted to compacted layers (measured at end-systole in a short-axis view), with a ratio > 2 diagnostic of isolated myocardial non-compaction. This technique allows for differentiation of the trabeculations of non-compaction from that observed with dilated or hypertensive cardiomyopathy.

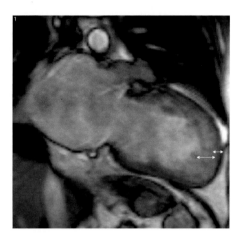

Figure 20.4 Vertical long-axis view of the heart in a patient with left ventricular non-compaction. The image shows marked trabeculation in the apex which is over twice as thick as the compacted layer in systole.

Following gadolinium, delayed enhancement reflecting fibrotic change may be seen at the trabecular level. The key advantage of CMR in non-compaction is the excellent apical visualization combined with differences in signal characteristics. See Video clips 35–37 ⊙.

Conclusions

CMR is well suited to the assessment of uncommon cardiomyopathies. Its strength lies in the range of methods for tissue characterization and the excellent resolution and visualization of all regions of the heart. For some of these conditions, such as iron overload, CMR techniques are well established but in sarcoid and amyloidosis larger multicentre trials with some histologic correlation are required to validate the exciting initial findings. A key challenge will be monitoring patients who undergo some form of device implantation.

References

1 Fattori R, Rocchi G, Celletti F, Bertaccini P, Rapezzi C, Gavelli G. Contribution of magnetic resonance imaging in the differential diagnosis of cardiac amyloidosis and symmetric hypertrophic cardiomyopathy. *Am Heart J* 1998;**136**:824–30.

2 Maceira AM, Joshi J, Prasad SK, *et al.* Cardiovascular magnetic resonance in cardiac amyloidosis. *Circulation* 2005;**111**:186–93.

3 Moon JC, Sachdev B, Elkington AG, *et al.* Gadolinium enhanced cardiovascular magnetic resonance in Anderson–Fabry disease: evidence for a disease specific abnormality of the myocardial interstitium. *Eur Heart J* 2003;**24**:2151–5.

4 Roberts WC, McAllister HA Jr, Ferrans VJ. Sarcoidosis of the heart. A clinicopathologic study of 35 necropsy patients (group 1) and review of 78 previously described necropsy patients (group 11). *Am J Med* 1977;**63**:86–108.

5 Skold CM, Larsen FF, Rasmussen E, Pehrsson SK, Eklund AG. Determination of

cardiac involvement in sarcoidosis by magnetic resonance imaging and Doppler echocardiography. *J Intern Med* 2002;**252**:465–71.

6 Nemeth MA, Muthupillai R, Wilson JM, *et al*. Cardiac sarcoidosis detected by delayed-hyper enhancement magnetic resonance imaging. *Tex Heart Inst J* 2004;**31**:99–102.

7 Vignaux O, Dhote R, Duboc D, *et al*. Clinical significance of myocardial magnetic resonance abnormalities in patients with sarcoidosis: a 1-year follow-up study. *Chest* 2002;**122**:1895–901.

8 Tandri H, Bomma C, Calkins H, Bluemke DA. Magnetic resonance and computed tomography imaging of arrhythmogenic right ventricular dysplasia. *J Magn Reson Imaging* 2004;**19**:848–58.

9 di Cesare E. MRI assessment of right ventricular dysplasia. *Eur Radiol* 2003;**13**:1387–93.

10 Anderson LJ, Holden S, Davis B, *et al*. Cardiovascular T2-star (T2*) magnetic resonance for the early diagnosis of myocardial iron overload. *Eur Heart J* 2001;**22**:2171–9.

11 Anderson LJ, Wonke B, Prescott E, *et al*. Comparison of effects of oral deferiprone and subcutaneous desferrioxamine on myocardial iron concentrations and ventricular function in beta-thalassaemia. *Lancet* 2002;**360**:516–20.

12 Weiford BC, Subbarao VD, Mulhern KM. Non-compaction of the ventricular myocardium. *Circulation* 2004;**109**:2965–71.

CHAPTER 21

Myocarditis and pericardial disease

Frank E. Rademakers

Introduction

Myocarditis and pericardial disease are two distinct clinical entities that share an often obscure etiology and a difficult differential diagnosis. They both show an acute inflammatory response to an infectious, non-infectious (toxic), or autoimmune agent that interferes with normal function and can evolve into a chronic phase with persistent inflammation or scar formation in the myocardium and/or stiffening of the pericardium with or without calcification. In the setting of an acute infectious or toxic event they can occur together with a variable clinical emphasis on myocardial or pericardial involvement.

The contributions of cardiovascular imaging are discussed, focusing on the content of information, rather than the imaging modality itself. Often, different modalities can provide similar information and it depends on cost, availability, and expertise which modality is chosen. The areas where some modalities can have a specific contribution are highlighted.

Myocarditis

In the acute phase, myocarditis can mimic acute myocardial infarction with respect to clinical presentation, ECG abnormalities, and concomitant arrhythmias and conduction disturbances. Elevation of troponin levels is often present and further obscures the differential diagnosis. In the chronic phase, the emphasis is on directing therapy and monitoring evolution and complications. Non-invasive imaging can contribute in several ways.

Myocardial dysfunction

The primary effect of acute inflammation of the myocardium is contractile dysfunction. This dysfunction is often not diffuse but can affect one or more defined regions of the left or right ventricle, further complicating the differential diagnosis with ischemic heart disease. Wall motion abnormalities can be identified by echocardiography, cardiac magnetic resonance imaging (CMR), multislice computed tomography (MSCT), or gated nuclear studies; regional function can be qualitatively assessed using a wall motion score (echocardiography, CMR,

MSCT) or quantitatively by measuring wall thickening (CMR, nuclear, MSCT) or myocardial strain rate/strain (velocity myocardial imaging [VMI]). Global function (EDV, ESV, and SV) can be determined by either technique but reproducibility (for follow-up) is better with CMR. The extent and severity of the dysfunction can vary widely from mild depression of pump function (borderline decreased ejection fraction) to an acutely dilated ventricle with a very low stroke volume and signs of heart failure or even cardiogenic shock. In cases of localized dysfunction, the unaffected regions can show compensatory hyperkinesia. Recovery can be spectacular in some cases but cannot be reliably predicted from the location or extent of the acute dysfunction.

If recovery is incomplete and patients present in this phase of the disease, a dilated hypokinetic ventricle is often present and the differential diagnosis of a dilated cardiomyopathy has to be made.

To differentiate from an ischemic origin, CMR with late enhanced imaging can be of help[1]: an ischemic origin typically produces subendocardial regions of late enhancement (subendocardial infarction and scarring), whereas a non-ischemic origin either does not show any late enhancement or a mid-myocardial or even subepicardial enhancement. Although the latter pattern has not been shown to be typical for a late evolution of myocarditis, it is compatible with the predominant epicardial affection of the myocardium in many cases.

Inflammation imaging

Tissue characterization can be obtained from ultrasonic backscatter analysis but few data exist in the setting of acute myocarditis. CMR uses different sequences[2] (T1-weighted with and without contrast gadolinium (Gd) administration; T2-weighted; cine imaging) to obtain tissue characteristics. High signal intensity with T2-weighting points towards edema but this finding is non-specific and also present in acute myocardial infarction. Increased signal intensity after Gd administration was shown consistently in the setting of myocarditis[3] and can be focal (probably earlier in the course of the disease) or more diffuse. Either the extent of contrast enhancement over time or the ratio between enhancement in the myocardium versus the peripheral muscles can be used. Again, such an enhancement—certainly if focal—is not specific for myocarditis. With serial follow-up, the remaining contrast enhancement 4 weeks after onset of symptoms was shown to be predictive for functional and clinical long-term outcome.[4]

Gallium-67 myocardial imaging can be used to identify inflammation of the myocardium and monitor the evolution and has compared favorably with endomyocardial biopsies. Indium-111 antimyosin antibodies bind specifically to damaged myocytes and were shown to give a more diffuse enhancement in myocarditis versus myocardial infarction. Although inflammation imaging is feasible with different techniques, the problem of non-specificity remains, so that this technique is currently more important for follow-up and prognosis than for diagnosis. However, it could be used to guide the site of endocardial biopsy and so improve the sensitivity and specificity of this diagnostic procedure.[5]

Complications

The different complications of myocarditis (pericardial and pleural effusion, congestive heart failure) can be visualized on chest X-ray, echocardiography, CMR, or CT. Echocardiography remains the modality of choice, because it can be used at the bedside and allows, in most cases, a good evaluation of these complications, including Doppler traces to identify the hemodynamic status, the presence of increased filling pressures, and the existence of valvular abnormalities. If echo Doppler is impossible or suboptimal for some reason, CMR is the best alternative.

Evolution towards scarring can be evaluated by CMR late enhanced imaging after Gd administration, where the high-intensity areas are typically subepicardial or mid-myocardial (Fig. 21.1, right, gray arrow) in contrast to ischemic subendocardial lesions (Fig. 21.1, right, white arrow) or lesions at the insertion of the right ventricle in hypertrophic cardiomyopathy (Fig. 21.1 left).

Prognosis

Although the end-diastolic volume, the ejection fraction, and the extent of inflammation[5] in the acute phase have all been proposed as predictive for outcome, none of these parameters can consistently predict the clinical evolution. Early follow-up (first month) is likely a better way of foreseeing the evolution,[4] but the impact on clinical management remains to be examined.

Future

Although non-invasive imaging has greatly enhanced our understanding of the impact and evolution of myocarditis, both with respect to the functional as well

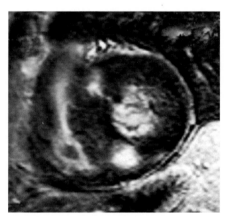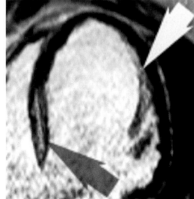

Figure 21.1 Cardiac magnetic resonance (CMR) late enhanced images after administration of gadolinium in hypertrophic cardiomyopathy (CMP; left) and in combined subendocardial, ischemic lesion (right, white arrow) and mid-myocardial (right, gray arrow) lesion which could be a late result of myocarditis or another non-ischemic etiology.

as the inflammatory changes, the differential diagnosis in the acute setting remains a challenge. Further evolution with molecular targeted imaging (echocardiography, CMR, nuclear) could help in identifying a specific agent as the cause of acute myocyte necrosis.

Pericardial disease

The main clinical pericardial syndromes are acute and relapsing pericarditis, pericardial effusion and tamponade, and effusive–constrictive and constrictive pericarditis (CP).Uncommon congenital pericardial abnormalities include pericardial cysts and the congential absence of the pericardium. Non-invasive imaging can contribute to the diagnosis by showing the morphologic abnormality (i.e. the presence of pericardial fluid), the absence or thickening of the pericardium, but also has the goal to evaluate the impact on cardiac function. To appreciate the different parameters used in the diagnosis and differential diagnosis of pericardial diseases, an understanding of the physiology and pathophysiology is important.

Pathophysiology

The normal human pericardium is a relatively stiff sac, enveloping the heart and the origins of the vessels and is attached to the adventitia of the arteries and to the sternum, vertebral column, and diaphragm (Fig. 21.2). The pressure in the pericardium, although still under debate, is between 0 and 3 mmHg and slightly less than right atrial pressure; as such it limits the distension pressure of the cardiac cavities and mostly so for the thin-walled, low-pressure right heart.

When fluid accumulates in the pericardium, the pressure in the pericardium increases, the transmural diastolic distending pressures of the atria drop to zero (tamponade sets in), and the increased atrial pressures equalize.[6] As the effect of a decreased distension pressure is more pronounced in the right heart, a compression of the right atrium and ventricle occurs at the time of lowest pressure (i.e. early diastole), impeding early filling and limiting stroke volume; with increasing pericardial pressures the atrium remains collapsed throughout diastole. Left ventricular (LV) filling and output become compromised by the decreased right heart output and the increased left–right interaction. The increase in pericardial pressure depends on the speed of fluid accumulation because the pressure–volume (P–V) relation of the pericardium is relatively flat in the first part, but becomes exponential thereafter. With slow accumulation, the pericardium can grow and adapt to accommodate large amounts of fluid with only a small increase in pressure. Every acute intervention that increases the venous return to the heart, increases total heart volume and as such intrapericardial total volume and pressure; if this occurs on the steep portion of the pericardial P–V relation this will ensue in an upward shift of the LV diastolic P–V relation. Significant hypovolemia with overall small heart cavities can mask the hemodynamic effects and clinical signs of tamponade.

Because the left and right heart occupy the pericardial sac together, ventricu-

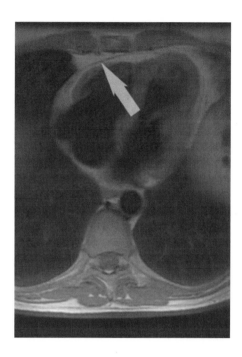

Figure 21.2 Transverse CMR image showing normal pericardium over the right ventricle.

lar interdependence or coupling exists (i.e. the more space one side of the heart occupies, the less is available for the other side), leading to increased diastolic pressures in the contralateral part. This interdependence is present in normal circumstances during breathing and is exaggerated by fluid accumulation in the pericardium or by pericardial stiffening. The depth and speed of respiration also significantly determines the size of the effect on cardiac hemodynamics and should be recorded during imaging. During inspiration, pressure in the thorax and the pericardium drops and flow towards (inferior vena cava) and from the right heart increases while the reverse occurs on the left side; during expiration the opposite changes take place.

While cardiac tamponade increases distension pressures throughout the entire filling period, the restraint in CP[7] is nearly absent during early filling but rapidly increases thereafter, giving rise to the characteristic square root sign on LV pressure traces. Another characteristic of CP is the belated transmission of changes in intrathoracic pressures to the intrapericardial structures, creating the exaggerated acute changes in filling gradients at the onset of the inspiratory and expiratory motions. During inspiration, the increased venous return is not coupled to the characteristic drop in right atrium (RA) pressure and systemic venous pressure may actually increase (i.e. Kussmaul sign in the superior caval vein [SVC]; Fig. 21.3). Because respiratory interdependence in CP decreases at higher absolute left atrium (LA) pressures and with the severity of constriction, examining a patient in the upright position (decrease of filling pressures) can unmask interdependence in such cases.

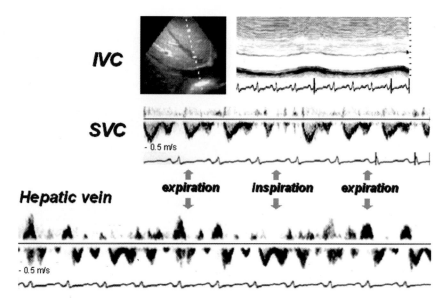

Figure 21.3 Diameter of the inferior vena cava (IVC), flow in the superior vena cava (SVC) and in a hepatic vein during inspiration and expiration in constrictive pericarditis.

In comparison with CP, tamponade exhibits a more marked pulsus paradoxus and a fall in RA pressure with onset of inspiration (no Kussmaul sign), as the intrathoracic pressure changes are readily transmitted to the intracardiac cavities. CP more than tamponade is mimicked by acute RV infarction.

CP must also be differentiated from restrictive cardiomyopathy (RCMP),[8] where the compliance problem resides within the myocardium, and from exaggerated respiratory variations and ventricular interdependence, occurring with increased intrathoracic pressure, swings in chronic obstructive pulmonary disease (COPD), marked obesity, recent thoracotomy, and marked dyspnea from another cause; hepatic vein and SVC flows can help to differentiate (Fig. 21.3).

CP and RCMP share the following features: non-dilated ventricles, ventricular filling limited to early diastole, high venous pressures with dilated inferior caval vein and reduced respiratory collapse, diastolic flow into the pulmonary artery and ventricular dip–plateau. Important differences are the larger atria in RCMP, the more pronounced respiratory changes in filling with increased interdependence in CP, the decrease of tricuspid deceleration time (DT) in RCMP, the early diastolic septal inversion in CP, and the hepatic vein reversal on atrial contraction which is more pronounced in expiration in CP (Fig. 21.3) and in inspiration in RCMP.

These pathophysiologic characteristics of pericardial syndromes can be studied with the different imaging modalities, but it is crucial to be able to register morphology, function, and flow during the different phases of the respiratory cycle.

Clinical syndromes
Congenital abnormalities
Pericardial cysts can be visualized by echocardiography, but CMR and CT are superior in identifying the extent and in their differentiation from tumors. Pericardial agenesis (complete or partial) can readily be identified by CMR or CT and the displacement of (parts of) the heart can be seen on the large field of view.

Pericarditis
The diagnosis of pericarditis is clinical (history, cardiac auscultation) and by typical ECG changes. Chest X-ray is normal in most cases but can point to causative pulmonary abnormalities. The presence of pericardial fluid can be shown most easily by echocardiography but epicardial and pericardial fat (which is not always proportional to subcutaneous fat) can be mistaken for fluid. Also, pericardial fluid is not synonymous with pericarditis nor is the absence of fluid a criterion to exclude the disease. CMR and CT[9] can show fluid quite well and can more easily make the distinction between fluid and fat. Increased signal of the pericardium after Gd administration on CMR is indicative of acute inflammation and can strengthen the diagnosis. Pericardial thickness (abnormal ≥ 4 mm) can be measured on transthoracic (if extensive) or transesophageal echocardiography, but is more reliable on CT and CMR (the latter is to be preferred if a pericardial effusion coexists).

Pericardial effusion and tamponade
The presence of fluid in the pericardial sac is normal and the effect on cardiac performance depends on the speed of accumulation: a rapid increase of 150–200 mL can cause symptoms, while a slow build-up of 2 L can go unnoticed until non-cardiac structures (lung, bronchi, trachea) become compressed. It is therefore more important to evaluate the impact on function and the evolution over time, than the amount of fluid at one given instance. In the differential diagnosis between pericardial and pleural effusion, the "separation" of the descending aorta from the LA in the parasternal long-axis echo view (pericardial effusion) can be of help.

Pericardial fluid can be identified with most techniques (see Pericarditis above) but it is important to report on the extent, location, and characteristics of the fluid (better with CMR; multiple sequences for fluid characterization) and to quantify the hemodynamic consequences.

Effusive–constrictive and constrictive pericarditis
Although thickening of the pericardium can be shown by CMR or CT, a normal thickness does not exclude CP because of increased stiffness without thickening.[10] Showing the typical hemodynamic features of constriction is therefore important. Calcification of the pericardium is best seen on X-ray or CT, because

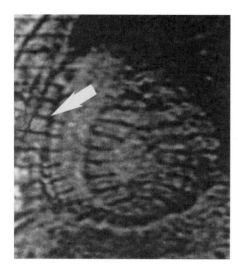

Figure 21.4 CMR striped tags during systole, showing the uninterrupted tags crossing the pericardium.

on CMR calcium is visualized as hypointense regions which can be mistaken for pericardial fluid or thickening only. A specific CMR application is the use of tagging, where lines or a grid are non-invasively enscribed on the heart: in non-CP (even with a thickened pericardium) the heart moves during the cardiac cycle independently from the pericardium, so the tags "break" at the pericardial interface, whereas in CP the tags cross the pericardium and remain uninterrupted from the myocardium to the pericardium during the cycle (Fig. 21.4).

Hemodynamic measurements both for tamponade and CP are most easily obtained by echocardiography because this real-time technique allows imaging during the different phases of the respiratory cycle. Registration of the respiratory trace is important because differentiation between changes occurring on the first beat after onset of inspiration or expiration (CP) should be differentiated from changes after two or three beats (COPD, exaggerated respiratory motion). With the advent of real-time imaging and flow measurements on CMR, this technique can also be used. Visualization of the abnormal septal motion with CP is often easier in a true short-axis image and can be well visualized on CMR.

The characteristics of tamponade, CP, and restriction are graphically summarized in Figs 21.5–21.7. Each figure shows the flow curves on the right (hepatic veins, SVC—if appropriate—and tricuspid) and on the left (pulmonary vein, mitral) during inspiration (left) and expiration (right), as well as some other hemodynamic characteristics (caval collapse, jugular vein, pericardial and intracavitary pressures).

In the differential diagnosis between CP and RCMP, nuclear studies and newer echo Doppler parameters can also help: in CP intrinsic systolic and early diastolic function are normal (certainly early in the evolution of the disease), whereas in RCMP intrinsic diastolic function is abnormal from the onset. Early

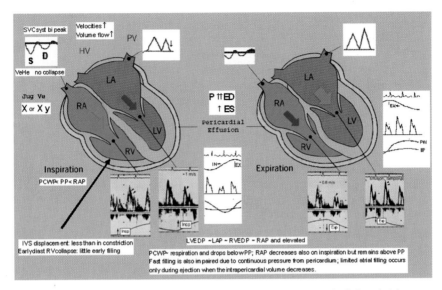

Figure 21.5 Tamponade with characteristics and flow patterns on the left and right during inspiration (left) and expiration (right).

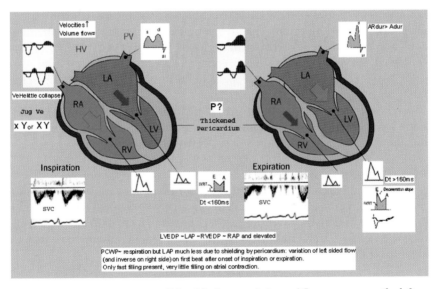

Figure 21.6 Constrictive pericarditis with characteristics and flow patterns on the left and right during inspiration (left) and expiration (right).

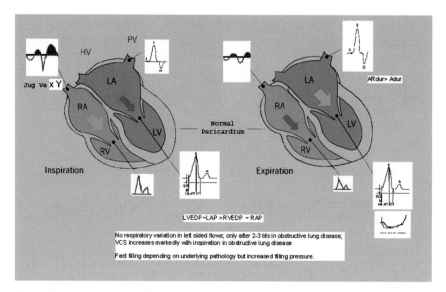

Figure 21.7 Restrictive cardiomyopathy with characteristics and flow patterns on the left and right during inspiration (left) and expiration (right).

filling velocity, as measured by nuclear techniques, is abnormal in RCMP but remains normal in PC. In a similar manner, long-axis shortening and lengthening, as measured by M-mode or VMI of the annulus, is normal in CP (Fig. 21.8), except when the valve annulus has become attached to the pericardium. Also color Doppler intracavitary flow propagation as measured by color Doppler M-mode remains normal in CP, whereas it is depressed in RCMP.

Diagnostic problems remain in cases with atrial arrhythmias (atrial fibrillation), a combination of COPD and LV myocardial restriction, and in the post-radiation patient, where constriction and restriction can coexist.

Regional tamponade and constriction

A regional fluid accumulation, pericardial adhesion, or a combination (effusive–constrictive) can be very difficult to diagnose with hemodynamic features limited to the underlying cavity rather then the entire heart and often occurring over the right ventricle (tubular-shaped). CMR is generally the best way to identify the localized thickening and adhesion (tagging).

Summary

Differential diagnosis in pericardial disease remains difficult and challenging to the clinician. When a discrepancy exists between clinical findings and hemodynamic evaluation with imaging, multiple modalities should be combined and if a very low or very high atrial pressure is suspected, an intervention to increase or lower this pressure can be required to unmask characteristic findings during respiration and with respect to ventricular interdependence.

Mitral flow velocity

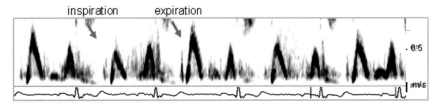

inspiration   expiration

Myocardial velocity, septum

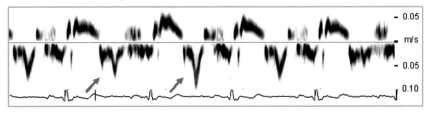

Figure 21.8 Mitral flow in constrictive pericarditis, showing a decrease with inspiration; myocardial velocity at the septum shows normal velocities, indicating preserved diastolic function, which follows the volume flow across the mitral.

Conclusions

Both myocardial and pericardial diseases often pose a diagnostic and therapeutic problem to the clinician. Not only a morphologic but also a functional hemodynamic evaluation is crucial in this respect. Echo Doppler remains the most comprehensive technique, but other modalities have increasing applications and offer additional information that cannot be obtained by echo Doppler alone. A multimodality, multidisciplinary approach, depending on availability, expertise and cost, has the best guarantee to arrive to the correct diagnosis and appropriate treatment.

References

1 McCrohon JA, Moon JC, Prasad SK, *et al*. Differentiation of heart failure related to dilated cardiomyopathy and coronary artery disease using gadolinium-enhanced cardiovascular magnetic resonance. *Circulation* 2003;**108**:54–9.
2 Laissy JP, Messin B, Varenne O, *et al*. MRI of acute myocarditis: a comprehensive approach based on various imaging sequences. *Chest* 2002;**122**:1638–48.
3 Friedrich MG, Strohm O, Schulz-Menger J, Marciniak H, Luft FC, Dietz R. Contrast media-enhanced magnetic resonance imaging visualizes myocardial changes in the course of viral myocarditis. *Circulation* 1998;**97**:1802–9.
4 Wagner A, Schulz-Menger J, Dietz R, Friedrich MG. Long-term follow-up of patients with acute myocarditis by magnetic resonance imaging. *MAGMA* 2003;**16**:17–20.
5 Mahrholdt H, Goedecke C, Wagner A, *et al*. Multimedia article. Cardiovascular mag-

netic resonance assessment of human myocarditis: a comparison to histology and molecular pathology. *Circulation* 2004;**109**:1250–8.

6 Spodick DH. Acute cardiac tamponade. *N Engl J Med* 2003;**349**:684–90.

7 Myers RB, Spodick DH. Constrictive pericarditis: clinical and pathophysiologic characteristics. *Am Heart J* 1999;**138**:219–32.

8 Hancock EW. Differential diagnosis of restrictive cardiomyopathy and constrictive pericarditis. *Heart* 2001;**86**:343–9.

9 Wang ZJ, Reddy GP, Gotway MB, Yeh BM, Hetts SW, Higgins CB. CT and MR imaging of pericardial disease. *Radiographics* 2003;**23**:S167–80.

10 Talreja DR, Edwards WD, Danielson GK, *et al*. Constrictive pericarditis in 26 patients with histologically normal pericardial thickness. *Circulation* 2003;**108**:1852–7.

CHAPTER 22

Congenital heart disease

Heynric B. Grotenhuis, Lucia J.M. Kroft, Eduard R. Holman,
Jaap Ottenkamp, and Albert de Roos

Introduction

Congenital heart disease (CHD) is rapidly growing in numbers and interest within adult cardiology because of great improvements in diagnostic tools, surgical techniques, and postoperative care for children with CHD over the last 40 years. However, postoperative abnormalities still frequently occur and a non-invasive imaging tool is desirable for the timely detection of morphologic and functional abnormalities. Transthoracic echocardiography is the most commonly used technique in the non-invasive assessment of CHD, especially in neonates and children whose small thoracic diameters provide an optimal acoustic window. In this chapter, the most frequently encountered pathologies in CHD (aortic coarctation, tetralogy of Fallot, transposition of great arteries, Fontan circulation) are discussed. Each pathology is illustrated by a representative case, focusing on the echocardiographic evaluation.

However, after surgical intervention the imaging quality is often restricted because scar, bone, or lung tissue may interfere with the acoustic window, while chest deformations may also be present. Catheter-driven angiography has clear advantages in imaging quality, but radiation burden and invasiveness are important drawbacks. Therefore, magnetic resonance imaging (MRI) is ideally suited for the non-invasive diagnosis and postoperative follow-up of CHD. MRI allows superior depiction of cardiac anatomy and highly accurate measurements of cardiac function. Accordingly, this chapter first provides a brief summary of the MRI techniques in the evaluation of CHD, before discussing the most frequently encountered pathologies in CHD. In each of these, the potential use of MRI is also addressed.

Magnetic resonance imaging techniques in congenital heart disease

A wide array of MRI techniques is available for detailed and quantified assessment of cardiac function and morphology. Black-blood imaging provides clear depiction of the cardiac anatomy because of its high tissue–blood contrast; spin-echo acquisition is used to increase the signal of static tissue and create a signal void (i.e. no MRI signal) for flowing blood. It provides two-dimensional (2D) images in three different directions (sagittal, transverse, and coronal) or in any other combined direction.[1]

Gadolinium-chelate-enhanced MR angiography (MRA) is well suited to detect morphologic abnormalities of the great vessels (e.g. coarctation of the aorta). With contrast-enhanced MRA, gadolinium-chelate shortens the T1 relaxation time of blood, resulting in high signal intensity. This allows rapid three-dimensional (3D) acquisition of the entire thoracic aorta within one breath-hold. After a bolus-timing acquisition to determine the delay between bolus injection and bolus arrival in a vessel, a 3D gradient-echo MRA sequence is performed. Then, 3D reconstructions can be acquired of the vessel, clearly depicting any region of interest.

Another rapidly advancing technique is coronary MRA for the depiction of the origin, course, and diameters of the coronary arteries. Congenital or acquired coronary anomalies such as after the arterial switch operation and Kawasaki disease can be detected without the need for conventional catheter-based coronary angiography.[2]

Gradient-echo balanced-TFE can be used to assess the function of both ventricles in a highly reproducible manner. A stack of consecutive slices in the transverse plane or along the left ventricular short-axis is applied, covering the complete myocardium of both ventricles. Endocardial and epicardial borders can then be traced by using dedicated software packages such as MASS®. Parameters such as end-diastolic and end-systolic volumes, stroke volume, cardiac output, and wall mass—the latter for the degree of myocardial hypertrophy—can be obtained. Cardiac function can be evaluated at rest, but also after dobutamine stress and even physical exercise.[3]

Delayed contrast-enhanced imaging of the myocardium can be used to determine viable and non-viable myocardium within regions of interest. After the administration of gadolinium, the non-viable cardiac regions reveal hyperenhancement on T1-weighted images compared with normal myocardium. This technique has already been proven useful in patients with coronary artery disease, but recent reports indicate that it can also be used in CHD, specifically in anomalies associated with perfusion defects and congenital coronary artery anomalies.[4]

Assessment of valvular function with phase-contrast MRI is another essential tool of cardiac MRI, allowing accurate measurement of regurgitation or stenosis. Shunt quantification is also possible by comparing the aortic and pulmonary flow. With phase-contrast MRI the flow velocity of blood can be measured, based on velocity-induced phase shifts of moving protons in the presence of a magnetic field gradient. In the area of interest, the flow volume of both the forward flow and the amount of regurgitation can be assessed, while peak velocities can be used to estimate pressure gradients over stenotic valves or vessels, using the simplified Bernoulli equation.[5] Flow mapping also provides information on the diastolic filling pattern of the ventricle and allows the construction of a ventricular time–volume curve. In patients with corrected tetralogy of Fallot and pulmonary regurgitation, the right ventricular time–volume curves have been used to demonstrate impaired relaxation and restriction to filling as markers of abnormal right ventricular diastolic function.[5]

Aortic coarctation

Coarctation of the aorta accounts for 5% of all CHD and is defined as a congenital narrowing of the aorta, most commonly located in a juxtaductal position just distal to the origin of the left subclavian artery.[6] Treatment can include surgical intervention or balloon angioplasty. Serial follow-up of these patients is necessary because of the considerable incidence of aneurysm formation and recoarctation, which varies between 8% and 67%, depending on the procedure of choice, the timing of follow-up, and the patient's age when the intervention was performed.[6] Black-blood MRI allows detailed visualization of the ascending aorta, the aortic arch, and the descending aorta by planning a stack of thin consecutive slices in the oblique sagittal direction through the plane of the aortic arch. It is sensitive for the detection and follow-up of recoarctation and aneurysms. Depiction of the aortic valve morphology—a bicuspid aortic valve is often associated with coarctation[6]—is also possible, using black-blood images perpendicular to the aortic root (Fig. 22.1). 3D MRA of the thoracic aorta can

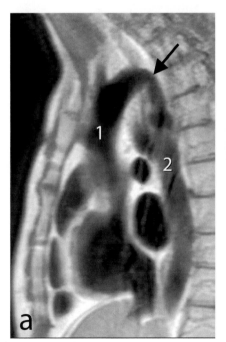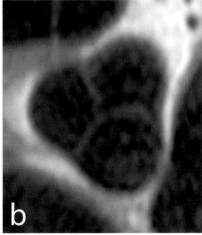

Figure 22.1 Recoarctation of the aorta after repair in a 42-year-old man with a right arcus. (a) One slice of a stack oblique sagittal black-blood spin-echo magnetic resonance imaging (MRI) slices showing the recoarctation (arrow). 1, ascending aorta; 2, descending aorta. (b) Double-oblique transversal image reveals a tricuspid aortic valve in this patient.

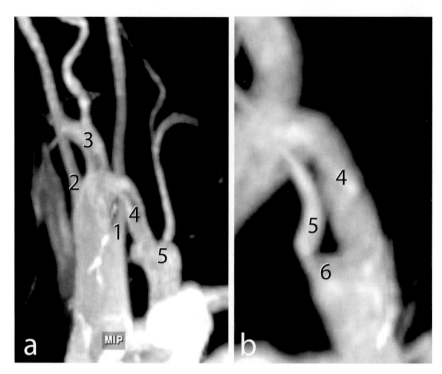

Figure 22.2 Maximum intensity projection (MIP) of magnetic resonance angiography (MRA) in the same patient, with a right arcus and aberrant left subclavian artery, and suspected recoarctation after repair. The sequence of branching can be clearly depicted (a, b). 1, left common carotid artery; 2, right common carotid artery; 3, right subclavian artery with right vertebral artery; 4, recoarctation; 5, small left subclavian artery with left vertebral artery arising from a small Kommerell diverticulum; 6, after the level of coarctation. Non-significant origostenosis of the left subclavian artery (arrow).

clearly show the spatial relationship between the stenosis, the ductus if patent, and the other arch vessels (Fig. 22.2).[7] Velocity-encoded studies enable the quantification of the pressure gradient across the narrowing and the magnitude of the collateral flow, by subtraction of the proximal aortic flow from the distal one (Fig. 22.3).[6]

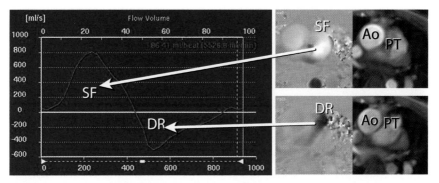

Figure 22.3 Quantification of pulmonary regurgitation by phase-contrast MRI in a 32-year-old man with corrected tetralogy of Fallot and a severely dilated right ventricle (end-diastolic volume 497 mL). The flow curve across the pulmonary trunk (PT) showed 183 mL systolic forward flow (SF) and 97 mL diastolic regurgitation (DR); calculated pulmonary regurgitation fraction was 53%.

Case Presentation 1

A 25-year-old man presented with Noonan's syndrome. At birth the coarctation was surgically corrected with a repair and patch interposition. At 20 years of age, significant recoarctation occurred with an associated left ventricular hypertrophy (Video clip 38 ⊙), and subsequently surgery was carried out during which dilatation and interposition with a Hemashield prosthesis of the stenotic region was performed. As an associated feature, a bicuspid aortic valve was found to be present (Video clips 38 and 39 ⊙).

Echocardiography at the age of 21 years revealed turbulence across the descending part of the aortic arch, with continuous flow across a narrowed part in the previously operated region (Video clip 40 ⊙). This was confirmed by cardiac MRI, showing kinking and slight stenosis (minimal diameter 1.5 cm) of the operated region, between the left carotid artery branch and the left subclavian branch. No pulmonary stenosis, ventricular septal defects, or asymmetric septal hypertrophy were observed in this patient that could be related to Noonan syndrome.

A recent echocardiographic examination showed a recurrence of pressure drop at the region of the previous coarctation and a saw-tooth shape of the continuous wave curve, indicating a recurrence of the coarctation (Figs 22.4 and 22.5). A cardiac MRI confirmed the new stenosis just proximal to the left subclavian branch with signs of collateral inflow into the descending aorta.

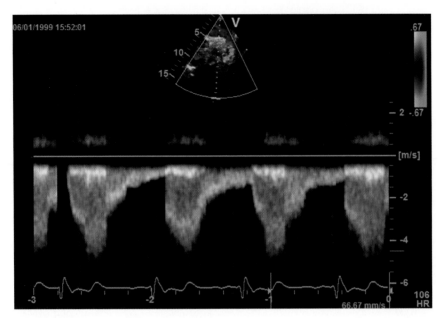

Figure 22.4 Spectral Doppler image (continuous wave) through the recoarctation. The peak gradient was calculated to be 87 mmHg. Note the saw-tooth shape of the curve, because of the wind kettle phenomenon during which the systolic and diastolic prestenotic pressure remains higher than the poststenotic pressure.

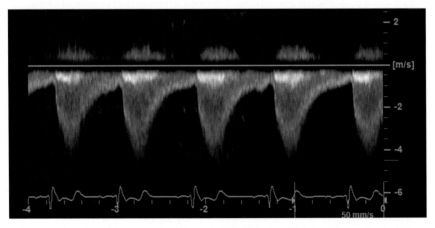

Figure 22.5 Same image as Fig. 22.4, except using the pencil probe. This type of probe does not produce two-dimensional images, but high-quality spectral Doppler curves (see caption for Fig. 22.4).

Tetralogy of Fallot

Tetralogy of Fallot (TOF) is the most common type of cyanotic CHD, occurring in approximately 5.5% of all CHD patients. It consists of four elements: a ventricular septal defect, overriding of the aorta, right ventricular outflow tract obstruction, and right ventricular hypertrophy. The intracardiac repair aims at closure of the ventricular septal defect and relief of the right ventricular outflow tract obstruction by resection of infundibular tissue and/or transannular patch placement. The resulting pulmonary regurgitation after transannular patch placement had initially been regarded as a relatively benign lesion, but recent reports have stressed the negative influence of pulmonary regurgitation on right and left ventricular performance. Pulmonary regurgitation-induced right ventricular volume overload may predispose for right ventricular failure and the development of ventricular arrhythmias and/or sudden death. Cardiac MRI is now frequently used for proper timing of replacement of the pulmonary valve, an important issue in the long-term management of TOF patients.[8] Other complications after TOF repair that can be detected and evaluated with MRI are recurrent or residual ventricular septal defects and central or peripheral pulmonary stenoses.[8]

Phase-contrast MRI can be used for the quantification of pulmonary regurgitation in postoperative TOF patients (Fig. 22.3) and for quantification of the pressure gradient across any pulmonary stenosis. Biventricular function can be obtained by the previously described gradient-echo technique, while clear depiction of (peripheral) pulmonary stenoses can be achieved best with gadolinium-enhanced MRA.

Case Presentation 2

A 39-year-old man presented with TOF. At the age of 2 years, a palliative operation was undertaken (aortopulmonary Potts shunt), and subsequent corrective surgery was performed at the age of 17 years. At the age of 37 years, he received a pulmonary homograft because of severe regurgitation of the native pulmonary valve (Fig. 22.6) and a tricuspid repair (De Vega method) was performed. During follow-up the patient received a cardiac defibrillator at the age of 40 years, because of ventricular arrhythmias with collapse. Recent echocardiography indicated a compromised systolic and diastolic right ventricular function and a slightly dilated aortic root (Video clips 41-44 👁, Fig. 22.8). The pulmonary homograft functions well without significant stenosis or regurgitation of the valve (Figs 22.7, 22.9 and 22.10). Despite the corrective surgery in the past, the tricuspid valve shows renewed regurgitation (Video clip 45 👁). Currently, the patient has a slightly impaired exercise performance (NYHA class II) and progressive signs of fatigue.

Atrial corrected transposition of the great arteries: Mustard and Senning procedure

Transposition of the great arteries palliatively corrected with the Mustard or Senning procedure illustrates the importance of assessing biventricular function on a regular basis with cardiac MRI. Intra-atrial venous pathways are constructed with these surgical procedures, redirecting systemic venous blood from the superior and inferior caval vein into the left ventricle, and pulmonary venous blood to the right ventricle (Fig. 22.11). Therefore, the right ventricle continues

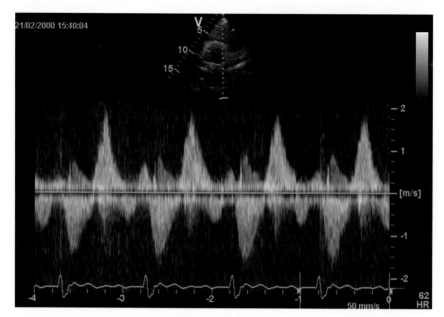

Figure 22.6 Continuous wave through the pulmonary valve before replacement with a pulmonary homograft. Note the severe regurgitation which occurs protodiastolic and the late diastolic forward flow.

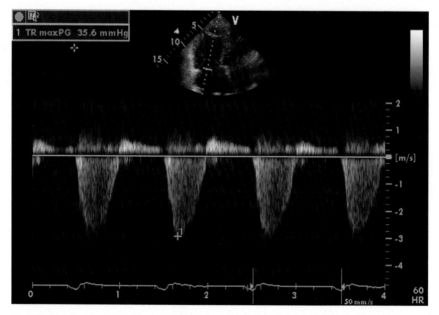

Figure 22.7 Spectral Doppler curve (continuous wave) showing slightly elevated systolic pressures between the right ventricle and right atrium. This indicates a non-significant gradient across the pulmonary arterial system.

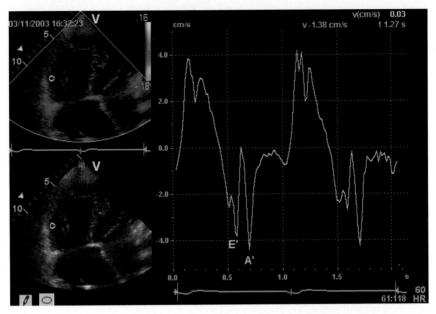

Figure 22.8 Tissue Doppler image of the right ventricle. Sample placed at the basal portion of the right ventricle. The velocity of the tissue at early diastole (E′) is low (3.8 cm s^{-1}). A′ is the tissue velocity during atrial contraction. This is compatible with diastolic dysfunction of the right ventricle.

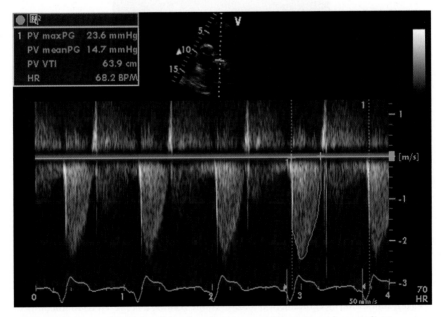

Figure 22.9 Spectral Doppler curve (continuous wave) depicting a low gradient between the right ventricle and pulmonary confluence.

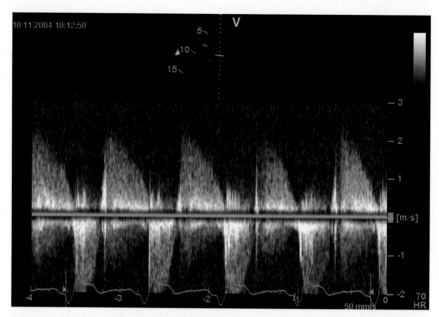

Figure 22.10 Spectral Doppler curve (continuous wave) depicting mild regurgitation, which is holodiastolic with high pressure half-time (236 ms). The maximal velocity depicts absence of pulmonary hypertension.

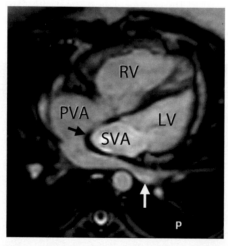

Figure 22.11 Gradient-echo "white blood" MRI (one slice, one phase) in a 26-year-old woman with transposition of the great arteries after Senning repair. Note the intra-atrial venous connection (black arrow) directing the blood from the pulmonary veins to the pulmonary venous atrium (PVA) and the right ventricle (RV). The left lower pulmonary vein is indicated by the white arrow. Note the RV hypertrophy as a result of the systemic load. Blood from the superior and inferior vena cava is directed through the systemic venous atrium (SVA) towards the left ventricle. This patient had some dilatation of the RV with subnormal ejection fraction (end-diastolic volume 241 mL, ejection fraction 43%), versus the left ventricle (184 mL and 60%, respectively). Parameters derived from multislice multiphase imaging with this MRI sequence.

to be subjected to systemic afterload. Although most patients are asymptomatic, numerous adverse effects have been described including systemic right ventricular failure, obstruction and leakage of the venous pathways, and atrial arrhythmias. These complications stress the need for close monitoring of the systemic right ventricular function and intra-atrial venous pathways.[3]

Black-blood images can provide insight in the morphology of atrial venous pathways, while evaluation of biventricular function can be performed with gradient-echo MRI. Delayed contrast-enhanced imaging can be used to identify ischemic myocardial injury. Turbulent flow patterns within the atria or ventricles, caused by stenosis of the intra-atrial venous pathways, leakage at the anastomosis of the intra-atrial venous pathways, or incompetence of the atrioventricular valves, result in signal voids on gradient-echo MRI. Differentiation between stenosis, leakage, or valve incompetence on gradient-echo MRI can be based on the location of the signal void within the atria or ventricles, together with phase-contrast MRI of the valves.

Case Presentation 3

A 37-year-old man presented with transposition of the great arteries. After birth a Rashkind septostomy was performed twice, with eventual Blalock–Hanlon septectomy. At the age of 3 years, the patient received a physiologic Mustard venous switch (Video clips 46–52 ⬥).

A pacemaker was implanted at the age of 17 years because of sick sinus syndrome and paroxysmal atrial tachycardia. Cardiac catheterization at the age of 36 years showed an abnormal site of origin of the right circumflex, with the right coronary artery originating from this right circumflex artery. Right ventriculography showed an enlarged right ventricle with moderate systolic function, and a non-significant tricuspid regurgitation. This picture is confirmed by recent echocardiography, showing right ventricular hypertrophy resulting from the systemic pressure load (Video clips 48, 53 and 54 ⬥). Unobstructed venous flow is depicted in Video clips 46–51 ⬥; Fig. 22.12. Also note the anterior position of the aorta compared with the pulmonary trunk in Video clip 55 ⬥.

Currently, the patient is asymptomatic without significant dyspnea or edema.

Fontan circulation

The Fontan procedure is most frequently carried out in the group of patients with a functional single ventricle (e.g. in the hypoplastic left heart syndrome and in tricuspid atresia). The procedure aims to establish a circulation in which the systemic venous return directly enters the pulmonary arteries. Different types of connections can be used: total cavopulmonary, atriopulmonary, and atrioventricular. In patients under consideration for a Fontan circulation, visualization of the pulmonary and systemic veins and pulmonary arteries is of particular importance. Black-blood MRI and MRA can visualize these structures

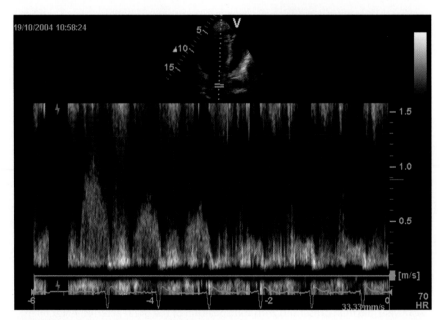

Figure 22.12 Spectral Doppler (pulsed wave) image, sample located in the conduit. The pressure gradient is low. Note the changing velocity during exhalation.

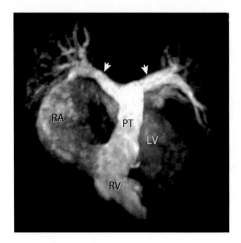

Figure 22.13 Follow-up MRA in a 27-year-old man with a Fontan circulation, obtained with a patch. Correction of tricuspid valve atresia with hypoplastic right ventricle (RV), infundibulary pulmonary stenosis, atrial septal defect, and ventricular septal defect. LV, left ventricle; PT, pulmonary trunk; RA, dilated right atrium. Note the open connection between the RA, RV, and PT. Normal pulmonary arteries (arrows).

with great accuracy. The postoperative management of patients with a Fontan circulation is concerned with evaluation of function of the systemic ventricle and the Fontan circulation itself. Black-blood MRI has proven to be successful in the detection of conduit obstruction.[9] The spatial relationship of the Fontan connections can be depicted by MRA (Fig. 22.13). Turbulent flow and increased flow velocity with phase-contrast MRI indicate the magnitude of any stenosis within the different types of Fontan connections. Other complications, including thrombosis, can also be visualized reliably.

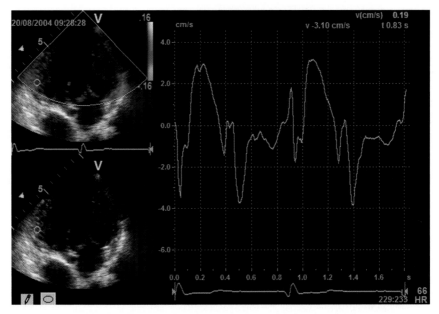

Figure 22.14 Tissue Doppler image with sample placed in the lateral wall of the left ventricle. Note the low systolic velocity (3.2 cm s^{-1}) and the low diastolic velocity during the early filling phase (3.8 cm s^{-1}), supporting the diagnosis of impaired diastolic function.

Case Presentation 4

This 25-year-old man has a double-inlet left ventricle and a rudimentary right ventricle, with double-discordant atrial–ventricle–arterial connections and severe pulmonary stenosis. Echocardiography showed situs solitus and levocardia.

At the age of 5 years, the patient received a modified Blalock (aortopulmonary) shunt, which partially obstructed 5 years later. At the age of 11 years, a modified Fontan system was constructed with a pulmonary homograft between the right atrium and pulmonary confluence. During the same procedure the ventricular septal defect was enlarged to secure aortic flow, as well as removal of the fossa ovalis to secure venous flow.

Echocardiographic evaluation showed hypertrophy and poor function of the single — morphologically left — ventricle (Video clip 56 👁; Fig. 22.14). Video clips 57–60 👁 depict the unobstructed flow through the ventricular septal defect and right ventricle to the aorta, despite some turbulence at the site of the ventricular septal defect. Video clip 61 👁 shows the pulmonary homograft (Fontan conduit). Currently, the patient experiences severe shortage of breath during minimal exercise, combined with cyanotic episodes.

Conclusions

Over the past few decades, the management of CHD has markedly improved. Transthoracic echocardiography is the mainstay for evaluation of CHD, as illustrated in the case examples. However, cardiac MRI can significantly contribute to the anatomic and functional evaluation of CHD. A wide array of different MRI imaging possibilities is available. Morphology of the heart can be clearly depicted with black-blood images from any angle, while MRA produces superior images of any vessel connected to the heart. Flow mapping provides information on valvular competence and/or stenosis. Finally, gradient-echo series provide quantified biventricular function and delayed contrast-enhanced imaging allows assessment of scar formation. The absence of radiation burden makes MRI especially for children with CHD a very relevant imaging tool, considering the fact that lifelong follow-up on a regular basis is necessary to provide optimal monitoring of the cardiovascular status and optimal timing of any (surgical) intervention.

References

1 Jara H, Barish MA. Black-blood MR angiography: techniques, and clinical applications. *Magn Reson Imaging Clin N Am* 1999;**7**:303–17.

2 Flamm SD, Muthupillai R. Coronary artery magnetic resonance angiography. *J Magn Reson Imaging* 2004;**19**:686–709.

3 Roest AA, Lamb HJ, van der Wall EE, *et al*. Cardiovascular response to physical exercise in adult patients after atrial correction for transposition of the great arteries assessed with magnetic resonance imaging. *Heart* 2004;**90**:678–84.

4 Prakash A, Powell AJ, Krishnamurthy R, Geva T. Magnetic resonance imaging evaluation of myocardial perfusion and viability in congenital and acquired pediatric heart disease. *Am J Cardiol* 2004;**93**:657–61.

5 Roest AA, Helbing WA, Kunz P, *et al*. Exercise MR imaging in the assessment of pulmonary regurgitation and biventricular function in patients after tetralogy of Fallot repair. *Radiology* 2002;**223**:204–11.

6 Konen E, Merchant N, Provost Y, McLaughlin PR, Crossin J, Paul NS. Coarctation of the aorta before and after correction: the role of cardiovascular MRI. *AJR Am J Roentgenol* 2004;**182**:1333–9.

7 Masui T, Katayama M, Kobayashi S, *et al*. Gadolinium-enhanced MR angiography in the evaluation of congenital cardiovascular disease pre- and postoperative states in infants and children. *J Magn Reson Imaging* 2000;**12**:1034–42.

8 Vliegen HW, Van Straten A, de Roos A, *et al*. Magnetic resonance imaging to assess the hemodynamic effects of pulmonary valve replacement in adults late after repair of tetralogy of Fallot. *Circulation* 2002;**106**:1703–7.

9 Sampson C, Martinez J, Rees S, Somerville J, Underwood R, Longmore D. Evaluation of Fontan's operation by magnetic resonance imaging. *Am J Cardiol* 1990;**65**:819–21.

Index